P9-DNK-866

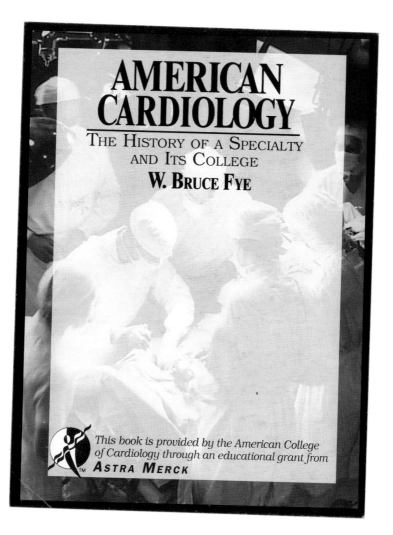

AMERICAN CARDIOLOGY

THE HISTORY OF A SPECIALTY AND ITS COLLEGE

W. BRUCE FYE

This book is provided by the American College of Cardiology through an educational grant from

ASTRA MERCK

AMERICAN CARDIOLOGY

AMERICAN CARDIOLOGY

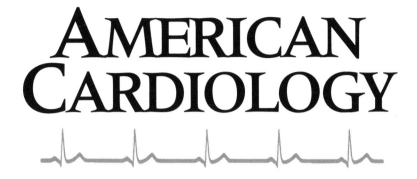

The History of a Specialty and Its College

W. BRUCE FYE

THE JOHNS HOPKINS UNIVERSITY PRESS
Baltimore and London

This book has been brought to publication with the generous assistance of the American College of Cardiology.

© 1996 The Johns Hopkins University Press
All rights reserved. Published 1996
Printed in the United States of America on acid-free paper
05 04 03 02 01 00 99 98 97 96   5 4 3 2 1

The Johns Hopkins University Press
2715 North Charles Street
Baltimore, Maryland 21218-4319
The Johns Hopkins Press Ltd., London

Library of Congress Cataloging-in-Publication Data will be found
at the end of this book.
A catalog record for this book is available from the British Library.

ISBN 0-8018-5292-7

For Lois, Katherine, and Elizabeth

Contents

Figures and Tables

Figures

Tables

Foreword

Upon the occasion of the fortieth anniversary of the founding of the American College of Cardiology (ACC), the officers of the college determined that the time was appropriate to record the history of the institution, while several early leaders were still active members. As president of the ACC, I was fortunate to be able to turn to one of the college's fellows, W. Bruce Fye, to undertake the history project. Bruce is chair of the cardiology department of the Marshfield Clinic in Marshfield, Wisconsin, as well as the author of many articles on the history of cardiology and a book on the professionalization of American physiology.

When I asked Bruce if he would write a history of the college, his response was an immediate and enthusiastic yes. But he wanted to write a book that would have broad appeal and that would make a significant and lasting contribution; a traditional organizational history would not do. Bruce proposed framing the college's story in terms of the development of cardiology as a specialty in the United States. The ACC leadership enthusiastically supported this approach and appointed him official college historian. While Bruce outlined an ambitious schedule of interviews and visits to libraries, the college's archives were reorganized to facilitate the project.

Bruce spent five years producing a seminal publication based on an exhaustive review of the literature, extensive archival research, dozens of oral history interviews, and his personal experience as a cardiologist. His book examines the complex roles played by individuals, organizations, academic institutions, and the federal government in the development of American cardiology and the specialty's professional society. The history of the ACC, from its humble beginnings in New York City to its present status as one of the nation's largest and most influential medical organizations, is fascinating.

The book describes the professionalization of cardiology in the United States during the twentieth century. It takes the reader from the early days, when a few self-designated heart specialists interpreted electrocardiograms and made house calls, to the current era, when nearly 20,000 board certified cardiologists deliver high-technology care to cardiac patients. In reading this book, I discovered how some general internists of previous generations came to be identified as cardiologists during the second quarter of the twentieth century: like many other aspiring heart specialists, my father spent two weeks with Paul Dudley White at the Massachusetts General Hospital and then bought an electrocardiographic machine. The process of becoming a cardiologist grew increasingly rigorous during the past half-century, though, as new technologies were introduced and formal training programs were created.

Bruce describes the implications of medical specialization for doctors, patients, and hospitals. Cardiology was shaped by many forces. There was no grand plan. Individuals and organizations exercised their options continuously in response to scientific advances, patient demand, economic incentives, and government initiatives. As a result, contemporary cardiology in the United States is exciting, effective, and expensive, but it is not available to everyone. In short, it reflects American medicine as a whole.

I salute Bruce for bringing the story of American cardiology and the ACC to life. Rich in detail and interpretation, his book illustrates the value of learning about our past as we reflect on the present and speculate on the future. Voltaire once warned that "the man who ventures to write contemporary history must expect to be attacked for everything he has said and everything he has not said." Bruce need not be concerned about Voltaire's admonition. His exhaustively researched and meticulously documented book should be required reading for everyone in the cardiovascular community and others interested in the development and present condition of American medicine.

WILLIAM L. WINTERS JR., M.D., F.A.C.C.
Past President of the
American College of Cardiology

Acknowledgments

I wrote this book on the professionalization of cardiology in the United States because it seemed like an ideal way to unite my historical and clinical interests. The concept arose in 1990 when William Winters, then the president of the American College of Cardiology (ACC), asked me if I would write a history of that organization. William Nelligan, then the executive vice president of the college, was enthusiastic about the concept. Subsequently, they and other ACC leaders agreed that the book would be more useful and interesting if it also addressed the development of cardiology as a specialty in the United States. I sincerely thank the officers, trustees, and staff of the ACC for their unwavering support, even when it became apparent that the project would extend well beyond the college's internal history.

Understandably, some scholars express concern about the objectivity of commissioned histories. I can assure readers that at no time did anyone at the ACC attempt to direct or influence my research or writing. This book reflects my interpretations of the events described; it was not subject to editorial review by the college. My conclusions are based on a careful analysis of numerous published, archival, and oral history sources as well as more than two decades of experience as a physician at the New York Hospital, the Johns Hopkins Hospital, and the Marshfield Clinic.

The ACC gave me free access to all of its records and provided generous grant support to assist in the research and writing of this book. Many college staff members contributed to this effort. I especially thank Helene Goldstein, director of the Griffith Resource Library, and her dedicated staff (Bernadette Artis, Kitty Kaschak, and Gwen Pigman) for their tireless efforts in tracking down obscure sources and facts. Sylvan

Weinberg graciously invited me to conduct oral history interviews in the ACCEL studio during national cardiology meetings. Kathi Rogers and Sidney Morton deserve my thanks for facilitating this effort.

Other college staff who contributed to the project in various ways include Sandy Beyer, Karen Collishaw, Dave Feild, Lawrence Ganslaw, Donald Jablonski, Marie Michnich, Penny Mills, Lisa Olson, Carolyn Thompson, Marcia Whitney, and Elizabeth Wilson. The late Philip Reichert, founder and longtime executive secretary of the ACC, deserves belated thanks for preserving so many documents that provide unique insight into the college's origins and history. I am also grateful to several former ACC presidents who sent me recollections of their terms of office and their impressions of important events in the history of the college and the specialty it represents.

This book could not have been written without the constant support and encouragement of my colleagues at the Marshfield Clinic. I am especially grateful to the other cardiologists who covered my practice during my "research days" and sabbatical. Chris Esser and Marilynn Tesmer, my secretaries, deserve my thanks for their many important contributions to the project. My medical assistants, Tami Roehl and Darla Schuld, also helped in many ways.

Marshfield Clinic president Richard Leer, medical director Frederick Wesbrook, medical education director Joseph Mazza, and the clinic's executive committee have consistently supported my historical activities, as have my colleagues in the Medical History Department at the University of Wisconsin. The staff of the Marshfield Clinic Library (Barb Bartkowiak, Jay Gawlikoski, Joann Gumz, Alana Ziaya, and Albert Zimmerman) obtained hundreds of articles on interlibrary loan and xeroxed hundreds more from the clinic's collection. Dieter Voss kindly translated several German papers. Amy Wilhelmi and the talented staff of the graphic arts department produced many of the charts, graphs, and photographs included in this book.

I thank countless other unnamed colleagues, friends, and staff members of the Marshfield Clinic and the American College of Cardiology who contributed to this project. Joseph Alpert and Bernard Gersh of the American Heart Association (AHA) Council on Clinical Cardiology deserve recognition for their support of my research into the history of the AHA. Susan Lucius and Leslie Austin of AHA headquarters in Dallas facilitated my use of the association's archives. Several people deserve my sincere thanks for encouraging my historical activities at critical points in my career. They include William Coleman, Milton Eisenhower, William Greenough, A. McGehee Harvey, Willis Hurst, Victor McKusick, Burton Sobel, and Myron Weisfeldt.

During the past five years, I discussed various aspects of this book with several historians, including Toby Appel, Saul Benison, Jack Berryman, Gert Brieger, Daniel Fox, Caroline Hannaway, Joel Howell, Saul Jarcho, Christopher Lawrence, Kenneth Ludmerer, Harry Marks, Sherwin Nuland, Ronald Numbers, John Parascandola, and Charles Rosenberg. I am grateful for their many astute observations and helpful suggestions.

Saul Benison and Charles Morrissey, my mentors in oral history techniques, deserve special thanks for introducing me to this indispensable tool. The subjects of the 45 formal oral history interviews I undertook are listed in the bibliography section of this book. I deeply appreciate their willingness to share their unique and candid insights into the history of cardiology and its organizations and institutions.

Jacqueline Wehmueller, my editor at the Johns Hopkins University Press, made many valuable suggestions regarding the content and style of this book. She also provided encouragement when it was needed the most. Two anonymous reviewers made many perceptive observations, asked several provocative questions, and challenged me to write a better book. I hope they are pleased with the final product. The first draft was also read by Howard Burchell, Lawrence Clouse, Joel Howell, Paul Kligfield, William Nelligan, Sherief Rezkalla, and William Winters. Arthur Hollman read the first three chapters and provided a valuable perspective on Thomas Lewis.

I also thank the archivists and librarians at several institutions for their assistance in discovering, retrieving, and copying the many manuscript sources used in researching and writing this book. Institutions and organizations that granted permission to quote excerpts from items in their collections include the American Board of Internal Medicine; the American College of Cardiology; the American Heart Association; the Bentley Historical Library, University of Michigan; the College of Physicians of Philadelphia; the Francis A. Countway Library of Medicine; the Franklin D. Roosevelt Library; the Johns Hopkins Medical Institutions; the Lane Medical Library, Stanford University; the National Heart, Lung, and Blood Institute; the National Library of Medicine; the New York Academy of Medicine; the New York Hospital–Cornell Medical Center; the Princeton University Archives; the Rockefeller Archive Center; the Rutgers University Libraries; and the Wellcome Institute for the History of Medicine.

Finally, and most importantly, I could not have written this book without the constant support and encouragement of my wife, Lois. She has shared me with medicine, history, and books for a long time; I am fortunate and grateful that she is so generous. I also thank my daughters, Katherine and Elizabeth, for their patience and their understanding.

AMERICAN CARDIOLOGY

Introduction

This book describes and interprets the invention of American cardiology as a specialty in the early twentieth century and its subsequent transformation into one of medicine's most significant fields. It also examines the origin, evolution, and significance of the American College of Cardiology (ACC), the specialty's professional society. The impact of heart disease—the focus of cardiology practice—can be measured in many ways. In the United States, almost 17 percent of the adult population has some cardiovascular condition, and cardiovascular diseases are the leading cause of death. Today, more physicians specialize in cardiology (about 17,000) than any other clinical, non–primary care, nonsurgical discipline.[1]

Heart disease is prevalent and serious, and the care of cardiac patients is an enormous economic enterprise. Money has influenced every aspect of American medicine; in recent decades it catalyzed heart care as an organized endeavor and cardiology as a specialty. Currently, one-fifth of total hospital charges are related to the diagnosis and treatment of cardiovascular disorders—$33 billion in 1987. Medicare alone paid cardiologists almost $3 billion in 1992. The annual budget of the National Heart, Lung, and Blood Institute (NHLBI), which helps to fund many academic cardiology careers, now exceeds $1 billion. Approximately 25,000 people (half of them scientists and physicians) attend each of the annual meetings of the ACC and the American Heart Association (AHA), the specialty's two major organizations. Academics and representatives of industry travel to them to share their knowledge and sell their products. Practitioners attend to learn about new diagnostic tests and innovative therapeutic approaches, to network, and to evaluate state-of-the-art equipment.[2]

The lure of specialization

Specialization is a major organizing principle of contemporary American medicine and society. Division of labor and the use of special tools is evident in almost every organized activity in our culture, from service industries to educational institutions, athletic teams, and assembly lines. Medical specialization developed gradually in the United States during the nineteenth century. Initially, the model was confined mainly to the nation's largest cities. For generations, individual doctors have chosen to narrow the scope of their practice (to specialize) for various reasons. Conventional wisdom frames medical specialization as a pragmatic response to the ever-expanding knowledge base that results from discovery, invention, and human experience. There is no doubt that many doctors choose to specialize for this reason. The intellectual content of medicine, like other organized fields of endeavor, has increased for centuries. Johns Hopkins internist William Thayer claimed in 1904 that the "enormous expansion" of medical knowledge "led naturally" to what he characterized as "ever-increasing specialism."[3]

There are other reasons, chiefly socioeconomic, that have fostered medical specialization. Market forces, which depend on the culture and context in which the doctor lives and works, may encourage or discourage career choices. Societies and individuals place distinct values, which vary over time and place, on different types of knowledge and skills. In American culture, rewards are traditionally measured in terms of income—dollars that can be traded for products and leisure. A century ago, some doctors thought they could provide better care, contribute more to their profession, earn more money, and have a better life-style by becoming specialists.

New York medical editor George Shrady was not surprised in 1875 that many new physicians planned to specialize, "considering the conventional understanding regarding the position and emoluments of specialists."[4] Patients who chose to see specialists were willing to pay a premium to get an opinion and receive care from an "expert." Describing factors that encouraged specialization, New York dermatologist Duncan Bulkley explained a century ago that "the public require and will pay for the highest attainable knowledge, experience, and success."[5] This custom conformed to the general economic order in which knowledge and talents commanded a premium if consumers thought they had particular value.

The boundaries of medical and surgical specialties have been drawn and interpreted in various ways. Some fields (such as ophthalmology and gastroenterology) are defined by a specific organ or organ system. Gynecology is focused on the reproductive system of women. Pediatrics and geriatrics are framed in terms of the potential patient's age. Other specialties (such as radiology and clinical pathology) are characterized by certain technologies and laboratory procedures. Specialists in tuberculosis (once a thriving field) devoted their careers to a specific contagious disease that affected people of all ages and could invade virtually every organ. Most cardiologists now define the boundary of their specialty quite narrowly, to disorders of the heart itself, although some include vascular diseases and high blood pressure.

Specialists have often found themselves embroiled in territorial disputes as they negotiated their claims to organs, procedures, and patients. Several organ systems are the professional focus of both medical and surgical specialists. For example, neurologists and neurosurgeons care for patients with disorders of the brain, and rheumatologists and orthopedic surgeons care for patients with joint diseases. Some specialties evolved so that a single practitioner integrated these medical and surgical roles (such as ophthalmologists and gynecologists). This diversity in the organization of specialties reflects traditions that have developed over generations. Nonsurgical specialists have long recognized that they were competing with surgeons for jurisdiction over some organs. Harvard internist Frederick Shattuck explained in 1900 that "the heart is practically the only viscus which remains the exclusive province of the physician."[6] This would remain true until the 1940s, when surgeons began to operate on the heart. Since then, medical and surgical heart specialists have cooperated in the management of cardiac patients.

Visual, verbal, and physical clues helped patients to distinguish various specialists when they entered a doctor's office. By the turn of the century, special techniques, technologies, and tools (such as diagnostic instruments, therapeutic devices, and even examination tables) differentiated ophthalmologists, gynecologists, and radiologists from other specialists and general practitioners. The questions specialists asked, the types of examinations they performed, the tools they used, and the treatments they provided or prescribed reinforced their distinctiveness. General changes in American culture (such as urbanization, improved transportation, and the invention and diffusion of the telephone) encouraged specialization because they made it easier for people to reach specialists and for consultants to contact physicians who referred them patients.

Until recently, American doctors derived most of their income from fees collected from private patients. To succeed as a specialist, a practitioner had to attract a critical mass of people willing (and able) to pay for his or her services. Before the expansion of health insurance, most people who sought specialists for themselves and their family members were affluent. Although specialization grew under fee-for-service financing, it expanded dramatically during the second half of the twentieth century as most Americans became covered by hospital insurance as a benefit of employment.

Historians and sociologists have interpreted the processes of professionalization and specialization for decades. Half a century ago, George Rosen investigated the origins and social meaning of specialization and characterized it as "an essential feature of modern medical practice."[7] Later, Rosemary Stevens published a seminal book on the influence of specialization on medical training and practice in the United States. Recent studies of American medical education by Kenneth Ludmerer and William Rothstein provide valuable perspective on how medical students during the twentieth century were trained to embrace science and technology as indispensable ingredients of the practitioner's art. During the second half of the century, specialists replaced generalists as the teachers and mentors of America's medical students because of educational reforms and government funding policies.[8]

Charles Rosenberg and Rosemary Stevens have written compelling books on how patients and doctors came to view the hospital as the appropriate context for acute care—the place where sick people were united with specialists, technology, and a corps of trained assistants.[9] Sociologist Paul Starr opens his perceptive interpretation of the history of the American medical profession by characterizing "modern" medicine as "an elaborate system of specialized knowledge, technical procedures, and rules of behavior."[10] These are the main themes of professionalization and specialty formation. The acquisition, use, and control of distinctive knowledge and procedures are at the heart of the process.

A medical educator wrote three decades ago, "If one wanted to pick out a single thing that has really changed the whole practice of medicine . . . it would be technology."[11] The innovation and diffusion of technology has had a profound influence on cardiology, as it has on many other specialties. Several authors (notably Stanley Reiser, Louise Russell, Audrey Davis, Joel Howell, and Harry Marks) have analyzed how technology has helped to define modern medical institutions and how it has affected patients and their doctors. Because some medical disciplines (such as cardiology and radiology) are more technologically intensive than others (such as endocrinology and rheumatology), the relative importance of technology and other shaping forces varies among specialties.[12]

Despite the significance of specialization as an organizing principle in medicine, there are very few book-length studies of individual medical and surgical disciplines (the American Medical Association currently recognizes more than thirty) that seek to integrate the scientific, technological, social, and economic forces that shaped each of them. Narratives of discoveries and discoverers abound, but only rarely have their authors gone beyond a superficial analysis of the context in which these people worked to explore the forces that shaped their careers and determined the responses of the public and the profession to their innovations. Russell Maulitz writes, "Few historians of modern medical specialties have sought to 'get inside' their material enough to pay attention to the technical *and* the social dimensions."[13]

Sociologists have published valuable perspectives on the emergence and growth of medical specialization, including books on the professionalization of pediatrics and rehabilitation medicine. Understandably, their works generally emphasize external social forces over internal technical developments. But it is difficult to achieve the proper balance between the science and sociology of medicine, the professionals and the patients—especially if an author seeks to write for a broad audience.[14]

Many heart specialists have chronicled the history of our current understanding of various forms of cardiac disease and innovations in diagnosis and treatment. Louis Acierno's recent book on the history of cardiology brings together a wealth of information on technical developments in the field. Joel Howell has published several papers on the development of American cardiology in which he skillfully analyzes both internal scientific and technical factors and external social forces in an attempt to explain the current content, structure, and significance of the specialty. This book is written from a similar perspective. In it, I explore in more detail several of the important events and dynamics that Howell has highlighted.[15]

Studies of specialization in other countries are valuable because they provide a means to separate generic medical, scientific, and technical factors from context-specific cultural forces. Roger Cooter's investigation of British orthopedics and George Weisz's study of specialization in France are useful in a general sense. These works demonstrate how unique historical, political, social, and economic forces shape specialty development in a particular national context.[16] Christopher Lawrence's papers on British cardiology, the definition of "new" heart diseases, and the adoption of medical technologies shed light on the complex dynamics that go on behind the scenes (sometimes unrecognized by the participants) as the boundaries of specialties are described, contested, and defended.[17]

Specialties are constantly defined and redefined, negotiated and renegotiated. They may subdivide or merge with other fields and may thrive or disappear. Two different medical specialties focused on organs within the chest exemplify this point. Following World War II, the once successful specialty of tuberculosis vanished with the advent of effective antibiotics. Tuberculosis experts transformed themselves rapidly into lung specialists—pulmonologists—so as to not be left without a specialty. Meanwhile, heart disease continued to increase, despite the introduction of antibiotics that promised to reduce the frequency and impact of rheumatic fever, once a major focus of cardiology practice. Cardiology blossomed as huge sums of money were pumped into the field in an attempt to find cures and (later) provide care for millions of cardiac patients. Yet the past and the present do not always predict the future—witness the sudden decline of the tuberculosis specialist and the disappearance of the sanatorium (and the more recent resurgence of the disease).

The invention and evolution of American cardiology

In this book on the origins and development of American cardiology, I emphasize organizational dynamics rather than the specific scientific and clinical content of the specialty. The focus is on interactions among individuals, organizations, and institutions (in the largest sense of the word). I intentionally term cardiology a specialty rather than a subspecialty of internal medicine (its traditional designation, especially in academic medical centers), because I believe this most accurately characterizes its present functional status. Today, cardiology possesses virtually all of the essential features that define a discipline: a distinct body of knowledge, unique diagnostic tools and therapeutic procedures, a formal career path that includes three or more years of fellowship training and a board examination, a large professional society (22,240 ACC members in 1995), a plethora of publications and meetings devoted to cardiology, and thousands of practitioners who consider themselves cardiologists rather than internists with a special interest in heart disease.

Cardiology's gradual and ongoing transformation into a functionally independent specialty has been problematic for philosophical and economic reasons. From an organizational point of view, cardiology is not an independent department in most American academic medical centers. There is no direct career path to cardiology. Before a doctor can begin cardiology training, he or she must complete a general internal medicine residency. In order for a cardiology graduate to take the official board examination in cardiovascular disease, he or she must have passed the general internal medicine examination. The origins and implications of these traditions are explored in this book.

American cardiology did not evolve simply as the result of a series of technological and procedural innovations, the accretion of new knowledge, or the activities of a few "great doctors." Although these components were all present, there was no predetermined course or predictable outcome. Doctors, patients, institutional leaders, and other interested parties were influenced by external factors such as market forces, regulations, research funding, and reimbursement schemes. Cultural attitudes, economic conditions, and political agendas also shaped cardiology and its institutions and organizations.

Shortly before World War I, a few doctors living in New York, Boston, and some other big cities began to focus their practices on heart patients. These urban centers provided ample clinical material and an economic base that made (at least partial) specialty practice feasible. If aspiring heart specialists were to succeed, their career choice required the cooperation of other people. Potential patients had to perceive that a self-designated cardiologist offered something beyond the care available from general physicians. At the turn of the century, most doctors were comfortable caring for cardiac patients when diagnosis relied on taking a history and examining the heart with a stethoscope, and treatment consisted mainly of rest and a few standard oral medications.[18]

Every medical student learned to examine the heart and to pre-scribe medicines for cardiac complaints. Possession and use of a stetho-scope became part of the content of general medicine during the nineteenth century. The electrocardiograph (a machine first used in 1902 to record the heart's electrical activity) gave aspiring heart special-ists a unique tool to differentiate themselves from other practitioners. During the 1920s, patients came to view the doctor who possessed an electrocardiograph and interpreted its tracings as a heart specialist. The cost of the machine limited its diffusion among practitioners, however, which helped those doctors who owned one to claim the status of a heart specialist. For more than a generation, general physicians seeking to transform themselves into cardiologists had to do little more than purchase an electrocardiograph and attend a brief postgraduate course to learn how to use it.

There were other paths to becoming a heart specialist in the era before formal cardiology training programs. Some aspiring American cardiologists studied with recognized heart specialists in Great Britain or on the Continent. Several of them returned home to become aca-demic cardiologists in the nation's largest teaching hospitals. America's first cardiologists were a heterogeneous group. The first chapter of this book includes brief biographical sketches of physicians who exempli-fied the various intellectual traditions that merged to constitute Amer-ican cardiology. Some of these doctors focused on science, others on practice, and still others on the social implications and economic conse-quences of cardiac disease.

Specialization challenges traditional relationships between doctors and their patients, among the doctors themselves, and between doctors and the institutions where they learn and work. The creation of profes-sional societies is one dimension in this process. A few of America's first-generation heart specialists began to organize cardiology during the second quarter of the twentieth century. They created a national organization (the American Heart Association, 1924), launched a peri-odical (the *American Heart Journal*, 1925), and established a board examination (in cooperation with the American Board of Internal Medicine, 1940).

Conflict was evident as individuals and groups sought to promote and institutionalize their own visions of cardiology. Some of these tensions led to the creation of America's second national heart organi-zation, at mid-century. The year after the AHA reinvented itself as a voluntary health organization in 1948, a group of New York City practitioners created the ACC. Chapter 4 describes and analyzes the formation of the ACC and the response of the AHA leaders. Both organizations succeeded because they served different purposes, the diseases they focused on were common, and the practitioners and academics they represented thrived during the final decades of the twentieth century as money poured into cardiology. The AHA devoted itself mainly to research funding and public education, while the ACC focused on continuing medical education for physicians. There was much to teach and to learn about cardiology during the second half of the century. Intellectual curiosity, ambition, and money were factors in the equation that resulted in many clinically relevant discoveries and innovations in cardiology.

The federal government inaugurated an ambitious campaign of research funding after World War II that fueled academic cardiology and transformed cardiology practice. Congress had both the discovery and the dissemination of knowledge in mind when it passed the National Heart Act in 1948. The American people—the taxpayers—would not benefit from their government's huge investment in academic medical centers and research unless they had access to the discoveries and innovations that resulted from it. Formally trained heart specialists were the solution to this problem of distribution. Federal grants partially subsidized the production of hundreds of practitioner cardiologists during the 1950s and thousands during the 1960s. These clinicians migrated to community hospitals across the country and took with them the latest diagnostic techniques and treatment approaches.

Three innovations introduced during the 1960s transformed the care of heart patients, the lives of cardiologists, and the structure of hospitals. The coronary care unit united high-risk heart patients, technology, and a specialized staff of nurses and doctors in a specific hospital environment. It also symbolized cardiology's growing independence from general internal medicine. *Selective coronary angiography* gave heart specialists a powerful tool to determine whether patients had significant narrowings in the body's most vital blood vessels. This information was critical for surgeons planning to perform *coronary artery bypass graft surgery*, introduced in 1968 to treat angina pectoris (chest pain caused by coronary artery disease). The potential market for coronary angiography and bypass surgery was huge: it was estimated at the time that at least three million Americans had angina.

As more people were insured against acute illness, the demand for heart care increased. Medicare reimbursement policies encouraged hospitals to purchase technology and specialists to use it. Many interested observers—practitioners, hospitals, and industry—sensed that cardiology had entered a "Golden Age" by 1970. Heart disease was prevalent, new technologies were abundant, and cardiac procedures were liberally reimbursed. Cardiology training programs grew dramatically during the 1970s and 1980s as the demand for trained heart specialists continued to increase.

Meanwhile, some people began to question whether America's specialist-dominated, hospital-based paradigm of medical care was sensible. The model focused on the treatment of acute flareups of chronic diseases and emphasized technology instead of prevention.[19] Epidemiology, technological and procedural innovations, and reimbursement policies placed cardiology in the center of the debate. As the federal government increased its involvement in medicine, the ACC, like other professional societies, began addressing the socioeconomic aspects of medical practice on behalf of its members.

The United States government's recent efforts to reduce the share of the federal budget spent on health care has implications for the future of specialization in general and for cardiology in particular. By reducing reimbursement to specialists (and for specific diagnostic and therapeutic procedures) and by other means, the government hopes to transform the current health care system, which emphasizes high-technology, specialty-based care into one that relies more on primary care physicians who stress disease prevention. The recent growth of "managed care" in the private sector has the same motivation: cost containment. Innovations in technology and health care delivery combined with liberal reimbursement catalyzed cardiology. Today, market forces have cooled the euphoria that characterized cardiology from the 1960s through the 1980s. The powerful financial incentives that, for a generation, led individuals and institutions to purchase and use technology and perform procedures to diagnose and treat heart disease are diminishing.

Over the course of the twentieth century, advances in medical science and technology, innovations in diagnosis and treatment, the emergence of the hospital as the central locus of acute care, the invention and expansion of health insurance, and a myriad of changes in American society transformed the way doctors evaluated and cared for their patients. These same things also changed the way patients viewed

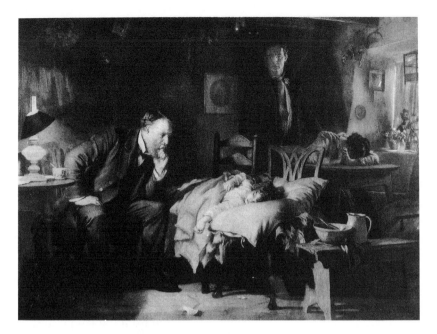

The Doctor by British artist Sir Luke Fildes (c. 1891).
SOURCE: Original in the Tate Gallery, London.

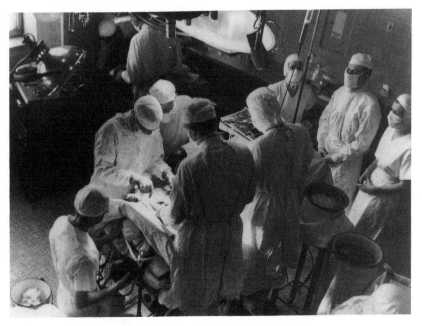

An early Blalock-Taussig "blue-baby" heart operation being performed at the Johns Hopkins Hospital (1947).
SOURCE: The Alan Mason Chesney Medical Archives of the Johns Hopkins Medical Institutions, Baltimore, Md.

their doctors. Cardiology prospered in this dynamic context. The following statements describe just a single aspect of the transformation of heart care that had occurred since the beginning of the century. Writing in 1965, a physician observed: "Once it took only one doctor to resign himself and the child's parents to the inevitable death of a 'blue baby.' It now takes a team of medical specialists and auxiliary personnel to correct the congenital abnormality of a baby's heart to insure the child a normal lifespan."[20] A writer in *Harper's Magazine* concurred: "The solitary practitioner has been replaced by an army of specialists whose skills must be integrated in the proper combination at the right time and place."[21]

Many people's lives spanned the eras described by these writers and depicted in the illustrations on these pages. These people lived during an age of intellectual and technological achievement, not just in medicine, but in society generally. They watched as intellectual curiosity, ambition, and money moved powered flight from the sand dunes of Kitty Hawk, North Carolina, in 1903 to the surface of the moon just sixty-six years later. Although cardiology is just one element of modern society and medicine, the dynamics of its invention and transformation into a major medical specialty provide useful insights into the organization and meaning of contemporary medical education, research, and practice.

CHAPTER 1

Defining a Discipline

In America, a few doctors began to invent the specialty of cardiology in New York, Boston, and other large cities just before World War I. The process drew, to a certain extent, upon European models of research and practice.[1] These doctors were a diverse group. Some focused on science, others on practice, and still others on the social consequences of cardiac disease. Each type played a role in defining cardiology as a discipline. Some doctors decided to become heart specialists, and some patients and practitioners thought they offered something useful and patronized them.

I distinguish four types of physicians who helped invent the specialty during the first quarter of the twentieth century. Admittedly, any scheme to categorize them is problematic. Labels suggest distinctions the individuals themselves may not have perceived. The approach is reasonable, however, because these doctors usually had a primary identity as perceived by their mentors, peers, and protégés. The terms chosen to identify them reflect the content and context of their main professional activity: _physiological cardiologist, practitioner cardiologist, academic cardiologist,_ and _public health cardiologist._ Brief definitions follow, to be amplified later. This scheme helps to illustrate how groups with distinct traditions and ideologies negotiated their claims to be part of a larger community of professionals concerned with the diagnosis, treatment, and prevention of cardiovascular disease.[2]

Physiological cardiologists were medical graduates with formal training in physiology. Their main professional interest was cardiovascular research, usually a combination of laboratory research and clinical investigation. They played a central role in transferring scientific instru-

ments and technologies from the physiological laboratory to the clinic and bedside—from animals to patients.

Practitioner cardiologists were doctors who chose to focus their practice on patients with known or suspected heart disease. During the first half of the century, most were so-called partial specialists whose practice was a blend of cardiology and general internal medicine. These cardiologists diffused the new diagnostic methods into patient care. They worked primarily in noninstitutional settings (private offices), which distinguished them from a third group of heart specialists who also cared for patients.

Academic cardiologists evaluated and treated cardiac patients as well as holding faculty appointments in teaching hospitals where they also taught and performed clinical research. They helped train the practitioner cardiologists who established the community-based clinical specialty.

The demand for heart specialists was catalyzed by the rhetoric and actions of the *public health cardiologists.* Although they were the smallest and most heterogeneous group, their impact was substantial. They shared an ideology rather than a common training experience or institutional context and were interested mainly in the socioeconomic implications of heart disease. Whereas the practitioner cardiologists cared for *individual* patients, the public health cardiologists developed strategies to enhance the care of cardiac patients *as a group.* Their first efforts were focused on rehabilitating working men with heart disease. Shortly thereafter they turned their attention to the prevention and early detection of cardiac disease.

These four types of heart specialists were distinguishable in the United States by 1920. Individuals within each of the first three categories shared common characteristics (e.g., training pattern, primary locus of activity, daily work, and peer group) that helped to differentiate them from members of the other groups. Still, there was overlap; the boundaries were never distinct. Some individuals functioned in more than one group simultaneously or moved sequentially from one to another. Their roles were complementary in many respects, but their different visions of cardiology created tensions as the specialty grew.

This chapter includes brief career summaries of a few individuals whose training, interests, and work patterns were typical of the groups I have distinguished. I chose this approach because, as Joel Howell states, "biography offers the historian certain advantages, particularly

when attempting to meld the internal content of a field with its social context."[3]

Physiological cardiologists: Ideology and instruments

By the twentieth century, physiology had replaced pathology as the science perceived as most relevant to the diagnosis and cure of disease. Physiology provided scientific instruments and an experimental approach that was especially useful in studying the heart, first in animals and later in patients. From the Renaissance until the mid-nineteenth century, illnesses were generally framed in terms of structural (pathological) abnormalities. During the nineteenth century animal experimentation replaced the autopsy as the primary method of attempting to interpret disease.[4] In this context, some researchers and doctors began to perceive (and portray) illness in a different way. A new paradigm, which attributed the signs and symptoms of disease to disordered function, gradually replaced the traditional pathological view of illness. The new approach was termed *pathological physiology*.[5]

The concept of pathological physiology can be traced to the second half of the nineteenth century, when several European physiologists invented a variety of measuring and recording devices, so-called instruments of precision, to study organ function in laboratory animals. As German clinical scientists like Friederich Müller and Carl Wunderlich espoused the experimental approach, the ideology of pathological physiology gradually began to influence the way clinicians viewed disease.[6]

Because the heart is fundamentally a pump, the organ was well suited for experimentation using new physiological techniques. By 1890 European and American physiologists had devised many elaborate experimental approaches to study the heart's electrical system, its pumping function, and its own circulation.[7] European and American physiologists championed animal experimentation as *the* method to advance medical knowledge. Increasingly, doctors and patients embraced this ideology of research and came to view disease as disordered function.[8]

German clinical scientist Ludolf Krehl, who taught at several universities (including Leipzig, Jena, Marburg, and Greifswald), first thoroughly articulated the concept of pathological physiology in his 1893 book, *Grundriss der allgemeinen klinischen Pathologie*.[9] Krehl and others

who shared his views wanted to integrate traditional clinical or "bed-side" diagnostic skills with newer approaches that relied on experimental techniques and scientific instruments such as the sphygmograph (a device that allowed them to record the form of the pulse wave). They emphasized the limitations of older methods of diagnosis and outlined the problems associated with viewing illness primarily as a manifestation of disordered structure.

Krehl taught or indirectly influenced several American physicians and clinical scientists (including Carl Binger, Albion Hewlett, Robert Loeb, and Joseph Pratt) who helped transfer the concept of pathological physiology to the United States around the turn of the century. There were other routes by which the European physiological tradition migrated to the United States. The earliest academic physiology departments in America (Harvard, Johns Hopkins, and the University of Michigan) were strongly influenced by Carl Ludwig of Leipzig and Michael Foster of Cambridge.[10]

Physiological cardiologists were scientists trained in physiology and medicine who worked in teaching hospitals. Their main interest was laboratory research on the cardiovascular system. By my definition, however, a physiological cardiologist must also have some involvement with patients; those who did not were pure physiologists. Often their clinical activities were limited to physiological diagnosis using instruments of precision such as the electrocardiograph. Their peers viewed them as clinical scientists whose work focused on the cardiovascular system.

The first Americans to fit this definition were educated around the turn of the century. Albion Hewlett's career illustrates the physiological cardiologist tradition.[11] After receiving his medical degree from Johns Hopkins and completing a residency at New York Hospital, he spent eighteen months studying in Germany with Krehl. Hewlett played a major role in transferring the ideology of pathological physiology to America, most notably by translating Krehl's book on the subject into English in 1905.[12] Hewlett's contemporaries viewed him as a clinical scientist; he was one of eight persons invited to be founding members of the American Society for the Advancement of Clinical Investigation in 1907. Two years later, British physiological cardiologist Thomas Lewis (discussed later in this chapter) invited Hewlett to be one of six coeditors of *Heart*, his new journal devoted to cardiovascular research.[13]

Hewlett's most productive years were spent at the University of Michigan Medical School, where he chaired the medical department from 1908 to 1916. His research resulted in dozens of scientific and clinical papers on the heart. Many publications dealt with disorders of the heartbeat and the effects of drugs on cardiac rhythm. Hewlett's other activities included making hospital rounds, teaching medical students and residents (including an elective course on the clinical physiology of the circulation), and seeing a few private patients.[14]

Hewlett's enthusiasm for instrumental and graphic methods of studying the heart (recordings on paper or photographic plates of physiological measurements such as pressure, pulse, or electrical waves) was shared by his friend and fellow Johns Hopkins graduate Arthur Hirschfelder. Another prototypical physiological cardiologist who had received advanced scientific training in Germany, Hirschfelder was hired in 1905 to organize and supervise the new "physiological laboratory" in the Johns Hopkins Hospital's medical clinic. The laboratory was designed to study individual patients and specific disease conditions "from the standpoint of function." There were, in fact, two separate laboratories, one for "the clinical study of patients by the special methods in use in physiological laboratories, particularly graphic methods" and the other "well equipped for animal experiment [where] . . . diseased conditions seen in the wards may be reproduced in animals and studied by physiological methods." One of the goals of this new physiological laboratory was pedagogical: to encourage medical students "to look upon their ward and dispensary patients from the physiological standpoint."[15]

Hirschfelder's most important contribution to the emerging physiological cardiologist tradition was his book *Diseases of the Heart and Aorta* (1910). It was the first American monograph on heart disease to reflect the ideology of pathological physiology. In it, Hirschfelder sought to "present side by side the phenomena observed at the bedside and the facts learned in the laboratory." He described and illustrated several tools and techniques to evaluate the cardiovascular system, including instruments to measure blood pressure (sphygmomanometer), record heart sounds (phonocardiogram) and pulse waves (sphygmograph), and assess the heart's size, shape, and motion (x-rays and fluoroscopy). The point of this 632-page hybrid physiology-cardiology text was to show how the principles and instruments of physiology could help practitioners evaluate and treat their cardiac patients.[16]

Hewlett mentored other heart specialists, including Frank Wilson, a recent Michigan medical graduate he hired to operate the electrocardiograph the institution acquired in 1913. During World War I, Wilson worked in England with Thomas Lewis and later became recognized as a world leader in the field of electrocardiography. Hewlett was also a role model for Carl Wiggers, who would become one of America's most influential physiologists.[17]

New tools and techniques that made it possible to objectively evaluate organ function in humans encouraged the acceptance of the ideology of pathological physiology. As laboratory instruments were adapted for use with patients, the intellectual approach took on a more practical dimension, especially for the doctors who had access to the new diagnostic tools and chose to use them. In the half-century before 1910, several sophisticated measuring and recording instruments were devised that eventually were used to evaluate cardiac function in patients. None had more impact on cardiology during the early twentieth century than the electrocardiograph.

The electrocardiograph: A cardiologist's "essential" tool

The physiological cardiologist tradition, already developing when the electrocardiograph was invented, was strengthened by the advent of this powerful research and diagnostic tool. In 1901 Dutch physiologist Willem Einthoven devised a new string galvanometer, which he used to record the heart's electrical impulse the following year. Because his instrument—an electrocardiograph—produced a graphic tracing of the heart's electrical activity, it was ideally suited for evaluating disorders of the heartbeat (arrhythmias). Whereas some people used the sphygmograph to evaluate arrhythmias, the electrocardiograph provided the first practical *direct* method to record the electrical activity of the human heart.[18] The electrocardiograph's tracings made it possible to measure and otherwise characterize the heart's electrical impulse. They could be stored and compared with recordings made at different times and in other people.

Within a decade, Einthoven's large and complicated instrument migrated from the physiologist's laboratory to the hospital, where electrical cables connected it to patients. Many cardiologists thought the electrocardiograph was useful—indeed indispensable—years before specific therapies were available to treat conditions revealed by the

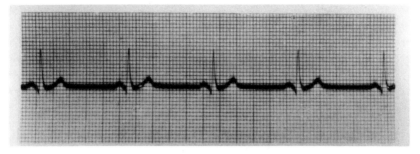

Einthoven's first published electrocardiograph tracing, recorded with his string galvanometer.
SOURCE: W. Einthoven, "Galvanometrische registratie van het menschelijk electrocardiogram," in *Herinneringsbundel. Professor S. S. Rosenstein* (Leiden: Eduard Ijdo, 1902), pp. 103–106, table 5.

machine (such as pacemakers for heart block). The test fit well with the ideology of pathological physiology, and self-interest was a factor for many of the individuals who promoted or used the technique.[19]

Physiological cardiologists oversaw the transformation of the electrocardiograph from a scientist's instrument to a clinician's tool. British physician and clinical scientist Thomas Lewis was the first person in the English-speaking world to acquire an electrocardiograph for clinical research. He installed one at University College Hospital, London, in 1909.[20] During the second decade of the twentieth century, Lewis's laboratory became a factory of new knowledge as a result of his passion for research and his possession of an electrocardiograph. In that brief period, he wrote or coauthored more than one hundred papers, most of them reporting studies using the machine.

Lewis was a role model for several Americans who became cardiologists.[21] They wanted to work with him because he offered them their first opportunity to learn how to operate an electrocardiograph and interpret the tracings it produced. These aspiring heart specialists could have studied with Einthoven or other Continental pioneers of cardiology, but working with Lewis had several benefits. He was a clinical scientist who also saw patients, whereas Einthoven was a pure physiologist. And Americans studying in London did not confront the language barrier they would in cities on the Continent.

In 1909 Lewis's American pupil Alfred Cohn installed the first electrocardiograph in the United States at Mount Sinai Hospital in New York. Soon, electrocardiographs were also in use at Presbyterian Hospi-

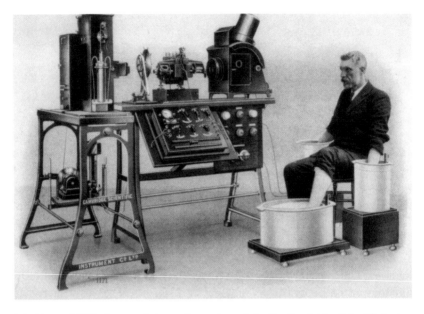

A "table-model" Einthoven electrocardiograph made by the Cambridge Scientific Instrument Company (London) in 1911.

SOURCE: Advertising leaflet tipped into front inside cover of *Heart* 4, no. 2 (1912). Author's collection.

tal in New York and Johns Hopkins Hospital in Baltimore. The chief of medicine at Johns Hopkins predicted in 1910 that the machine "will doubtless form a part of the instrumental armamentarium of the larger general hospitals."[22] Lewis shared this view and became an influential advocate of the practical utility of the electrocardiograph. His writings encouraged its diffusion into the clinical world of doctors and patients.

After just four years' experience with the technique, Lewis published a primer on it in which he declared that an electrocardiographic "examination has become essential to the modern diagnosis and treatment of cardiac patients." He advocated its widespread use: "Those cardiac patients are few in whom an electric examination is superfluous." The machine could not only help patients but also offer the institutions caring for them a competitive edge: "The time is not distant, when no hospital which undertakes the care of many of these patients may neglect the string galvanometer, if it is to rank amongst institutions whose design is proficiency." It must be acknowledged that self-interest may have influenced Lewis's views, as he was publishing books on the electrocardiograph, and his career centered on the technique at this time.[23]

The electrocardiograph contributed to tensions that had been developing in medicine for more than a generation. Physiological cardiologists were part of a scientific tradition whose influence in medicine was increasing. But some practitioners and medical professors were skeptical of (or openly hostile to) the growing emphasis on technology and laboratory tests. In 1907, just before the electrocardiograph was introduced into clinical medicine, an internist at the Massachusetts General Hospital denounced the artificial distinction between the "laboratory diagnostician" and the "clinical diagnostician."[24]

Writing eight years later, physiological cardiologist Carl Wiggers conceded that he was reluctant to undermine the credibility of "the master minds of medicine" whose reputations derived from their superior clinical diagnostic skills. But he stressed that the physiologists' tools could help them and ordinary doctors recognize "many phenomena of the circulation" that were undetectable by their "unaided senses." This had practical implications: instrumental methods of diagnosis had "led to the elucidation of many obscure conditions, to the recognition of new diseases, and to the institution of new forms of treatment."[25]

Recent medical school graduates were more receptive to medical technology than most of their predecessors; they had seen it used and were better prepared to make use of it. The efforts of a generation of educational reformers were coming to fruition. By World War I their agenda, to make medicine more scientific and to produce better-trained doctors, was widely accepted. The transformation was catalyzed by Abraham Flexner's detailed exposé of the nation's medical schools, by the campaign of the American Medical Association (AMA) to elevate educational standards, and by vast sums of money from philanthropists like John D. Rockefeller, who endowed medical schools that embraced the ideology of research. Throughout the nation, physician-owned medical schools closed or merged with universities, entrance requirements were raised, terms lengthened, and curricula standardized.[26]

Eventually, the physiologists and physiological cardiologists had a profound impact on medical practice as doctors came to rely on their tools and techniques to assess the heart's electrical and hemodynamic functions. Speaking of the early twentieth century, Joel Howell believes that "the dissemination of physiology from the scientist's laboratory to the practitioner's office . . . [was] one of the most significant transformations (social or otherwise) of medical practice." By this time, most American medical students were learning the complex facts of cardiovascular physiology and the ideology of pathological physiology from textbooks, lectures, and laboratory exercises.[27] The polygraph, sphygmomanometer, and electrocardiograph were developed by physiologists and introduced into clinical practice by physiological cardiologists. Soon, they were adopted by community-based doctors—practitioner cardiologists—who chose to focus their internal medicine practice on patients with heart disease.

Practitioner cardiologists put science to work

"To-day medicine is a science," declared Chicago surgeon Arthur Bevan, who chaired the AMA's Council on Medical Education in 1910. Rhetoric like this was not new; the same claim had been made for decades. The difference was that the tools and tests of science were becoming indispensable for ambitious practitioners and more evident to patients. New scientific techniques made their organs more visible and their symptoms more comprehensible to doctors. Increasingly, when people sought medical advice (especially for cardiac complaints) they encountered scientific tools that measured and recorded things they did not even perceive, such as their blood pressure and heartbeat.

This linkage of medicine with science also had implications for the nation's practitioners. Although some tensions persisted between the proponents of clinical diagnosis and those who embraced the new laboratory tests and scientific tools, doctors believed their profession was scientific, and they wanted their patients to think so as well. Bevan put it this way: "The individual citizen, if he is wise, can secure for himself and his family the benefits and the protection of modern scientific medicine by securing the services of a well-trained scientific physician." This rhetoric reflected the "regular" medical profession's concern about "irregular" practitioners like homeopaths and osteopaths—sectarians they portrayed as unscientific.[28] Another writer told practitioners that the appearance of their office could help to instill confidence in their patients. It should be equipped to convey the impression of "an earnest, working, scientific physician, who . . . makes full use of the instruments of precision, and the various methods that science has devised for doing different kinds of medical and surgical work."[29]

One kind of medical work that a few American doctors began to choose just before World War I related to the evaluation and management of patients with heart disease. They inaugurated a process by which cardiology gradually became distinct from general internal medicine. Internal medicine, itself, was a new specialty that had begun taking shape, intellectually and organizationally, in the 1880s. The American interpretation of it adapted the German concept of *innere Medizin* to a practice structure based on the British model.[30]

In the United States, internal medicine came to be defined as a field whose practitioners (internists) cared for the nonsurgical illnesses of adults. Internists also avoided obstetrics and gynecology, leaving those areas to general practitioners or specialists. Still, internal medicine was a broad domain that included several major organ systems. In 1897 William Osler, the most prominent internist in the English-speaking world, expressed the view that internal medicine embraced "at least half a dozen" specialties.[31] Because so many people had complaints that they, those around them, or their doctors attributed to gastrointestinal or cardiovascular dysfunction, some physicians saw these organ systems as intellectually interesting and potentially lucrative fields for specialization.[32] At the same time, gastroenterology and cardiology were at the forefront of the pathological physiology movement; almost half of Krehl's book was devoted to these organ systems.[33]

Gastroenterology was organized as a specialty before cardiology in the United States. The American Gastro-Enterological Association was formed in 1897, the same year Osler delivered an address entitled "Internal Medicine as a Vocation." The first gastroenterologists (like the first practitioner cardiologists) became specialists only gradually. As more specialized work came their way, they reduced the amount of time they devoted to general internal medicine. But it was a slow process, both at the individual and at the specialty level. When Samuel Meltzer presided over the American Gastro-Enterological Association in 1904, he acknowledged that the "practical activity" of a "goodly number" of the members was in "the field of general medicine."[34]

America's first practitioner cardiologists, like the nascent gastroenterologists, entered the field through general practice or internal medicine. They were not scientists or academic physicians; they were office-based doctors trained in an era when science was increasingly emphasized. Aspiring cardiologists progressively focused their practice on patients who had known cardiac disease or whose complaints

suggested a heart problem. The balance between general internal medicine and cardiology was determined both by the practitioner's interests
and by market forces. Were there enough paying patients to support
specialty practice? Did the specialist have any extra training, unique
diagnostic instruments, or innovative therapeutic procedures to distinguish himself from general practitioners or other specialists? Were
there regulations that limited entry into specialty practice?

Scientists and physiological cardiologists were creating new knowledge that excited some doctors about the prospects of heart disease as a
specialty early in the twentieth century. It also provided them with
tools like the electrocardiograph that helped to differentiate them from
other practitioners. There were no regulations; any licensed physician
could claim to be a specialist. But paying patients were another matter.
Most specialists worked in larger cities where they could draw upon the
middle and upper classes to support their focused practice.

Most practitioner cardiologists have no historical voice. They left
little or no trace, because their focus was on patient care rather than on
research and writing. One New York physician who exemplifies the
practitioner cardiologist tradition left a rich historical record, however.
Louis Bishop was one of the first American physicians (arguably the
first) to specialize in cardiology. His career can be traced by reviewing
his many publications and consulting his biography, which includes
excerpts from his correspondence. Bishop did not hesitate to call himself a cardiologist rather than an internist with a special interest in heart
disease, and he was an early proponent of forming a national cardiology specialty society. His writings reveal the ambitions and concerns of
a doctor trying to carve out a niche as a specialist, and the attitudes and
ailments of the patients who sought his services.[35]

Bishop was an office-based internist who transformed himself into
a cardiologist at a time when heart disease was not viewed as a distinct
specialty. He followed a pattern that had emerged in the United States
during the second half of the nineteenth century whereby ambitious
medical graduates got some additional training and declared themselves specialists. Bishop's career path shared common features with
other internists who became America's first heart specialists: most
possessed college degrees, attended leading medical schools, took medical internships, received some postgraduate training at home or
abroad, and embraced the ideology of pathological physiology. Most of
America's general practitioners were less educated and less likely to

have received laboratory instruction in physiology during medical school or postgraduate training.

Historian Charles Rosenberg has noted how difficult it is to "reconstruct the texture of a past practitioner's career as construed and lived."[36] Although this is true for Bishop, his many writings and an abundant literature about medicine in New York City at the turn of the century provide useful clues. Like many specialists of his era, Bishop had certain social advantages that made it possible for him to get a better education and more extensive medical training. He came from a patrician background, and his preliminary education and medical training represented the best America had to offer in the 1880s. He entered private practice in Manhattan in 1892 after graduating from Rutgers College and the College of Physicians and Surgeons of New York and completing a two-year internship at St. Luke's Hospital.[37]

Initially, the scope of Bishop's practice was broad, like that of most of his contemporaries. It was centered in the homes of his patients or in his office in his Manhattan townhouse. Bishop cared mainly for adults, but he also saw some children and delivered babies. In 1893 he was appointed assistant physician in the outpatient department of the new Vanderbilt Clinic of the College of Physicians and Surgeons. This facility, designed to supply "a fully equipped dispensary service to the poor," provided its staff physicians with enormous clinical experience. In 1901 "an army of 47,156 patients" was treated there. Bishop's contemporaries viewed appointments in outpatient departments as stepping-stones to scarce hospital posts and more specialized practice.[38] Few New York doctors had hospital privileges when Bishop was appointed attending physician to the Colored Home and Hospital on East 65th Street in 1898.[39]

By this time Bishop had decided to specialize in internal medicine. He hoped other doctors would recognize him as a medical consultant, a position that promised a better schedule and more income. A contemporary writer explained, "a successful specialist has many advantages over the hurly-burly life of the general practitioner. . . . He has short hours and is seldom or never called out at night. . . . His fees are always good, sometimes fat."[40] During the first decade of the twentieth century, Bishop progressively narrowed his focus *within* internal medicine. Initially, he was classified as a specialist in "diseases of the chest (heart and lungs)." His identity as a heart specialist was affirmed in 1907, when he got a part-time teaching appointment as "clinical professor of diseases of the heart and circulation" at the Fordham University School of Medicine. Bishop sensed the novelty of his career choice. Three years later, he told a friend that he was the only doctor in New York City *"frankly* devoting himself to this line of work as a specialty."[41]

Charles Rosenberg characterizes the era in which Bishop entered practice as one of "dramatic transition" for the American medical profession.[42] When Bishop began seeing patients in 1892, doctors did not have the diagnostic tools that would shortly foster the advent of cardiology as a specialty. A quarter of a century later, Lewellys Barker declared, "A physician that went to sleep in 1890 and woke up yesterday would find himself a disoriented Rip Van Winkle in diagnosis, with utterly antiquated ideas and information. The diagnostician that sleeps longer than eight or nine hours at a stretch in these days runs a risk!"[43]

Barker's Rip Van Winkle would have slept through things that helped transform Bishop into a heart specialist: the discovery of x-rays, the invention of the electrocardiograph and the sphygmomanometer, and the introduction of a multitude of laboratory techniques. In 1916 the dean of the University of Michigan School of Medicine told a Colorado doctor, "the diagnosis of disease depends now largely upon laboratory tests."[44] Bishop, like most other practitioner cardiologists, was quick to adopt the diagnostic tools that had migrated from the laboratory into clinical practice, some of which helped to distinguish them as specialists. He was among the first to use a sphygmomanometer routinely and to describe the clinical manifestations and adverse consequences of abnormally high or low blood pressure.

For decades, ambitious doctors had traveled abroad to supplement the meager opportunities for clinical training available in the United States. They hoped to learn skills or gain knowledge that would make them more competitive when they returned home. Many aspiring specialists of Bishop's era sought training in Germany, which was characterized as "the most attractive country in the world for medical men" in the 1912 *Handbook to Medical Europe*. Its author thought that European postgraduate training was "so well organized, the clinical material so abundant, as to offer splendid opportunities for this kind of work."[45]

Bishop spent the summers of 1908 and 1910 at Bad Nauheim, Germany, a world center for the treatment of heart patients. By going abroad, he was following a career path to specialization that had evolved over several decades. In 1913 one writer explained that the common route to specialization was to "announce your intention and spend a few months in studying the Great Principles that are of special interest to you, and also to see practice and gain experience in some noted American or European hospital." All that remained was to return home "and make your change to your specialty" which "will be of tenfold benefit to you *in more ways than one.*"[46]

Bishop's postgraduate training at Bad Nauheim shaped his views of the diagnosis and treatment of patients with heart disease. The other experience that molded his vision of cardiology was a brief meeting in 1908 with James Mackenzie, who was just becoming recognized as a leader of contemporary cardiology thought and practice. From Mackenzie, Bishop gained a greater appreciation of how pulse tracings might be useful in practice by helping to correlate heart patients' symptoms with their physical findings. When he returned home, he used a Mackenzie polygraph in his routine evaluation of heart patients.[47]

During subsequent prewar visits to Bad Nauheim, Bishop was impressed with how some heart specialists there used the x-ray and the electrocardiograph to objectively evaluate their patients. By 1915 he had incorporated fluoroscopy and electrocardiography into his office practice. Bishop could afford such expensive machines because his patients were affluent and he was independently wealthy. Most doctors would not have been able to buy them.[48] Bishop's enthusiasm for instruments of precision was typical of heart specialists in private practice or in teaching hospitals. Their emphasis on technology helped distinguish them from general internists.

Eventually, Bishop advocated the routine use of the electrocardiograph, x-ray, and fluoroscope as part of a "complete cardiologic examination of every patient" with known or suspected heart disease. By the end of World War I, Bishop's "complete examination" consisted of a history, physical examination, chest x-ray, cardiac fluoroscopy, electrocardiograph, pulse tracings, Wassermann test for syphilis, blood count, and urinalysis.[49] This aggressive use of technology was deplored by some internists, and some practitioner cardiologists urged caution. Heart specialist Selian Neuhof had installed an electrocardiograph and an x-ray unit in his New York office by 1917. He emphasized their value but urged doctors to use them as a supplement to, rather than a replacement for, traditional methods of physical diagnosis.[50]

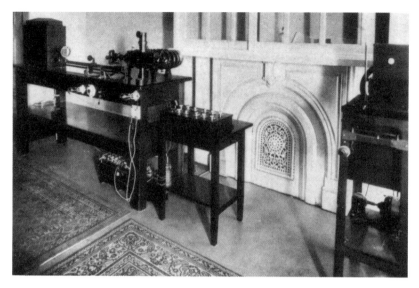

Bishop's electrocardiograph installed in his office.
SOURCE: L. F. Bishop, *Heart Troubles: Their Prevention and Relief,* 2d ed. (New York: Funk & Wagnalls, 1921), facing p. 152.

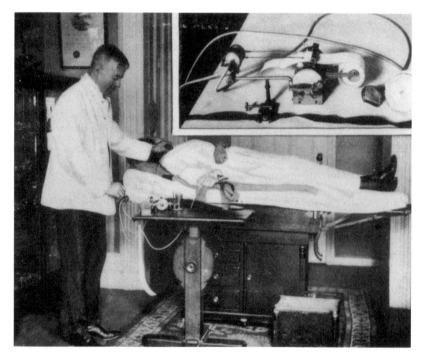

A Mackenzie polygraph used to record the jugular venous pulse and the radial artery pulse set up in Bishop's office.
SOURCE: Bishop, *Heart Troubles,* facing p. 312.

But there were incentives to use technology. Bishop and other aspiring heart specialists could claim that the special instruments they used gave them a diagnostic advantage over general practitioners and internists. It was harder to demonstrate an objective advantage in therapeutics, however. In the early twentieth century, doctors treated cardiac disease with a combination of drugs and "hygienic" measures like diet and exercise. Their treatment strategies varied depending on when and by whom they were trained—and their enthusiasm for adopting new therapeutic approaches.

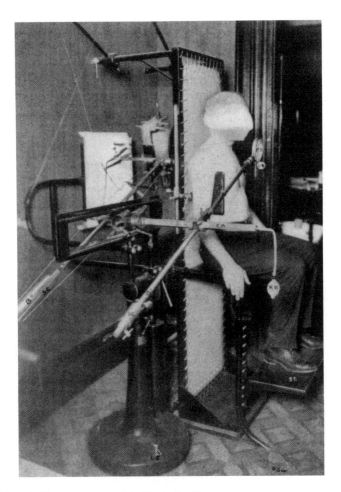

Groedel Orthodiascope x-ray unit in Neuhof's office.
SOURCE: S. Neuhof, *Clinical Cardiology* (New York: Macmillan, 1917), plate 17, facing p. 110.

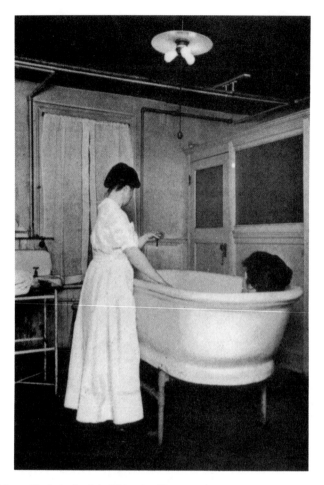

Nurse giving a Nauheim bath in Bishop's office.
SOURCE: Bishop, *Heart Troubles,* facing p. 228.

Most doctors followed the advice of recognized experts like William Osler, author of the most popular medical textbook in the English-speaking world. His book provides insight into contemporary approaches for treating cardiac patients (Table 1-1). Bishop's writings indicate that his treatment strategies were similar to those advocated by Osler.

There was growing controversy about the value of the "Nauheim" approach, which combined hot saline baths with a program of diet and special exercises. Despite mixed reviews from doctors—some of whom

TABLE 1-1
Therapy of Heart Disease—William Osler (1909)

Pericarditis: Absolute quiet; application of an ice bag to the chest wall or "local" bloodletting. (p. 782)

Acute rheumatic fever: Six weeks of bed rest; salicylates (such as aspirin) were known to reduce joint pains and fever and were thought to "protect the heart, shorten the course, and render relapse less likely." (pp. 227–228)

Decompensated valvular heart disease—accompanied by symptoms (such as shortness of breath) and signs (such as arrhythmias or edema): Rest; bloodletting for vascular congestion; cathartics and a salt-free diet for edema; direct draining of excess fluid by puncturing the skin of the legs using Southey's tubes for severe edema; digitalis for "weakness of the heart-muscle." (pp. 816–820)

Myocardial disease (of diverse etiologies, most poorly understood at the time). The most problematic cases were those with "marked cardiac arrhythmia, with a feeble, irregular, very slow pulse, and syncope or angina." Treatment of decompensated patients: Complete bed rest and a "carefully regulated" high-protein diet. The Schott treatment, a "combination of baths and exercises at Nauheim," was most suitable for patients "with myocardial weakness from whatever cause" except for those with decompensated valvular disease. (pp. 828–829)

Simple palpitations: "Hygienic measures" consisting of moderate exercise; ten hours in "the recumbent posture" daily; a tepid bath each morning; and avoidance of coffee, tea, alcohol, smoking, and large meals. If these measures are ineffective: Iron, strychnia, and nux vomica. (pp. 838–839)

Angina pectoris: Amyl nitrite for acute attacks and nitroglycerin taken regularly between episodes. (p. 842)

SOURCE: Adapted from W. Osler, *The Principles and Practice of Medicine*, 7th ed. (New York: D. Appleton, 1909).

denounced the Nauheim treatment out of self-interest—patients flocked there. In 1908 more than 425,000 baths were given to 30,000 people. James Mackenzie condemned it, but Bishop and several of his contemporaries were impressed with the results in selected patients. Bishop incorporated the treatments into his practice (he installed a special bathtub in his office) and urged other American doctors to do so as well.[51]

Although Neuhof did not share Bishop's enthusiasm for Nauheim-style baths and exercises, he could not ignore his patients' interest in them. The issue was relevant for practitioner cardiologists, whose patients were more affluent than most city dwellers. Neuhof wrote in

1917, "The question frequently and insistently arises in private practice" as to what types of cardiac patients should be sent to the Continent for the "Nauheim treatment." He mentioned Nauheim because "it is the most popular and best known among the patients themselves." The patients who benefited most, in Neuhof's opinion, were those with "mild decompensation" and others who were "nervous, high-strung, and worried." The European spas allowed them to "quickly divorce their minds and thoughts from domestic and business cares." This rhetoric reflects the lingering influence of the "rest cure" approach for treating patients suffering from "nervous exhaustion" introduced by American neurologist S. Weir Mitchell in 1875.[52]

During World War I, Americans formerly treated in Germany were forced to seek alternatives, which increased the demand for heart specialists in New York and other cities. By this time, Bishop's identity as a cardiologist was secure. In 1913 he claimed that his practice was "devoted exclusively to the practical care of heart patients."[53] Bishop promoted himself as a specialist in several standard ways. Contemporary specialists attempted to enhance their reputations and attract referrals by lecturing or publishing on topics in their area of interest. In 1913 ambitious doctors were told that if they were "ever offered a professorship" they should accept one that reflects their interests, "relates directly to the sick, and . . . is likely to increase your skill and get you special work of that kind or otherwise advance your reputation and your private practice." This same author urged doctors not to "hesitate to put pen to paper . . . both for the benefit of others and to enhance your own personal value and professional reputation." Presenting lectures at medical meetings would also be an "aid in having you discovered, or . . . will be an addition to your fame."[54]

Bishop used all of these methods to enhance his reputation as a sophisticated practitioner cardiologist. Although he wrote many articles, he wrote them as a practitioner for other practitioners, some of whom might refer patients to him. Early in his career, Bishop protested that "the trouble with much of the medical literature in the past is that it has been written chiefly by teachers of medicine rather than by practitioners." Although his main audience was general practitioners and internists, he also wrote for laypersons (some of whom were potential patients). Bishop's career demonstrated that it was possible, by World War I, for a doctor in a traditional, office-based setting to become a heart specialist whose "chief duty is the care of the individual."[55]

During the 1920s practitioner cardiologists began to appear in many of America's largest cities. Most, like Bishop, started their careers as general practitioners and internists who gradually built up a practice that focused on heart disease. As self-designated, office-based heart specialists, they saw self-referred patients and helped other doctors care for people with cardiac problems. Very few physicians were able to confine their practice to cardiology; there simply was not enough specialty work. Most remained partial specialists who practiced some general internal medicine. Although most practitioner cardiologists completed an internship and a year of medical residency, few had any formal cardiology training. Some had taken brief postgraduate courses in the few teaching hospitals with an academic cardiologist on staff.

Academic cardiologists: Clinicians in an institutional context

A few teaching hospitals had appointed heart specialists to their staffs by the mid-1920s. These were part-time appointments; there were virtually no full-time academic posts for cardiologists until after World War II. In this era academic cardiologists earned most (or all) of their income by seeing private patients and interpreting electrocardiograms. They were differentiated from practitioner cardiologists by their academic appointments and the fact that some of their professional activities took place in a teaching hospital. Their identity depended on the context and content of their work.

An academic cardiologist was more likely to have served as an assistant to an established academic cardiologist or to have had some formal cardiology training abroad than the average practitioner cardiologist. Some had begun their academic careers as physiological cardiologists but had shifted their focus from laboratory research to patient care. In contrast to physiological cardiologists, who were *scientists* who spent part of their time in a clinical context, academic cardiologists were *clinicians* who spent part of their time in an academic context. In addition to delivering care to patients in their hospital and its cardiac clinic, or supervising its delivery, they taught medical students and trained internal medicine residents and aspiring heart specialists.[56] Academic cardiologists published papers based on clinical observations or clinical investigation rather than basic research. Many used the electrocardiograph as their primary research tool, and they were often viewed as their institution's expert in the technique.

The influence of academic cardiologists on the development of cardiology was substantial. They helped shape the specialty as lecturers and authors, as organizers of cardiac clinics and local heart associations, as consultants, and as role models. Through informal networks and, after 1924, through the American Heart Association (AHA), they had greater influence on the character of the emerging specialty than the much larger group of practitioner cardiologists.

For more than a generation, Boston cardiologist Paul Dudley White was America's most influential academic cardiologist.[57] He was a prolific author and respected teacher who mentored dozens of heart specialists. White's institutional base was the Massachusetts General Hospital (MGH), an elite Harvard teaching institution. He was the first Boston physician to focus exclusively on heart disease. Unlike Bishop (twenty-two years his senior), White began his medical career as a cardiologist. He never practiced general internal medicine, mainly because of singular institutional circumstances. His career path was typical of the nation's first academic cardiologists who came on the scene after World War I. He chose to become a heart specialist at a time when job opportunities were just beginning to appear in teaching hospitals as a result of the advent of cardiac clinics and the electrocardiograph.

An institutional decision facilitated White's entry into the emerging field of cardiology. The son of a general practitioner in Roxbury, Massachusetts, White graduated from Harvard Medical School in 1911. He spent the next two years as an intern on the pediatric and medical services at the MGH. In 1913 White's chief, David Edsall, decided to purchase an electrocardiograph for the hospital, the first machine of its type in Boston. Edsall wanted a physician who was a clinical scientist like himself to use the instrument as part of a new program that acknowledged the growing clinical significance and research potential of heart disease. He was also addressing a concern he had raised a year earlier: that American medical schools "have done practically nothing systematic to provide for the training or the careers of their future clinical teachers and investigators." Edsall sent White abroad for just this purpose.[58]

White wrote in his diary in 1913, "[I have] been offered a remarkable opportunity by Drs. Edsall and W. H. Smith to be an expert on *hearts.* To go abroad in Fall with expenses paid, to study in London with [Thomas] Lewis for six or nine months, then back to MGH next year to run the new electrocardiogram for two years and then—." Joseph Pratt, one of White's mentors at the MGH, encouraged him to study cardiology in London.[59] White warned Lewis that he would "come with merely a general medical school training supplemented by two years medical work in the Mass. General Hospital—my knowledge of hearts is extremely limited though I am trying to pick up a few rudiments."[60]

By autumn, White was working in Lewis's laboratory at University College Hospital and rounding with him and James Mackenzie at the London Hospital. White thought Lewis would soon be "the world's greatest cardiologist." He told his brother, "Mackenzie still is regarded as the foremost heart-man but his day is done. From what I have seen of the two men, I think there is no comparison." Other Americans like Alfred Cohn shared White's opinion of Lewis and encouraged aspiring heart specialists to study with him.[61]

White bought an electrocardiograph for the MGH from the Cambridge Scientific Instrument Company for $1427.37 and installed it in the basement of the MGH in August 1914.[62] Later that year, at Edsall's request, he organized a formal clinic for cardiac patients at the hospital. White was optimistic about his (and cardiology's) prospects. In 1915 he told his brother, "The field I'm in is fertile. . . . Never can I regret having gone into it. The clinical side alone is inexhaustible."[63] White's career at the MGH was disrupted by World War I, when he served in Europe with other MGH staff members.[64] He returned to Boston in the fall of 1919 to spend a year as a research resident at the MGH, after which he began his career as the institution's first cardiologist.

During the 1920s White divided his time between clinical research, patient care, and teaching. "At the present time," he wrote in 1925, "my chief interests are two: first, clinical research, and second, the practice of medicine. A small amount of my time I devote to teaching and administrative work." Most of White's patients were sent to him "in consultation in order to study the condition of their hearts." They were evaluated in his office and electrocardiographic laboratory at the MGH. Between 1920 and 1925, White saw approximately fifteen hundred private patients. He enjoyed teaching medical students and characterized the work with his cardiology residents as "stimulating and delightful."[65]

A prolific author, White published more than one hundred papers on a wide range of heart-related topics between 1920 and 1930. During that decade, he trained fourteen cardiology residents, three of whom—H. M. (Jack) Marvin, Howard Sprague, and Duckett Jones—became influential in the AHA. More than a dozen students worked with White on various research projects during the decade. Between 1920 and 1960, White trained 238 cardiology residents and research associates. They represented an informal but influential network of cardiologists throughout the nation and the world. During the 1920s, a few other teaching hospitals added heart specialists to their (part-time) staffs who functioned as academic cardiologists. They included Samuel Levine at Boston's Peter Bent Brigham Hospital, George Nelson at Ohio State University, Stewart Roberts at Emory University, and William Stroud at the University of Pennsylvania. These individuals had academic appointments, but they (like White) earned their income from private practice.[66]

Before 1920 there were few opportunities for cardiologists of any type in America. During the next decade, the situation would change dramatically as more than two hundred cardiac clinics opened in larger cities and more hospitals sought trained electrocardiographers. At the same time, more patients sought out heart specialists as public health cardiologists generated concern about the frequency of heart disease and the possibility of preventing it.

Public health cardiologists and the socioeconomic consequences of heart disease

After World War I, public health cardiologists influenced patterns of care for heart patients in several large and medium-size American cities. Their influence was exerted not by their numbers but by their innovation (the cardiac clinic) and their ideology (the prevention of heart disease). I chose the term *public health cardiologist* as a convenience; it is meant to convey a concept rather than to imply that there was a specific group of individuals who defined themselves as narrowly as the phrase suggests.

The public health cardiologists' careers were diverse in content and context. Unlike most practitioner and academic cardiologists, they had no desire to limit their activities to heart disease. Indeed, most of them did not view themselves as heart specialists *or* public health physicians. The most influential public health cardiologists were, in fact, academic internists like Lewis Conner of New York Hospital and Cornell University Medical College and John Wyckoff of Bellevue Hospital and New York University College of Medicine, public health physicians like

Haven Emerson of New York City, and medical scientists like Alfred Cohn of the Hospital of the Rockefeller Institute, who was deeply interested in cardiovascular epidemiology.[67]

When they began their organizational activities just before World War I, their vision of cardiology was framed around the provision of both medical and *social* services to cardiac patients. By the end of the war, their agenda had expanded to include the prevention of heart disease, a new concept they aggressively promoted. William Robey told members of the AHA in 1928, "Some time ago, at a meeting of cardiologists, a doubt was expressed that we could do anything to prevent heart disease."[68] Meanwhile, public health cardiologists also established a new social institution, the cardiac clinic, where a team of professionals (heart specialists, nurses, and social workers) focused on the socioeconomic consequences of heart disease in addition to delivering medical care to cardiac patients.

Public health cardiologists also played a major role in establishing and setting the agenda of the first major organizations in the United States devoted to cardiac disease: the New York–based Association for the Prevention and Relief of Heart Disease (1915) and the AHA (1924). The public health cardiologists influenced the attitudes and actions of practitioner and academic cardiologists and other doctors who cared for heart patients. Their emphasis on preventive medicine contributed to a significant change in the care-seeking behavior of cardiac patients and healthy persons who feared heart disease. This stimulated the demand for heart services during the 1920s.

By the turn of the century, the public health movement had expanded beyond its original focus on sanitary engineering. A broad spectrum of professionals—doctors, scientists, nurses, social workers, and government officials—now concentrated on the health needs of specific types of patients (e.g., those with tuberculosis or venereal disease) or defined populations such as infants. Their efforts were supported by public funds, private gifts, and grants from philanthropic foundations. This expanded public health agenda reflected growing concern about—and a broader definition of—social problems, a feature of the Progressive Era.[69] It was also the product of the impact of bacteriology on medical practice. According to historian John Duffy, the "bacteriological revolution . . . immeasurably strengthened the position of the medical profession" and put physicians "in charge of public health."[70]

Several prominent American physicians championed the cause of preventive medicine. In 1904 William Thayer of Johns Hopkins told a group of internists that "the enforcement of scientifically planned . . . prophylactic measures has become to-day one of the main duties of the practitioner of medicine." He was also optimistic about treatment: "To-day from the study of the *pathological physiology* [emphasis added] of bacterial and cytotoxic intoxications, we are rapidly evolving scientific preventive and curative measures." His comments reflected the fact that, for Thayer and most of his contemporaries, the concept of prevention was restricted to communicable diseases—those attributed to bacteria and viruses.[71]

The public health cardiologists adopted the prevention of heart disease as the centerpiece of their agenda. But this was not the first concern of those people who began to address the social consequences of cardiac disability around 1910. Their original goals were modest and pragmatic. A team of social workers and doctors established a new organizational model—the cardiac clinic—to expand the definition of cardiac care beyond diagnosis and treatment. The first cardiac clinics in the United States were established in New York and Boston shortly before World War I. Although some factors leading to their creation were unique to each setting, there were common themes. The innovators shared a concern about the financial implications of heart disease and a conviction that something should be done to improve the efficiency and quality of care of working-class and poor cardiac patients.

These specialty clinics were an extension of the dispensary concept that evolved during the nineteenth century. Dispensaries began in cities as freestanding institutions where one or more doctors evaluated indigent patients, wrote prescriptions or dispensed drugs, and performed minor procedures. Dispensaries served two purposes: the urban poor received care, and medical students and ambitious practitioners gained experience. They also played an important role in establishing the social hierarchy of physicians in America's cities. A dispensary appointment "served as a step in the career pattern of elite physicians," according to Charles Rosenberg.[72]

During the late nineteenth century, many hospitals established outpatient clinics that competed successfully with the freestanding dispensaries. This development was part of a larger movement in which hospitals assumed a greater role in medical training and in caring for patients with acute illnesses. At the same time, some doctors and hospitals established clinics (or reorganized existing ones) for patients with specific types of diseases.

In 1907 Richard Cabot, director of the MGH outpatient department, characterized the work done there as "usually slipshod." In part, this was a manifestation of the "tradition of hurry" in outpatient departments. Because there were too few doctors for the number of patients, "no thorough diagnosis is possible." Cabot also attributed the poor quality of care in outpatient departments to a lack of incentives for physicians who worked in them. He knew that most doctors viewed the post as a "stepping-stone to something higher." Because they were not paid for their outpatient work, most doctors were inclined to devote more time and energy to activities (like office practice) for which they received income.[73]

Cabot advocated changes to make the MGH outpatient department more efficient and the care delivered there more comparable to that provided by private practitioners. Although he thought the MGH had "succeeded in raising the standard of diagnostic work in the dispensary nearly as high as it is in private office practice," Cabot conceded that "in treatment we are still woefully far behind."[74] He saw another reason to reorganize outpatient care. Like many physicians of his day, Cabot was troubled by the wholesale use of empiric remedies. He wanted to know which drugs and other forms of treatment were most effective and thought this knowledge could be "gained by following up the patient in his home." At the same time, Cabot's MGH surgical colleague Ernest Codman was developing his concept of "end-results" for patients operated on at the institution. Cabot and Codman thought patient follow-up was critical if one hoped to prove that medical or surgical therapy had been effective.[75]

Doctors were not trained (nor were most of them interested) in the kind of follow-up Cabot envisioned. So, in 1905 he introduced an innovation: a trained social worker was hired to help evaluate patients in the clinic, deliver home care, and monitor their response to treatment.[76] Cabot implemented other changes in the MGH outpatient department in an attempt to improve efficiency and the quality of care. The changes affected staff as well as patients: new types of assistants (nurses, technicians, clinical clerks, clinic secretaries, and therapeutic assistants) were hired to help the doctors who worked in the clinics. This division of labor meant that a team of health workers replaced the traditional model in which the doctor was "wont to try to do, himself, everything or nearly everything."[77]

One of Cabot's innovations in the MGH outpatient department was the introduction of medical subspecialty clinics. By 1904 organic heart disease was the most common problem seen in the MGH's medical dispensary, even more common than tuberculosis. Three years later, Cabot pointed out that just two groups of patients, infants and those with tuberculosis, "now get first-class treatment" in most dispensaries. He thought outpatient departments should be reorganized so this would be the case for "every other disease."[78]

Cabot's program for reorganization was implemented gradually. Although some cardiac patients were grouped informally in the MGH general medical clinic by internist Joseph Pratt in 1910, Paul White established a structured cardiac clinic four years later. Despite multiple commitments, Pratt had considered getting more involved in heart disease, but in 1907 Mackenzie discouraged him: "It involves a lot of drudgery and wearisome work that will take up a lot more time than you can spare." Pratt's decision not to develop cardiology at the MGH left the field open for White a few years later.[79]

The first formal outpatient clinic for cardiac patients was established at Bellevue Hospital in New York in 1911. Like the less structured program at the MGH, the Bellevue clinic was designed to enhance the outpatient care of cardiac patients. But its focus on the social implications of heart disease reflected the fact that it was inspired by a social worker rather than a physician. Stimulated in part by Cabot's example, Bellevue Hospital established a social service department in 1906. The department was organized by Mary Wadley, a Bellevue nursing graduate who had worked for the Department of Health.

Five years later, Wadley encouraged Hubert Guile, an internist with a special interest in heart disease, to help her develop and supervise a new clinic specifically for cardiac patients.[80] The original name of Wadley and Guile's cardiac clinic reflected its narrow purpose. Called the "Bellevue Experiment in Preventive Work for 'Cardiacs'," it focused on the employment consequences of heart disease in adult men. Guile and a hospital social worker saw patients one evening a week. Working men (the population that especially concerned the social service workers) were unable to attend the regular daytime general medical clinic without missing work (and possibly losing their jobs).

Public health cardiologist Lewis Conner explained the concept to a group of Philadelphia doctors a decade later. He told them that the Bellevue clinic had been organized to help "workingmen" who had suffered a "heart breakdown" but were unable or unwilling to follow their doctors' advice to get a less physically demanding job. "These [men] never found the light work. They knew only one trade, as a rule, and they could get a living wage at their occupation—longshoremen, hod-carriers, truck drivers and what not—and they always went back to that trade, and within a few weeks came back to the hospital in the same dreadful plight as before." With each relapse, their recovery time was longer. Within a "year or two the breakdown was complete."[81]

The original focus of the Bellevue clinic was not on the *prevention* of heart disease in any broad sense but on *rehabilitation* and assistance in finding suitable employment for working-class men with cardiac disease. The clinic organizers believed the right job would prevent relapses, repeat hospitalization, and loss of employment. Indeed, cardiac disease was not viewed as preventable when the Bellevue cardiac clinic was established. There is no mention of heart disease or even acute rheumatic fever in Milton Rosenau's 1074-page book *Preventive Medicine and Hygiene* published in 1913.[82] A 1914 report on the Bellevue clinic experience is explicit on this point: "Because heart disease is not contagious or even, in the strict sense of the word, preventable, the social bearing of the matter has been almost entirely overlooked. Anyone, however, who follows the career of the cardiac patient after his discharge from the hospital must know that this is a disease which calls, above all things, for social treatment."[83]

Initially, this "social treatment" was focused on vocational rehabilitation of male cardiac patients. The Bellevue group was concerned about the medical and financial consequences of heart disease, especially the cost to society of the unemployed "laboring class" cardiac patient. Contemporary public policies "accept his decline (often from comparative health and usefulness) to misery and dependency as inevitable, not realizing that even from the economic point of view this is a wasteful attitude."[84]

Their innovation was to get trained social workers involved in the post-hospital care of "workingmen who had had a breakdown." The social workers could evaluate them in the clinic, could "go to their homes and educate them and their families in their limitations; could go to the workshops and investigate the work they were doing; could

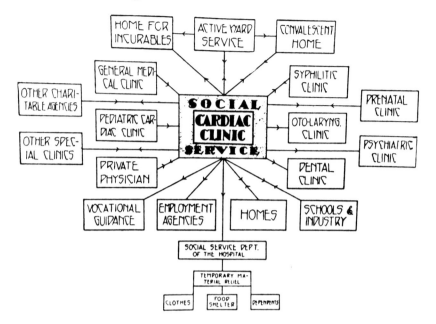

Wyckoff's schematic drawing of the cardiac clinic's relationship to "outside agencies" reflects the public health cardiologists' emphasis on social service and disease prevention. SOURCE: J. Wyckoff, "The organization of the cardiac clinic," *N.Y. State J. Med.* 25 (1925): 995–1001, figure 1, p. 997.

go to their homes and bring them back to the clinics for regular monthly or biweekly examinations." According to Conner, "the success of the clinic rested very largely upon this social service side of it."[85]

During its first three years of operation, 232 patients were seen in the Bellevue cardiac clinic. The organizers reported some dramatic successes and framed them in economic terms. Six patients, hospitalized for a total of almost 36 weeks the year before they began attending the clinic, required no hospitalizations the following year. This resulted in "a saving of 251 days of misery" as well as "a saving of $439.25 to the city." This experience led other New York institutions to imitate the Bellevue clinic program.[86]

Shortly after the Bellevue experience was reported, Conner helped develop another type of program that focused on the convalescence of working men with cardiac disease. He supervised the "Sharon experiment," which allowed men (the program "was only for workingmen") to go to Sharon, Connecticut, for several months of vocational training.

They were taught a "sedentary trade," hoping this might mean "some chance of maintaining them as wage earners."[87]

The cardiac clinic model flourished. In 1915 there were just four in New York City. Two years later there were twenty-four. Conner explained that some were "devoted to children solely, some for adults, some for workingmen, some were held in the afternoon, and some at night."[88] New York's public health cardiologists, noting the success of the model, wanted to organize (and help raise funds for) the clinics that were springing up all over their city. With Haven Emerson, Conner coordinated the creation of the Association for the Prevention and Relief of Heart Disease in 1915. Conner was elected president and chaired a twenty-five-person board of directors that included eight laypersons. This new organization brought together physicians and laypersons who shared a concern about the frequency and social consequences of cardiac disease. Its name reflected the public health cardiologists' commitment to a new notion they helped frame: that heart disease could be prevented.[89]

Public health cardiologists adopted some of the rhetoric and organizational structures of the tuberculosis movement as they developed their agenda and planned how to implement it. At the turn of the century, tuberculosis was the leading cause of death in the United States. One million Americans suffered from the disease, and one in ten deaths was attributed to it.[90] The tuberculosis movement gained momentum during the early twentieth century. In 1902 Hermann Biggs of the New York City Health Department, tuberculosis specialist Adolphus Knopf, and ten other doctors had organized the Committee for the Prevention of Tuberculosis of the Charity Organization Society of New York. By the time World War I began, according to historian Barbara Bates, "Physicians, nurses, politicians, social leaders, officials of the tuberculosis societies, and doubtless much of the public all believed that the tuberculosis movement was scientific, socially justified, and somehow effective." Public health cardiologists tried to capture some of this momentum for their cause.[91]

The agenda of the Association for the Prevention and Relief of Heart Disease reflected the founders' conviction that some forms of cardiac disease might be preventable and their frustration about the general lack of concern about the social consequences of these illnesses. Conner, the association's first president, explained that it would not "do actual heart work" but would be a "coordinating" and "propaganda" organization. The cardiac clinics that the association would help to organize would deliver medical care and social service support to heart patients.[92] The New York group had national ambitions: one of their original (1915) goals was to "encourage the setting up of branch (or like) associations elsewhere."[93]

World War I and the organization of American cardiology

World War I retarded the cardiac clinic movement, but it stimulated more American doctors to become heart specialists. Wartime experiences influenced attitudes about the organization of medical care and led to the development of informal networks of doctors who shared an interest in heart disease. The care of injured Allied soldiers reflected growing acknowledgment of the advantages of specialization. Citing the "modern development of specialism," the Surgeon General established a Division of Internal Medicine in June 1917, which included a cardiovascular section.[94]

Conner was appointed chief of the Army Medical Corps Division of Internal Medicine in 1917. He explained that the Surgeon General defined a "cardiovascular specialist" as an officer with "adequate training in the modern aspects of cardiac diagnosis, including familiarity with the use of the polygraph and the electrocardiograph." Conner hoped to assign one to each large base hospital, but he experienced "considerable difficulty" in "securing a sufficient number of properly qualified cardiovascular examiners."[95] By September forty-five examiners were stationed in various military facilities, including "a number of the best consultants and heart men in the country," according to Theodore Janeway, a medical consultant to the Surgeon General's Office.[96]

America's specialists benefited from a military policy "that officers highly qualified in any special branch of medicine or surgery should be assigned to the corresponding professional division." This directive helped the Army build an experienced staff of specialists. Conner explained that the strategy enabled the Army to recruit many "highly trained internists" who would not have applied for a commission "unless they could be assured that their work in the Army would be of the kind to which they were accustomed and to which they were especially qualified."[97]

In the fall of 1917, several Americans with an interest in heart disease were assigned to the 700-bed Military Heart Hospital at Colchester, England. This facility offered unprecedented opportunities for the care and study of heart patients. It also meant that several dozen American doctors were exposed to Thomas Lewis, who supervised one of the hospital's four services.[98] Some Americans, like aspiring cardiologist Thomas McMillan of Philadelphia, were impressed by the Military Heart Hospital. He remarked in 1924, "In the four years of the World War more was learned about heart disease than centuries of haphazard individual study had yielded. The reason was that large numbers of cases were being studied by trained persons, and the various units of the system worked as a systematized, standardized whole, using standard methods."[99]

The war ended the annual pilgrimage of hundreds of American doctors to Germany. In 1914 the New York Post-Graduate Medical School had a record number of matriculants. School officials knew that the war was the main reason, but they boasted that aspiring specialists could "get from us what they want quite as well as in Europe." The quality of clinical training was improving rapidly in the United States. By 1919 the Continent was in shambles. Lingering anti-German sentiment after the war kept most Americans from going to Germany for training.[100]

Conner had made many contacts during the war, and he used this network to promote his public health agenda. Speaking to a group of Philadelphia physicians in 1921, Conner acknowledged that most doctors and lay people would view "the idea of including diseases of the heart as among that group of preventable diseases . . . [as] novel and perhaps chimerical." But he, Emerson, and other public health cardiologists would work hard to promote this concept during the 1920s. Conner argued that heart disease was "preventable," even though it was not an epidemic disease like diphtheria and typhoid fever or a traditional communicable disease like tuberculosis and syphilis. He cited organized efforts to prevent industrial accidents, blindness, and cancer as models for the prevention of heart disease. Before the public would embrace the concept of preventing heart disease, Conner thought it would be necessary to prove to them that "heart disease is sufficiently important in its social and economical effects to justify such special consideration."[101]

The strategy of the public health cardiologists included the use of statistics to impress American doctors and laypersons with the incidence and socioeconomic implications of heart disease. This approach

TABLE 1-2
Deaths in the United States (1917)

	ALL AGES		40 YEARS AND OVER	
	No.	*Percent*	*No.*	*Percent*
All causes	1,066,711	100.0	566,323	100.0
Heart disease	128,719	12.1	110,426	18.8
Kidney disease	82,657	7.7	70,725	12.1
Cerebral vascular accident	62,417	5.9	59,822	10.2
Cancer	61,429	5.8	55,929	9.5
Lobar pneumonia	74,577	7.0	43,236	7.4
Pulmonary tuberculosis	93,290	8.7	35,151	6.0

SOURCE: Adapted from L. A. Conner, "The value to the community of organized effort to control heart diseases," *Trans. Coll. Phys. Phila.*, 3d ser., 43 (1921): 53–63, p. 54.
NOTE: Arranged in descending order for people aged 40 years and older. Miscellaneous other causes account for the remainder of the mortality.

had been used previously by the social hygiene campaign against venereal disease as well as the antituberculosis and child welfare movements. Conner showed his audience data that proved more Americans died from heart disease than any other cause—more than from tuberculosis, kidney disease, stroke, cancer, or pneumonia (Table 1-2). Another graph demonstrated the increasing incidence of heart disease. He cited the Bellevue cardiac clinic experiment as evidence that the social and economic effects of heart disease were profound.

Conner reported two other recent studies showing that heart disease was more common than anyone thought. He explained that the Army's special cardiovascular examiners had detected evidence of heart disease in 4 percent of drafted men who had already passed the general health screening. Given the number of men examined (five million), the program had detected 200,000 adult males with signs suggesting some cardiac abnormality. Conner also reported the results of a school screening project that found 1.6 percent of 250,000 New York City pupils had evidence of heart disease. Extrapolating these findings, he explained, "There must be approximately 20,000 children of school age in New York with heart defects of greater or less degree."[102] These studies, as well as insurance company statistics, led Conner to conclude that 2 percent of any population "suffer from some form of heart disorder." This had major economic implications, because patients with advanced cardiac disease were dependent on their families or "public charities." The solution? Prevention—a concept "constantly in the minds of the leaders of the Association [for the Prevention and Relief of Heart Disease].[103]

Conner then explained his group's strategy for preventing cardiac disease. He divided organic heart disease into three groups: rheumatic diseases "found chiefly in childhood and adolescence," syphilitic cardiovascular disease "seen chiefly in the middle years of life," and a "somewhat miscellaneous group" of "degenerative diseases" occurring in older people. He thought that rheumatic heart disease offered the greatest hope of prevention—by preventing tonsillitis and throat infections. Conner thought hygienic measures were useful and hoped that tonsillectomy would reduce the number of throat infections. He recommended prolonged convalescence after throat infections to lessen the risk of heart damage.[104]

Another innovation of the public health cardiologists was the notion that heart specialists and social workers should be involved in the care of *potential* cardiac patients as part of their strategy of prevention. "Every syphilis patient is a potential heart patient," according to Conner. He explained, "by watching these patients in the heart clinics . . . something has been accomplished in the way of prevention." He did not elaborate. Turning to "degenerative" heart diseases, Conner conceded, "I cannot say that we have accomplished anything in the direction of prevention." The campaign was built on rhetoric and hope. Public health cardiologists could not prove their claim that heart disease could be prevented.[105]

Conner and his group promoted the value of *organizing* the care of cardiac patients. He had gone to Philadelphia to stimulate the city's doctors to adopt the philosophy and structure of the New York cardiac clinics. They already had. Joseph Sailer embraced the ideology and was Philadelphia's most influential public health cardiologist. One doctor told Conner that "some fifteen of us have been meeting. We have in operation about five clinics following your lead."[106] Another doctor thought Conner's paper proved that "proper organization is a tremendous advantage" in handling a problem as large and socially important as heart disease. He explained, "Many of us have been carrying on work of this kind for years in individual clinics in a spasmodic way and there is no question of the advantage of cooperation of all the hospitals in a given community."[107]

Conner's message resonated with several of his listeners, but money was needed to establish the clinics that were the centerpiece of the public heath cardiologists' agenda. One doctor thought Conner's presentation should "act as a marked stimulus" for the medical profession and for the public, whose contributions were necessary to "supply many of the facilities [clinics and convalescent institutions] that are absolutely requisite." This doctor thought that "a good deal can be accomplished in the way of prevention by societies" such as those organized in New York.[108] Another Philadelphia physician told Conner that his paper "will serve as a sort of Gideon's trumpet, the sound of which will cause not only Philadelphia, Boston, and Cleveland, where beginnings have already been made, to follow the excellent example in New York, but all other large communities throughout the country."[109]

Gideon's trumpet: Promoting preventive cardiology

Haven Emerson helped Conner promote the public health cardiologists' innovation; he titled a 1921 lecture "The Prevention of Heart Disease—a New Practical Problem." Emerson told his audience of Massachusetts doctors that it was "within the reach of present day medical and social knowledge and resources to make as much reduction in sickness and premature death from heart disease as has been obtained by teaching, by diagnosis, by organized medical services in the control of tuberculosis." But success depended on more than delivering medical care to the sick; there was a larger social agenda. For Emerson, "disease control depends on a general elevation of the health of all people, and . . . no age, sex, occupation or race group can long maintain an advanced position of healthfulness without the assistance of all the rest."[110]

The public health cardiologists adopted some elements of the antituberculosis movement as they framed their campaign against heart disease. In America the large-scale, organized effort against tuberculosis was a recent phenomenon. The first dispensary devoted to patients with tuberculosis was established by Edward Bermingham in New York City in 1894. The model thrived, and by 1918 there were nearly five hundred tuberculosis clinics.[111] Seeing how quickly many members of the public and the medical profession had embraced the ideology and approaches of the antituberculosis movement, the public health cardiologists enlisted scientists and social workers to help practitioners and patients deal with heart disease. This coalition promised earlier diagnosis, new cures, less disability, and the hope of prevention. As they sought to organize the care of cardiac patients and plan for their rehabilitation, the public health cardiologists recognized the shortcomings of traditional approaches for classifying heart disease. This was another area that required organization.

At the turn of the century, Ludolf Krehl, the German framer of the concept of pathological physiology, had decried the traditional pathology-based classification of heart disease. He hoped that the "sad state of affairs" would stimulate someone to develop a new approach that also addressed the "clinical phenomena" or symptoms of disease.[112] Richard Cabot, a disciple of the ideology of pathological physiology and an advocate of organization, published a new scheme for classifying heart disease in 1914. It emphasized pathophysiology rather than the traditional approach based on "naming the region affected or the function disturbed." Cabot explained that the simple diagnosis of mitral regurgitation, for example, was inadequate because it failed to differentiate the various causes of this functional problem—a leaking valve. The issue of classification was not simply philosophical, it had "many practical aspects." He thought that "sane prognosis and treatment" depended on understanding the etiology of the disease. The availability of new diagnostic tests and procedures made this new pathophysiological and etiological approach to classifying cardiac disease possible.[113]

The wartime experiences of some heart specialists and other doctors convinced them that a standardized and more complete system for classifying cardiac disease was desirable, indeed essential. Tait Mackenzie, a rehabilitation specialist, explained that "when men came back with all sorts of symptoms connected with the heart, there were various attempts made to classify these cases." The limitations of traditional approaches became apparent: "You may remember they were divided into various classes and given cryptic letters, like D.A.H., for disordered action of the heart, and then there were others added, not yet diagnosed, ending up with G.O.K., God only knows."[114]

Paul White found Cabot's classification scheme very useful in his MGH cardiac clinic. In 1921 White published an enhanced version that included three parts (etiology, structural change, and functional condition). He hoped this new approach would be used in "medical centers" as well as "in distant rural communities" because he thought it provided unique information that would help doctors give a more accurate prognosis. Patients and their families wanted a reliable prognosis, but so did social workers who were charged with arranging convalescent care and job retraining. The new approach also spoke to the prevention movement.

White explained that by emphasizing the cause of the patient's heart disease, it would "forward the prevention of heart disease, about which the medical world is beginning to take more action than in the past."[115]

The public health cardiologists espoused the new etiological and functional classification scheme. In 1922 Alfred Cohn launched a major project on behalf of the Association for the Prevention and Relief of Heart Disease in New York. It incorporated White's classification system into a series of data forms designed to collect detailed information about patients seen in cardiac clinics. As an incentive, the association offered to supply the cards at cost to cardiac clinics across the nation. Doctors (used to keeping minimal records) must have been amazed (and amused) when they saw the complex forms reproduced in the *Journal of the American Medical Association* in 1922. There was a form with hundreds of questions about the patient's general medical history, physical findings, and laboratory results; one specifically for the cardiac history; one for summarizing hospitalizations; and one for the social service record. The charts were printed in duplicate, and a carbon copy was to be sent to the AHA. Cohn acknowledged that what they were attempting to do was "difficult" and "complicated."[116]

These ambitious public health cardiologists wanted to influence attitudes about heart disease by educating the profession and the public. They also wanted to reorganize the way care was delivered to many cardiac patients. In 1923 the New York group published a detailed position statement, "Requirements for an Ideal Cardiac Clinic and a System of Nomenclature." Their system classified each patient's illness in terms of etiology, structural abnormality, pathological physiology, and functional capacity. This was supplemented by a special category for patients with "potential disease," an acknowledgment of the concept of prevention.

Their plan had implications in terms of job opportunities for heart specialists: the ideal clinic should have at least one physician for every fifty active patients. It would also employ nursing, social service, clerical, technical, and administrative personnel. Cardiac clinics became a significant step in the career path for doctors seeking recognition as heart specialists.[117] During the 1920s, the public health cardiologists' influence expanded as more doctors and laypersons adopted their social agenda. Soon, they would be organizing more than cardiac clinics: they would form a coalition with academic cardiologists that put them in a position to shape the emerging specialty.

CHAPTER 2

~~~~~~~~~~~~~~~

Organizing the American Heart Association

Professional opportunities for heart specialists were limited, between the world wars, almost exclusively to private practice. The organization and marginal financial status of most of the nation's medical schools and hospitals provided few opportunities for aspiring physiological or academic cardiologists. Almost all practitioner cardiologists were partial specialists who combined cardiology with general internal medicine practice. Their training consisted of an internship, a year (or two) of internal medicine residency, and a variable amount of time spent as an assistant to a recognized cardiologist or as a physician in a cardiac clinic. Most practitioner cardiologists had taken one or more brief postgraduate courses that a few teaching institutions began offering in the 1920s. They established themselves in many large American cities between 1920 and 1940.

The demand for heart specialists was fueled, in part, by two innovations the public health cardiologists adapted from the antituberculosis movement. One was organizational (cardiac clinics) and the other was ideological (heart disease was preventable). Working in a cardiac clinic was an important step in the career path of many aspiring heart specialists. There, they helped recognized cardiologists care for large numbers of heart patients while they gained clinical experience. They also became more proficient at examining the heart using the stethoscope, electrocardiograph, and fluoroscope—cardiology's main diagnostic tools. Meanwhile, the activities and rhetoric of the public health cardiologists and their circle changed the way doctors cared for cardiac patients and the way people thought about heart disease.

This chapter examines several developments between the world wars that helped define cardiology as a specialty. Public health and academic cardiologists collaborated to create programs that formed the elements of the discipline. They organized a national society, the American Heart Association (AHA), in 1924. The next year they introduced a specialty journal (the *American Heart Journal*) and an annual meeting that enhanced communication among the various types of cardiologists and provided academicians with outlets for their research findings, epidemiological studies, and clinical reports.

Members of a discipline typically claim some special knowledge or expertise that distinguishes them from others. For more than a generation, electrocardiography played this role for most cardiologists. They professed expert knowledge of this specialized tool, which provided unique information to those who could interpret its tracings and understand the jargon developed to describe them. By 1940 a certifying examination was being designed for heart specialists, and some claimed that cardiology was a distinct specialty. But it remained a heterogeneous field reflecting the traditions described in Chapter 1.

Public health cardiologists extend their influence

By the early 1920s, the New York public health cardiologists had helped to stimulate doctors in more than a dozen cities to develop cardiac clinics and to form local heart organizations modeled after their own Association for the Prevention and Relief of Heart Disease.[1] Paul White took the lead in organizing Boston's cardiac clinics along the lines of the New York program. With the help of other interested doctors and social workers, he formed the Boston Association of Cardiac Clinics in 1921. The following year White and his circle established the Boston Association for the Prevention and Relief of Heart Disease to educate the public about cardiac disease and to raise funds for their clinics.[2]

Philadelphia joined the movement in 1921, when public health cardiologist Joseph Sailer and a few other doctors organized the Philadelphia Society for the Study of Heart Disease. After Lewis Conner's visit that year, they restructured their society along the lines of the New York group and incorporated it as the Philadelphia Association for the Prevention and Relief of Heart Disease. The New York and Philadelphia societies cosponsored a scientific exhibit at the 1922 American Medical Association (AMA) meeting (5,174 attendees), which helped to stimulate the development of similar local heart associations around the nation.[3]

The experience in Chicago shows that not all doctors embraced the public health cardiologists' agenda and their clinic model. When James Herrick and other heart specialists organized the Chicago Association for the Prevention and Relief of Heart Disease in 1922, they were attacked by the Chicago Medical Society. The general practitioners, who cared for most heart patients, worried that the new cardiac clinics and the specialists who worked in them would compete with them for patients.[4] For years practitioners had sensed that they were losing some business to dispensaries and hospital outpatient clinics. This concern intensified as the number of clinics increased. By the end of the decade, Haven Emerson estimated that "one-fourth of the entire population of our large cities applies at out-patient departments for diagnosis and treatment," and the average patient made three visits each year.[5] Even if most of the patients seen in clinics could not afford a private physician, some could. John Wyckoff explained that "public patients, so-called, seek medical aid not only from medical clinics but also from physicians in private practice."[6]

There were other tensions between office-based practitioners and recognized public health physicians (especially those employed by public health departments) who sought to reorganize care. Some doctors resented the whole public health movement, which occasionally portrayed them as inadequate. The authors of a 1919 book on public health officers argued that "public health work is a new specialty in medicine. . . . It calls for more skill and knowledge than the average doctor possesses." While this type of exclusionary rhetoric was common to groups seeking to delineate a new specialty, there was more: "A family doctor frequently owes his success to his ability to please his families, regardless of his ability and knowledge." Attitudes like this surely alienated some practitioners from the expanding public health movement.[7]

This was the context in which the Chicago Medical Society investigated charges that Herrick's new heart association was soliciting patients by advertising their clinics, a move portrayed as unethical and unfair to practitioners. Although the effort to establish a heart association in Chicago was successful, it was controversial. Herrick recalled that the critics of this attempt to organize cardiac care "charged us with intent to take the bread and butter away from the underdog, the struggling family doctor, who, they said, could just as efficiently give digitalis to a heart patient or prescribe rest in bed as the doctor who claimed to be a specialist." Herrick probably expected the attack, which he saw as a "battle between high-brow and low-brow."[8] One year earlier, he described the "oft heard rancorous protest on the part of the practitioners against the smaller privileged class of specialists who seem to them to be reaching out more and more after the glory and the major portion of the financial returns."[9]

In 1922 Alfred Cohn remarked that America "possesses a large and increasing number of physicians who have had special training and who are especially interested in circulatory diseases."[10] During the 1920s and 1930s more doctors chose to become heart specialists. They were a diverse group: most were practitioners, some emphasized science, and a few were interested primarily in public health. As the numbers of heart specialists increased, the public health cardiologists launched a campaign to encourage them to adopt their vision of heart disease—one that emphasized its socioeconomic implications.

Lewis Conner, Haven Emerson, and Robert Halsey invited approximately one hundred physicians to attend a luncheon during the 1922 annual AMA meeting in St. Louis, where they would present a proposal to establish a "National Association for the Prevention and Relief of Heart Disease."[11] As they developed their program, these public health cardiologists drew upon the experience of the antituberculosis movement. The model was useful, but Cohn admitted that "from the view of public health, the problem of heart disease is not as simple as that of tuberculosis." He explained that unlike tuberculosis and other "bacterial" diseases, heart disease did not consist of "a single entity but of diseases etiologically as distinct as the acute rheumatic affections, syphilis and arterial degenerations."[12]

Almost fifty doctors attended the St. Louis meeting, including Louis Bishop and John Wyckoff of New York; William Thayer of Baltimore; William Stroud and Joseph Sailer of Philadelphia; and James Herrick of Chicago. Emerson outlined the organization's purpose: "co-ordination of efforts, development of research, collection and distribution of information, public health and industrial education, to develop sound public opinion as to the true meaning and seriousness of the problem."[13] After two years of planning, the AHA was incorporated on 14 March 1924. Conner was elected president and chair of the board of directors (composed of fifteen physicians, mainly academic cardiologists).[14]

The simple name—American Heart Association—the founders eventually chose for their new organization was more inclusive than the working version, the National Association for the Prevention and Relief of Heart Disease. The dynamics of inventing and naming the AHA affirm Joel Howell's observation that "the definitions of cardiology have been negotiated and renegotiated."[15] The individuals who took the first steps in creating this national organization framed cardiology mainly in terms of the social and economic dimensions of heart disease. But they had to convince other doctors to cooperate with them in institutionalizing their concepts and methods. The founders succeeded because they were willing to incorporate programs that addressed the interests of other constituencies—the academics, scientists, and practitioners.

Still, the AHA's agenda emphasized the interests of public health cardiologists; the mission statement was based on the plan Conner and Emerson had developed nine years earlier for their New York association. It stressed data collection, public education, and the improvement of patient access to various specialized services (Table 2-1). The focus of the nation's first national heart organization would have been different if it had been created by physiological cardiologists like Carl Wiggers or practitioner cardiologists like Louis Bishop.

Conner, Emerson, and their circle spent two years launching the AHA. According to Sailer, "Whilst we groped and wondered what to

---

TABLE 2-1
The Purposes of the American Heart Association

1. The study and dissemination and application of knowledge concerning the causes, treatment, and prevention of heart disease
2. The gathering of information on heart disease
3. The development and application of measures that will prevent heart disease
4. Seeking and provision of occupations suitable for heart disease patients
5. The extension of opportunities for adequate care of cardiac convalescents
6. The promotion of permanent institutional care for such cardiac patients as are hopelessly incapacitated for self-support
7. The encouragement and establishment of local associations with similar objects throughout the United States

SOURCE: W. M. Moore, *Fighting for Life: The Story of the American Heart Association* (Dallas: AHA, 1983), pp 17–18. Reproduced with permission. Copyright William W. Moore and the American Heart Association.

do, others suggested work that we had not foreseen." They were encouraged "to establish a journal for heart disease," but this was not an innovation, since periodicals devoted to cardiology had been published in Europe for more than a decade.[16] In 1925 Conner explained in the inaugural issue of the *American Heart Journal* that the periodical had been established in response to the "very widespread interest in circulatory diseases which is now so apparent." He attributed the field's vitality to "the truly revolutionary advances made in our knowledge of the normal and pathological physiology of the heart and its beat, along with the advance in understanding of its diseases and their management." Conner also articulated the AHA's main agenda; he told readers that the association was "dedicated to the prevention and public health aspects" of heart disease.

The journal's purpose was to meet the "increasingly evident demand by physicians throughout the country for a periodical covering the field of diseases of the heart and circulation." One goal was to educate the "medical profession in matters relating to the diagnosis, treatment and prevention of heart diseases." The intended audience was not a "limited group of heart specialists," but a "very much larger class of intelligent well-trained general practitioners who aspire to keep abreast of the rapidly growing knowledge of the heart and its disorders." Conner knew that most cardiac patients received their care from general practitioners, and he envisioned a journal that would be "primarily clinical in character." At the same time, it would provide physiological and academic cardiologists with an outlet for their research findings.[17]

Although there were no physiological cardiologists on the AHA's original board of directors, they were represented on the editorial board of the journal. Albion Hewlett, Carl Wiggers, and Frank Wilson shared editorial responsibilities with nineteen other board members, mainly clinical investigators and academic cardiologists.[18] Despite a pledge to publish papers for clinicians, many articles were rather esoteric. For several years, the transactions of the AHA's annual scientific meeting were published in the journal. These records reveal something about the character of the meetings. During the 1920s and 1930s, fewer than ten papers were presented and commented upon. The emphasis was on research to elucidate the pathophysiology of various types of heart disease and to evaluate new diagnostic and therapeutic approaches.

Approximately two hundred "representative physicians and laymen from all parts of the country" attended the first annual meeting, held in Atlantic City in 1925. They heard reports of Samuel Levine's study of the value of the sympathectomy operation in angina pectoris (some patients "strikingly helped"), Frederick Willius's review of heart disease in severe hypothyroidism (no evidence that such a specific entity existed), and Emanuel Libman's investigation of elevated white blood cell count in acute coronary thrombosis (a useful confirmatory finding).[19] The programs of the AHA's meetings and the contents of its journal prove that several American medical schools and teaching hospitals were sponsoring productive research programs by 1930.

The AHA's public health agenda was more visible in the journal, which included papers on the epidemiology of heart disease, occupational health issues (such as pre-employment examinations and vocational training of cardiac patients), and the economic burden of heart disease. For example, one writer (summarizing the experience at two clinics in Chicago in 1925) concluded that "the economic loss, private and public, covering only a fraction of the patients with heart disease in one of our large cities must be estimated in hundreds of thousands of dollars annually."[20]

Joel Howell has emphasized the important link between the AHA and the antituberculosis movement "conceptually and organizationally." This reflects the dominant role of New York City public health cardiologists in inventing the AHA. In 1927 five of the seven members of the association's executive committee could best be classified as public health cardiologists (Conner, Emerson, Halsey, Sailer, and Wyckoff). The other members (Herrick and Stroud) supported the AHA's public health agenda. That year they published a table that drew parallels between tuberculosis and heart disease as an aid to individuals "considering the organization of cardiac work with the cooperation of tuberculosis associations." The AHA founders embraced the ideals of the antituberculosis movement and marveled at its success; they also hoped to capture some of its momentum and resources to assist patients with heart disease.[21]

Heart disease presented certain challenges that tuberculosis did not. Although tuberculosis could affect many organs, it stemmed from a single infectious agent, the tubercle bacillus, which could be identified microscopically and grown in culture media. There were several distinct types of heart disease, and little was known about their causes.

The following outline shows some of the parallels that may be drawn between tuberculosis and heart disease. This outline should prove of interest to those who are considering the organization of cardiac work with the cooperation of tuberculosis associations.

Tuberculosis	Heart Disease
Medical Aspects	*Medical Aspects*
1. Communicable disease	1. Ditto (Rheumatic & Syphilitic)
2. Involves childhood chiefly	2. Ditto (Rheumatic & Congenital)
3. Chronic infection	3. Ditto
4. May become active	4. Exacerbations occur
5. Handicaps physical efficiency	5. Ditto
6. Treatment chiefly hygienic with emphasis on rest	6. Ditto (except for Syphilitic)
Social Aspects	*Social Aspects*
1. Influenced profoundly by economic conditions	1. Probably influenced by economic conditions
2. Requires guidance of P. H. nurse and social worker	2. Ditto
3. Handicaps but does not necessarily destroy efficiency	3. Ditto
4. Usual methods of quarantine useless	4. Ditto
5. Control of carrier through hospitalization and education important	5. Ditto (communicable types)
Public Education	*Public Education*
1. Accomplished through all publicity channels reaching individuals, home, school	1. Ditto
2. Channels of reaching people well developed	2. Channels not yet developed
3. Training in health habits important	3. Ditto
4. Both knowledge and motivation necessary	4. Ditto
Equipment and Facilities	*Equipment and Facilities*
1. Sanatoria necessary and well developed	1. No Sanatoria. Heart cases need similar facilities
2. Preventoria growing in popularity	2. Preventoria needed but not now generally available
3. Preventorium class rooms being established	3. Heart cases would profit by similar equipment
4. Health camps, especially when regarded as training camps, are valuable and popular	4. Similar opportunities valuable for heart cases
5. Tuberculosis clinics universally accepted	5. Chest clinics easily care for tuberculosis and heart cases

Similarities between tuberculosis and heart disease.

SOURCE: *Bull. Am. Heart Assoc.* 2 (1927): 22. Reproduced with permission. Copyright American Heart Association.

The AHA leaders viewed accurate classification of cardiac disorders as a necessary prerequisite to understanding the causes and finding cures for the various kinds of heart disease. The AHA supported the ongoing efforts of the New York Heart Association (NYHA), the new name of their 1915 organization, to refine its classification scheme. Robert Halsey, an influential person in both groups, explained: "Where there is now a babble of medical terms there might be a common language. In place of a confusion of expressions there might be systematic, orderly, concise statements which would be more correctly understood."[22] The AHA endorsed a detailed classification scheme, which the New York group published in book form in 1928. To be complete, each cardiac diagnosis now required four components: etiology, anatomy, physiology, and functional capacity. Technology had become central to their classification scheme; more than half of the section on physiological criteria dealt with the electrocardiographic findings in various cardiac disorders.[23]

The growing influence of the electrocardiograph

By this time, cardiology was becoming a technological medical field. Heart specialists were dependent on the electrocardiograph, chest x-ray, and fluoroscope to help them detect and characterize heart disease. Meanwhile, they helped to define a specialty and encourage its growth. The advent of cardiac clinics staffed by doctors interested in heart disease encouraged the diffusion of these new technologies. When a children's cardiac clinic was formed at the Johns Hopkins Hospital and staffed by Edwards Park, a pediatrician with a "particular interest" in heart patients, the number of x-rays and electrocardiograms "increased tremendously."[24]

In 1926 Arthur Hirschfelder told a group of Philadelphia doctors, "We are living in an era of diagnosis. When we speak of a good clinician, we say he is an excellent diagnostician."[25] Practitioner cardiologists, who wanted to be viewed as the group best able to diagnose (and treat) heart conditions, knew the electrocardiograph gave them an advantage over other doctors. This machine assumed greater importance as doctors, patients, employers, and insurance companies sought objective measures of the heart's functional capacity. But this trend toward technology disturbed some doctors, especially older ones who had been taught that a heart murmur was a powerful predictor of cardiac disease. James Herrick acknowledged the "great value" of the electrocardiograph, but he protested the "tendency nowadays to attack the stethoscope." He thought "the stethoscope, the x-ray and electrocardiograph should be allies not enemies."[26]

Increasingly, cardiologists championed the electrocardiograph as an aid to diagnosis. Some manufacturers went further: one claimed it could change people's lives. A 1934 advertisement recounted the case of a doctor's son "condemned to inactivity" after his father detected abnormal heart sounds and took him to several "well-known pediatricians." Because he followed their advice, "Jimmy became wizened." But "luckily," Jimmy's father consulted "a competent cardiologist . . . who took tracings with his 'Hindle Electrocardiograph'. The heart muscle proved to be in good condition even though abnormal sounds were heard." The boy's activity restrictions were lifted, and "today Jimmy is not wizened." The advertisement sent a clear message. A doctor—a cardiologist—armed with an electrocardiograph was a better diagnostician than the traditional experts, and accurate diagnosis was the key to prognosis and treatment.[27]

The electrocardiograph would not become the twentieth-century equivalent of the stethoscope—a diagnostic tool carried by all physicians. The machine's high cost (about one-third of the average general practitioner's annual income in 1931) limited the market.[28] Doctors who spent this much money on a machine assumed it would enhance their status as well as their diagnostic ability. Joel Howell notes that some physicians "justified their expertise in a specific area of medicine by claiming a special ability to operate a medical tool, thus using medical technology to define their specialty."[29] This was true for a generation of doctors who sought recognition as heart specialists before there were formal cardiology training programs or board examinations. For many patients in this era, a practitioner who possessed an electrocardiograph was, de facto, a heart specialist.

Brooklyn cardiologist Edwin Maynard "was able to learn something about reading electrocardiograms" as an intern and resident at Presbyterian Hospital in New York from 1919 to 1921. After he set up Brooklyn Hospital's electrocardiograph in 1921, Maynard found that some doctors viewed him as a heart specialist. He later recalled that when staff physicians received his electrocardiographic reports, "they called on me to ask what I thought about their patients' hearts." This led to consultations: "I was forced to tell them truthfully that I could give no opinion from the electrocardiogram alone. Whereupon I was often asked to examine their patients."[30] Maynard had completed two years of postgraduate education in internal medicine and had learned to use the electrocardiograph, but he had no formal cardiology training. This career path was typical of practitioner cardiologists until after World War II.

The ability of the electrocardiograph to transform a general practitioner (who had even less training in internal medicine) into a heart specialist worried some cardiologists. A Philadelphia heart specialist who identified himself as "formerly special cardiovascular examiner, United States Army," expressed this concern in 1923. He thought that any doctor hoping "to make a success of electrocardiography" must "be prepared to devote all his time" to learning the "art" which "must be practiced regularly, systematically and faithfully, day after day, week after week, before proficiency is obtained." The bottom line: "The mere possession of electrocardiographic equipment no more makes a person

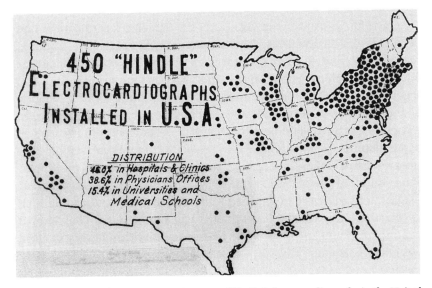

Location of Cambridge Instrument Company "Hindle" electrocardiographs in the United States (1925).
SOURCE: *Am. Heart J.* 1, no. 3 (1925): ads, p. 1.

a cardiologist than the possession of Shakespeare's volume makes the owner a *littérateur.*"[31] But this idealistic view did not retard the diffusion of the technology. But a Mayo Clinic heart specialist had just published a book on electrocardiography because of its "constantly increasing use" by "clinicians, especially in hospitals and clinics."[32] The machines promised to improve diagnosis and elevate the status of individuals and institutions; they generated additional income for the doctors that used them and the hospitals that owned them.[33]

Doctors and hospitals were not the only parties interested in the electrocardiograph. Patients were becoming aware of its perceived value. In 1922 a Brooklyn physician claimed that "the patient of today has read and heard much about the electrocardiograph, and if he suffers from heart disease is very apt to have an electrocardiographic tracing in his possession."[34] Harold Segall, a trainee of Paul White, began practicing cardiology in Montreal in 1926. He purchased a portable electrocardiograph the following year and later recalled that the machine "did much to make the medical profession and the laity aware of the new specialty of cardiology."[35]

By 1926, just seventeen years after the first electrocardiograph had been installed in the United States, there were nearly five hundred machines in the nation: 46 percent were in hospitals and clinics, 38.6 percent in physicians' offices, and 15.4 percent in universities and medical schools. Their location reflects the distribution of cardiologists at the time, because the persons responsible for the machine were recognized as heart specialists by their patients and peers.[36] The market was expanding rapidly. Within two years after they began selling electrocardiographs, General Electric claimed to have installed more than three hundred around the world.[37] In 1930 readers of the popular magazine *Hygeia* were told, "The electro-cardiograph has become such an efficient and valuable instrument that almost every well known heart specialist includes one in his office equipment, and every modern hospital boasts one."[38]

The ideology of prevention and its implications for cardiology

Although diagnosis and treatment were the main concerns of practitioner cardiologists, public health cardiologists remained committed to their concept of preventing heart disease. Their approach stressed the importance of periodic examinations of presumably healthy people as a means of detecting asymptomatic heart disease. They collected and published statistics about the incidence and economic consequences of heart disease that heightened the public's concern. Various AHA publications prepared for doctors and laypersons stressed that morbidity and mortality from communicable diseases (especially tuberculosis) was declining. Meanwhile, heart disease, already more frequent than tuberculosis, was increasing.[39]

In 1926 the Metropolitan Life Insurance Company's statistician reported that 20 percent of Americans who survived to the age of ten would die of heart disease, three times as many as would die of tuberculosis. He considered heart disease "the outstanding problem in contemporary preventive medicine."[40] Public health cardiologists used these statistics to advance their cause. Haven Emerson argued that the decline in mortality from tuberculosis had "left heart disease in a position of single eminence" as the leading cause of death. He challenged doctors to "take an active part in the attack upon heart diseases. . . . Your Hippocratic oath requires this of you."[41]

Laypersons also had a responsibility: they must get periodic examinations. As early as 1915, Emerson had helped launch a "campaign" to encourage "all classes of the community" to get annual medical examinations "by competent physicians." He thought the program would appeal to general practitioners who "noted a falling off of their incomes" as a result of the declining incidence of communicable and childhood diseases. Emerson framed the periodic examination program as a means to make up for this decrease in traditional medical work: "We are creating a demand for the services of physicians as diagnosticians and practitioners of preventive medicine."[42]

By 1920 Emerson had extended the prevention philosophy to cardiac disease, focusing on the association between tonsillitis and acute rheumatic fever. The goals included the "prevention of infection, prevention of cardiac damage, prevention of extension of lesion or disability, and postponement of death from heart diseases."[43] The discovery of asymptomatic heart disease in New York City schoolchildren and World War I recruits gave impetus to the campaign for periodic medical examinations of presumably healthy people. The AMA officially sanctioned periodic health examinations in 1922, and people heard about them on the radio and read about them in the popular press and in public health pamphlets. This ambitious program represented a paradigm shift for doctors and healthy citizens alike—especially once the focus went beyond communicable diseases. In 1923 public health physician Charles Winslow declared that "the control of the degenerative diseases requires nothing less than the systematic medical examination of presumably normal individuals." He acknowledged that this philosophy represented "a complete reconsideration of the function of the physician in modern community life."[44]

For (potential) patients one message was clear: have a competent doctor examine your heart! In 1925 the *American Mercury* advised, "Every sensible person should go at least once a year to a reputable physician . . . and have a complete appraisal." Why? "Periodic health examinations serve to detect heart disease in time for something to be done about it." And no one was safe: "No layman can ascertain the condition of his heart merely by the way he feels or thinks he feels." Life insurance companies and their agents reinforced the message by encouraging or requiring health examinations that emphasized the heart and lungs.[45]

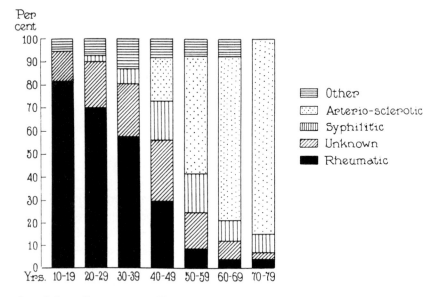

Organic heart disease (arranged by age and etiology) in 1,001 patients from the Bellevue Cardiac Clinic and John Wyckoff's private practice.
SOURCE: A. E. Cohn, "Heart disease from the point of view of the public health," *Am. Heart J.* 2 (1927): 291.

The AHA embraced this philosophy to help achieve their goal of preventing heart disease. In May 1925 they inaugurated the *Bulletin of the American Heart Association*, a newsletter aimed not just at doctors but also at social workers, nurses, and laypersons who might be interested in (and support) the association's programs. The first issue reaffirmed the founders' commitment to preventive medicine. The "great public" was urged to get periodic examinations to help reduce the incidence and consequences of heart disease. This approach implied that conditions (such as tonsillitis) thought to cause rheumatic heart disease could be "discovered and eliminated." At the same time, "heart damage may be detected in its earliest stages when most can be done for its alleviation."[46]

The AHA leaders realized that most American physicians did not share their intense concern about rheumatic heart disease or their preoccupation with prevention. In 1928 AHA vice president William Robey told association members that "the incidence of acute rheumatic fever was so slight in the southern and southwestern states that an interest in its cardiac sequelae was negligible."[47] Twelve years later, rheumatic fever expert May Wilson explained that "interest" in the disease in the United States "was aroused through the efforts of the New York Heart Association," while the AHA "directed attention to the public health aspect of rheumatic fever throughout the United States."[48]

Compared to the diagnosis and treatment of heart disease, prevention received very little attention during the first quarter of the century. This claim is supported by data derived from an exhaustive bibliography of publications on heart disease that appeared between 1901 and 1925. There were forty times as many articles on diagnosis and treatment as there were on prevention (which was covered on one-half page of this 115-page bibliography).[49] Public health cardiologists kept up their campaign and gradually expanded their focus to include the prevention of arteriosclerosis and coronary artery disease.[50]

John Wyckoff articulated the AHA's new strategy. The first step was to repudiate the traditional view that "arteriosclerosis, like a fate, must attack us all." He realized that the etiology of arteriosclerosis was unknown, although various theories attributed it to hypertension, infection, toxic substances, and disordered metabolism. Wyckoff acknowledged that until etiology was understood, prevention was problematic. Although he encouraged additional laboratory research, Wyckoff emphasized that "still greater information can be learned from the properly organized clinic" where physicians could chart the natural history of the disease as it affected patients systematically followed there.[51] Using data Alfred Cohn had collected from New York cardiac clinics, he explained that arteriosclerotic heart disease was significantly more common (40 percent) than rheumatic heart disease (25 percent) in this sample. Meanwhile, there was growing recognition of a distinct and disturbing clinical syndrome—coronary thrombosis or acute myocardial infarction. This condition, popularly known as "heart attack," posed a threat of sudden death to people previously thought to be healthy.[52]

Heart murmurs helped identify asymptomatic rheumatic heart disease that affected the heart's valves, but there were no consistent physical findings to help doctors detect asymptomatic coronary artery disease. A normal cardiac examination, electrocardiogram, and chest x-ray did not prove that a middle-aged or older patient had normal coronary arteries. As the serious implications of coronary disease were recognized, heart specialists sought new ways to evaluate the functional capacity of the heart. Early approaches focused on heart rate and blood pressure responses to exercise and the measurement of vital capacity, a breathing test that assessed heart and lung function.[53] By the mid-1930s "tests of myocardial function" had become "a common procedure in physiological and medical institutions and also in the office of the medical practitioner."[54]

Increasingly, Americans were urged to get periodic health examinations and cautioned about the dangers of unrecognized heart disease. Readers of the popular magazine *Hygeia* were warned about the risk of heart attack and sudden death (there was no mention of rheumatic heart disease) and told "no business man who expects to succeed would think of neglecting to take inventory of his stock once a year." Readers were urged to get an annual examination supplemented by "instruments of precision" because "you can't get another heart." The same message was repeated on the radio.[55]

Given all the rhetoric, it is not surprising that patients undergoing routine medical examinations expressed concern about their hearts. Through their many publications and programs directed at laypersons, the AHA contributed significantly to the public's growing awareness of, and anxiety about, the risks of undetected heart disease. "There can be no doubt," cardiologist Albert Hyman declared in 1929, "that the lay public, as well as the physician, is becoming more and more conscious of the fearful toll exacted by the rheumatic and degenerative diseases of the circulatory system; widespread publicity and organized propaganda for enlightenment have made these facts known to all."[56]

Three years later, Hyman claimed that "intense publicity" had "swept into many a physician's consulting room individuals who had never before sought medical advice." And they were especially worried about their hearts. "Many persons have besieged their doctors to examine them and to allay their fears of sudden death from heart failure."[57] This growing demand for cardiac evaluations (including an electrocardiogram) encouraged more doctors to specialize in heart disease. Patients who sought care from practitioner cardiologists were not the same as those who went to cardiac clinics. They were members of America's growing middle class and urban professionals who talked about their health in settings that reflected their affluence: "the club, the golf course, the Turkish bath, the lunch hour."[58]

But these concerns were not limited to patients who could afford a private physician. Wyckoff was impressed that "the need for treatment by a specialist in heart disease" was becoming "increasingly felt . . . as more and more cardiac patients are referred to cardiac clinics." The desire to provide care to cardiac patients unable to afford private doctors and the ideology of prevention led to the organization of more cardiac clinics. Meanwhile, more doctors and clinics bought electrocardiograph machines. By the late 1920s, the *American Heart Journal* was filled with advertisements for them.[59]

Practitioner cardiologists and the rise of a clinical specialty

Cardiology was becoming a distinct specialty, although some internists regretted it.[60] The trend toward specialty practice in the United States was continuing to gather momentum. In 1925 AMA president William Pusey observed that "our present graduates show a preponderant tendency to go into the specialties. They are not going into general practice."[61] Three years later, after surveying nearly four thousand recent medical graduates of fifty-seven "class A" American medical schools, the dean of Syracuse University College of Medicine concluded that the progressive trend toward specialization was "undoubtedly in response to opportunities offered and demands made by society on the medical college graduates."[62]

The growth of cardiology as a specialty was encouraged by an expanding knowledge base and by new technologies like the electrocardiograph. But, like other specialties, its character and rate of expansion were shaped by social and economic factors. Fifty years before the AHA was founded, a New York physician explained that he was not surprised that many medical graduates were inclined to specialize "considering the conventional understanding regarding the position and emoluments of specialists."[63] In 1926 James Herrick expressed the view that most doctors worked "for gain, recognition, opportunity, power."[64] And those rewards were more likely to go to specialists. The following year, a government economist reported that general practitioners were "most likely to have difficulty in earning an adequate income" and were "also losing prestige."[65] Academic surgeon Hugh Cabot called the differential in average net income between specialists ($10,000) and general practitioners ($3,900) "striking" in 1935.[66]

This income differential reflected the willingness of patients to pay a premium for specialty care. Herrick was impressed with the "tendency on the part of the laity to demand and secure first hand, i.e., over the head of the family doctor the services of the expert, i.e., what in their view are the best services."[67] Meanwhile, many types of specialists were becoming more accessible. There were more of them, and they were no longer confined to large cities. Herrick explained, "Telegraph, telephone, good roads, the automobile, and the small-town hospital makes specialists easily and increasingly available."[68]

The number of practitioner cardiologists (almost all of them partial specialists) increased during the 1920s and 1930s as a result of the growth of electrocardiography, the creation of more cardiac clinics, and increased patient demand. Gradually, some cardiac patients and asymptomatic people who feared heart disease and who lived in or near larger cities began gravitating to cardiac clinics or to practitioner cardiologists. They were self-referred or sent by other doctors. In this context, aspiring heart specialists sought institutional appointments to affirm their status as experts in the eyes of potential patients and as consultants in the opinion of doctors who might refer cardiac cases to them. Doctors selected to head a cardiac clinic or supervise a hospital-based electrocardiography unit could point to these institutional activities to validate their identity as heart specialists. The quest for positions and privileges created tensions in some contexts because the public health and academic cardiologists exercised control over some of these appointments, especially those affiliated with more prestigious institutions.

In 1923 the New York Association for the Prevention and Relief of Heart Disease published a position paper in the widely read *Boston Medical and Surgical Journal* detailing the "requirements for an ideal cardiac clinic." Aspiring heart specialists who read it discovered that this ambitious group was planning to organize New York's cardiac clinics—with implications for their careers. The association's white paper included criteria for selecting "chiefs" for cardiac clinics: the doctor had to be a specialist (an internist or pediatrician) with "broad clinical training and a special knowledge of the cardiac problems." Ultimately, the association's leaders would choose whom they wanted to head a cardiac clinic that sought to affiliate with them. Anyone wishing to head a cardiac clinic had to have "sufficient experience with patients having heart disease to meet the approval of the Executive Committee of the Association."[69]

This policy, which empowered a small committee to select the heads of New York's official cardiac clinics, was symbolic of a larger trend in American medicine. Increasingly, doctors worried that they might lose the right to chose where and how to practice medicine. In 1931 the president of the New York Academy of Medicine articulated the concern: "Much fear is at present expressed that the doctors are losing control of their own destiny . . . that our freedom of action is being taken away from us."[70] Other tensions were in the air; some doctors thought their profession was under siege. The Committee on Costs of Medical Care, sponsored by several philanthropic foundations, "blamed American doctors for the problems of medical care on almost every page of their report," according to Daniel Fox.[71]

Meanwhile, relations between academic physicians and office-based practitioners were becoming increasingly strained—the "town-gown" problem. American academic medicine was in the midst of a revolution when the AHA was founded, and many urban practitioners felt threatened by the increasingly influential teaching centers.[72] Some office-based doctors who had formerly taught the clinical subjects resented their declining influence in medical education as the numbers of university-based clinicians increased. In 1922 an Ohio doctor argued that practitioners had lost control of training student physicians when medical schools merged with universities in an effort to win philanthropic support. He protested that the ensuing "scramble for the Rockefeller-Carnegie millions" had resulted in "worship at the shrines of two fetishes—research and full-time teachers." Six years later, Harvard physician Joseph Pratt acknowledged that "it is openly lamented among some influential groups of clinicians that scientific workers trained in the laboratory and with little clinical experience are elected to clinical chairs. The old days are recalled when 'practical men' instead of 'scientists' occupied these positions."[73]

The issue was not simply who taught the medical students; it also had to do with status—and patients. Doctors who held part-time faculty positions could use their titles to affirm their status as self-designated specialists. Academic appointments sent a signal to other doctors and patients, but elite teaching institutions excluded most practitioners. They were also denied entry into most academically oriented medical societies, since they lacked the proper credentials or interests. For example, many academic, physiological, and public health cardiologists joined the elite Association of American Physicians in the 1920s and 1930s. Reflecting their academic status, two-thirds of the original AHA board were members of the society. Practitioner cardiologists were not invited to join this organization, whose members shared an interest in research.[74]

Although they shared an interest in the heart, the four types of cardiologists had distinct interests and needs. They were representatives, in one specialty, of the ideological and functional diversity that now existed in American medicine. In the late 1920s, New York public health physician Sigismund Goldwater told a friend, "The research worker and the university medical teacher look upon themselves first as scientists and only incidentally as clinicians." The medical scientist "concentrates on aspects of disease rather than upon the whole patient." It is not their purpose "to study the patient as a human being in all his physical and social relations."[75]

The fifteen men appointed to the AHA's original board of directors were representatives of two main groups: academic and public health cardiologists. With one exception, they were affiliated with major teaching institutions. They did not represent the interests of the practitioner cardiologists who, with internists and general practitioners, cared for most cardiac patients. In 1928 AHA vice president William Robey predicted that the association would play a major role in cardiology because it had brought together "most of the outstanding workers in this field." Despite this elitist rhetoric, he acknowledged that "cardiac disease belongs pre-eminently to the family practitioner and it is for him that we exist."[76]

When they wanted to expand their organization, the AHA leaders looked first to their peers—academically oriented physicians. A 1927 membership drive targeted "(1) professors and assistant professors in Grade A medical schools; (2) all physicians who have submitted papers on the subject of heart disease during the past two years from a list secured from the Index Medicus; (3) all subscribers to the *American Heart Journal.*"[77] Seven years later, H. M. (Jack) Marvin, an academic cardiologist at Yale who chaired the association's executive committee, told Howard Sprague, a cardiologist at the Massachusetts General Hospital, that "the members of the advisory council and committees are carefully selected men of high standing, who are familiar with the work and aims of the association."[78] This philosophy excluded ordinary practitioner cardiologists from positions of influence in the AHA.

The creation of the AHA demonstrated that there was no single vision of cardiology or of cardiac patients. Practitioner cardiologists were first and foremost clinicians; they were not especially interested in the social implications of their patients' heart problems. In 1922 one writer explained that the "over-worked hospital doctor cares nothing for [social] 'case work,' his interest lies in curing disease."[79] Practitioners focused on the diagnosis, treatment, and prognosis of heart disease in middle- and upper-class patients. The people they saw in their offices or in the hospital were unlike the patients followed in the AHA-affiliated cardiac clinics or admitted to public wards. Louis Bishop recognized the distinction: "By public practice I mean all that work done in hospitals, dispensaries and teaching institutions and upon the poor or pauperized classes. By private practice I mean work that is carried on with people with whom the relationship of private physician is established."[80]

The different social class origins of public and private patients had implications for the type of heart disease they had, their care-seeking behavior, and the treatment options available to them. According to Bishop, patients in public practice developed heart disease "under conditions of irregular living and the strain of continuous labor, or . . . lived under bad hygienic conditions." Among the patients in this group, "severe organic disease" was "very conspicuous." They tended to ignore "minor discomforts" and were "in a great measure fatalistic in their outlook upon life." Bishop thought the situation in private practice was "just the reverse." More affluent patients were more likely to develop "functional" cardiac disease "under conditions of luxury and indolence." They did "not disregard any personal discomfort" and would "carry out any reasonable plan of treatment or change in environment."[81]

Most physiological and academic cardiologists were less concerned with individual patients. They were more interested in extending the boundaries of knowledge about heart disease. For them, patients were more than sick people who needed care or the "worried well" who required reassurance; they were an integral part of their academic medical center's mission of education and clinical research. Finally, public health cardiologists saw the entire population as potential cardiac patients, and they used statistics, the rhetoric of prevention, and the ideology of periodic examinations to convince people of their vulnerability.

Bishop and many other practitioner cardiologists supported the idealistic goals of the NYHA and the New York–based AHA. Indeed, he dedicated his book *Heart Troubles, Their Prevention and Relief* to "all those who are concerned in the development of modern cardiology and in public health education."[82] But Bishop and other office-based practitioners had needs that those organizations were not meeting. Aware that they had no influence within the NYHA or the AHA, a group of practitioners in the Northeast created a *clinical* cardiac society in the fall of 1926. They wanted a forum where they could discuss diagnostic techniques and clinical problems they encountered in individual patients. Eighteen men met in the Park Avenue office of Albert Hyman, a New York practitioner who had recently worked under British cardiologist James Mackenzie. Hyman chaired the meeting, which was attended by several other practitioner cardiologists (including Louis Bishop), two radiologists, a pediatrician, a surgeon, a few recent medical graduates, and a medical student. Some of them had met "from time to time during the past few years to discuss the recent developments in the study and treatment of heart disease."[83]

These clinicians decided to form "a special medical organization which would foster clinical study of the various new types of physiologic apparatus." They named it the "Sir James Mackenzie Cardiological Society" in honor of the influential British cardiologist, who had died one year earlier. Their society would make a political statement in addition to providing its members with a forum for discussing interesting electrocardiographic tracings and patients. Hyman thought it should be "dedicated to the advancement of heart disease as a distinct specialty of internal medicine and I would prefer to use the word, CARDIOLOGY, which has recently been suggested by Dr. Bishop." The founders knew there was resistance to their vision of cardiology as a special clinical field; institutional policies and politics had retarded or blocked the creation of cardiac clinics in several hospitals. Although Hyman had organized a cardiac clinic at New York's Beth David Hospital, he was aware that "many hospital staffs [had] refused to acknowledge that heart disease should be treated as a separate entity."[84]

The cardiac clinics these practitioner cardiologists sought to establish were different from those being created by the AHA. These clinicians wanted clinics "devoted exclusively to the examination and treatment of patients with heart disease." There was no mention of social workers or of the socioeconomic aspects of heart disease—the main concern of the public health cardiologists. The practitioners envisioned cardiac clinics like those created by James Mackenzie at the

London Hospital and Karel Wenckebach in Vienna that focused on clinical and instrumental diagnosis and medical treatment. Hyman, Bishop, and their circle were ambitious, and they thought other doctors would join them to make the Mackenzie Society a "large and important group."[85]

A few months later, Bishop publicly revealed his vision for a new national cardiology society. Without mentioning the Mackenzie Society (or the aspirations of its founders), he told an audience of physicians at a medical history meeting in Atlantic City, "There are some signs that make me believe that very soon there will be a group of men devoted to cardiology, large enough to form their own national society where they can confer with each other on their intimate problems." When AHA founder Joseph Sailer heard Bishop's speech he must have been chagrined. Wasn't the AHA a national society for cardiologists? Yes, but more so for some types of heart specialists than others. The issue was the association's mission and the elitism of its leaders.[86]

Most of the Mackenzie Society founders were from New York, although physicians from Boston, Philadelphia, Baltimore, and Washington, D.C., were present at the organizational meeting. It functioned as a local society; nineteen meetings were held at various hospitals in the metropolitan New York area during 1927 and 1928. Although it was unincorporated, the mere existence of the Mackenzie Society raised tensions between some of New York's practitioner cardiologists and the men who ran the NYHA and the AHA. In 1928 Walter Bensel told fellow society members that the NYHA "has not been too friendly and we must write off any cooperation from this group."[87]

In this context, the active members of the Mackenzie Society changed the name of their group to the New York Cardiological Society (NYCS). Hyman explained that they did so because the organization had "outgrown a number of our original concepts. Among these are the qualifications for membership, type of program, and our relationship with other medical organizations." Bensel explained that at least five other James Mackenzie societies had been founded since their namesake died in 1925, and "we seem to be losing our identity here in New York." He thought the new name was "more descriptive of our work and interests."[88] It was unambiguous; their organization was a *cardiological* society. Even their seal conveyed this message: it incorporated an electrocardiographic tracing of the heartbeat. The society's mission was education: it sought "to further the progress of cardiology by postgraduate instruction."[89]

In 1934 Hyman, Bishop, and fourteen other doctors—almost all New York practitioner cardiologists—met to begin a process that led to the formal incorporation of the NYCS the following year.[90] This group of sixteen men will be termed the "incorporators" to distinguish them from the individuals who had created the Mackenzie Society in 1926 and the original (unincorporated) NYCS two years later. The reorganized NYCS was more homogeneous than these precursor societies. Only five of the original eighteen Mackenzie society founders participated in the 1934 "[re]organizational" meeting of the NYCS. Gone were the recent medical graduates, radiologists, and other doctors who were not practitioner cardiologists. The members of the reorganized NYCS also had a narrower geographical focus: all were from the New York metropolitan area.[91]

This transformation of the NYCS acknowledged the emergence of a distinct community of practitioner cardiologists in New York City during the two decades since Bishop declared himself a heart specialist. In preparation for their 1934 meeting, Hyman had surveyed New York heart specialists and "found that practically all of them were dissatisfied with the present organizations" devoted to heart disease.[92] Russell Burton-Opitz, a former physiologist who had transformed himself into a practitioner cardiologist, chaired the organizational meeting. He claimed that "no existing organization or society was primarily concerned with the problems and practice of cardiology as a specialty." In an obvious reference to the NYHA and the AHA, he argued that "other societies which professed to be interested in heart disease were either under lay domination or were concerned with the public health aspects of the problem."[93]

This rhetoric reflected the tensions between the NYCS incorporators and the NYHA and AHA leaders. Elitism was also an issue: it was an acknowledged factor when groups selected new members or leaders in this era.[94] Seven of the incorporators were graduates of Columbia University's College of Physicians and Surgeons (one of the nation's leading medical schools), and most held hospital appointments as cardiologists. But they were not affiliated with New York City's elite teaching institutions, and none had served on the board of directors of the NYHA or the AHA.[95] More than half of the incorporators were Jewish, which partially explains their hospital affiliations. During this era, most Jewish physicians found it difficult or impossible to get academic posts or admitting privileges at most of New York's elite teaching hospitals.[96] They were marginalized to lesser institutions that focused on patient care rather than education and research, the activities that NYHA and AHA leaders most valued. Although it was undoubtedly a factor (given the time and cultural context), anti-Semitism was not the primary reason the NYCS incorporators were invisible in the NYHA. At the time, the NYHA's board of directors included Jewish physicians (e.g., Ernst Boas, Alfred Cohn, Harry Gold, Robert Levy, Arthur Master, and Bernard Oppenheimer). But they were viewed as academics because they held appointments at New York's leading teaching or research institutions.[97]

The NYCS incorporators were not especially interested in public health activities, so they limited their society to *doctors,* especially other practitioner cardiologists. Bishop thought the "lay public" should be excluded from their meetings, which should be restricted to physicians "with a knowledge of cardiology or particular interest in it." He thought the society "should be organized purely for the mutual cultivation of its members in cardiologic knowledge." It "should be a body to which we could carry our ignorance without the unfair criticism of those who do not understand and of that large group of men who know so many things that are not true!"[98]

The local New York name and membership roster of the newly incorporated NYCS obscured the ambitions of some members who hoped one day to create a new national organization. Hyman had already received requests "from many cardiologists in other cities to develop a national association." After receiving letters from Joseph Wolffe of Philadelphia and Allen Sussman of Baltimore (former members of the unincorporated NYCS), the incorporators voted unanimously in 1934 that their group "would cooperate with other local cardiological societies in the formation of the American Cardiological Association."[99] This goal would be achieved fifteen years later, when (as discussed in Chapter 4) several NYCS members founded the American College of Cardiology.

During the mid-1930s NYCS members held monthly meetings at hospitals where they had privileges: Cumberland Hospital, Gouverneur Hospital, Manhattan General Hospital, Bellevue Hospital, Beth El Hospital and Jewish Hospital in Brooklyn, and Lebanon Hospital in the Bronx. Printed programs were circulated, and the medical staff members of the host hospitals were invited to attend.[100] Their meetings consisted of brief clinical presentations (supplemented by electrocardiographic tracings and pathological specimens where relevant) followed by discussion. New York's practitioner cardiologists now had a forum for meeting regularly with their peers to discuss innovations in the diagnosis and treatment of heart patients. The society also sponsored an annual clinical meeting featuring a visiting professor.

Although new diagnostic instruments and classification schemes helped Bishop and other practitioner cardiologists to detect and characterize heart disease, they still had few effective treatments to offer their cardiac patients. In 1928 James Herrick told a group of doctors, "The cynic said to me, when he heard that I was to discuss the treatment of heart disease: 'Why not condense and say there is no treatment for heart disease save rest and digitalis?'" Herrick admitted, "Really, the cynic is not far wrong. The great majority of our heart cases are treated along these lines."[101]

Paul White's four-and-one-half-pound, 931-page book on heart disease published in 1931 reveals much about contemporary cardiology theory and practice. New classification schemes and diagnostic instruments had helped doctors distinguish various types of heart disease and estimate their frequency. White separated cardiac disease into three main groups in order of frequency: coronary, hypertensive, and rheumatic heart disease were common; syphilitic and thyroid heart disease were fairly common; and bacterial endocarditis and congenital heart disease were uncommon. The sections on treatment show that practitioners used a wide variety of medicines and nonpharmacologic approaches to treat heart patients. But a close reading of the text reveals the limitations of contemporary therapeutics—something that White, like Herrick, acknowledged.

Although the sphygmomanometer made it possible for doctors to detect high blood pressure and monitor it over time, White conceded that treating hypertension was a "difficult and almost hopeless task." The electrocardiograph had greatly enhanced awareness of a spectrum of disorders related to coronary artery disease. But despite growing understanding of angina pectoris and acute myocardial infarction, he conceded, "there is no specific treatment for coronary disease." In this preantibiotic era, infective endocarditis was invariably fatal and there were no curative therapies for syphilis or streptococcal infections (which some scientists now linked to acute rheumatic fever). Valvular heart disease defied treatment despite heroic attempts to operate for mitral valve stenosis. Between 1913 and 1928, surgeons reported a total of twelve valve operations, but only one patient survived. Aware of this, White concluded that there was "no treatment" for aortic or mitral valve disease.

Digitalis, quinidine, morphine, and nitroglycerin are the main cardiac drugs available to practitioners in the 1930s that are still used today. There were no antibiotics, potent diuretics, or antihypertensive agents. Congestive heart failure was treated with digitalis and diuretics (mercury compounds or purine derivatives like theophylline), but doctors knew these remedies had significant side effects or had to be administered by injection. Rest was a mainstay of therapy for heart failure and angina pectoris.[102] Despite this rather meager armamentarium, White and other heart specialists were optimistic. Shortly before his book appeared, White stated, "Although we have not yet reached the Golden Age of therapeutic discoveries, there are many indications that we are approaching the threshold of it."[103]

Discovery was the main business of the physiological cardiologists who designed experiments to unravel the heart's mysteries and find cures for its diseases. Like the New York practitioners who created the NYCS, some physiological cardiologists wanted to form a group that acknowledged their identity as scientists especially interested in the cardiovascular system. As their parent discipline (physiology) flourished during the 1920s and 1930s, the number of physiological cardiologists increased.[104] The ongoing movement to make medicine more scientific provided a nurturing environment in medical schools and university hospitals for the small but growing band of physiologists and physiological cardiologists. Most of them held full-time faculty appointments in physiology departments of medical schools where they had scientific apparatus, assistants, and protected time for research. This was a financial necessity before the expansion of the full-time faculty system to the clinical branches in America's medical schools during the middle third of the twentieth century. Johns Hopkins physiological cardiologist Cowles Andrus (who studied with Thomas Lewis) entered practice in 1934. "The financial limits of the 'cloister' make it necessary for me to increase my income," he told Alfred Cohn. Andrus hoped to maintain his teaching and research activities, however. His career path exemplifies how some cardiologists migrated from one heart specialist category to another based on their individual needs or institutional circumstances.[105] During the first half of the century, many academic and physiological cardiologists became practitioners because they lacked predictable or adequate financial support from institutional or other sources.[106]

Physiological cardiologists were primarily interested in science, and their professional activities reflected this. Typically, they presented their research papers at meetings of the American Physiological Society (APS), the Society of Experimental Biology and Medicine, or the American Society for Clinical Investigation, and they published in the official journals of those organizations. Their more clinically oriented papers appeared in periodicals like the *Journal of the American Medical Association*, the *Archives of Internal Medicine*, and the *American Heart Journal*. Frank Wilson contributed many papers on electrocardiography to the AHA's journal, but he thought its readers "as a class are not engaged in clinical investigation, but in medical practice."[107]

Like other medical and scientific fields, physiology was becoming progressively subspecialized. By the 1930s, some American scientists using physiological techniques to study specific organ systems formed new groups with peers who shared their professional interests. Physiologist Wallace Fenn noted that the APS was "very eager to represent all kinds of physiology" and did not encourage the formation of "special interest groups." Nevertheless, between 1932 and 1935, APS members interested in circulation, metabolism, and coagulation started informal groups that met in conjunction with the society's annual scientific meeting.[108] By this time, physiological cardiologists were branching into two groups: those primarily concerned with basic research and those interested in applied cardiac physiology. In 1932 a few APS members met to discuss forming a circulatory physiology group within the society. Carl Wiggers's protégé Louis Katz played a major role in establishing this "circulation group." The following year, he invited forty-two society members to join a "small group of those individuals interested in circulation."[109]

The APS circulation group represented the formalization of a network of individuals who worked in different institutional contexts but shared an interest in the scientific study of the cardiovascular system. Their only formal activity was an annual dinner during the APS meeting which included a scientific presentation and discussion period. The goal was to "promote frank discussion between active investigators and to arouse interest in the physiology of the circulation among the younger [APS] members."[110] Like the practitioners who formed the

NYCS, these physiological cardiologists sensed that the AHA did not meet all of their needs.

The members of the APS cardiovascular group shared a commitment to laboratory research—something that was not yet part of the AHA's mission. As early as 1927, Harold Pardee of New York Hospital and a few other academic cardiologists urged the association to "take a more active part in fostering the scientific investigation of various aspects of heart disease." The AHA's executive committee, led by Conner and Emerson, concluded it did not have enough money to support scientific research. They chose instead to use their limited resources to fund statistical research, which related more directly to their public health mission.[111]

The AHA's historian claimed recently that "research was farthest from the minds of the heart leaders in the 1930s," but the cardiovascular physiologists' influence in the association would increase dramatically during the middle of the century.[112] As discussed in the next chapter, this small but vocal constituency joined a coalition that reformulated the AHA's mission shortly after World War II, placing scientific research at the center of its agenda.

Tensions within the AHA

During the 1930s it became apparent that a significant number of AHA members—mainly practitioner cardiologists and internists—resented the fact that the organization was controlled by an academic clique from the Northeast. Their discontent increased when the association, like every other segment of American society, confronted unprecedented challenges during the Great Depression. In December 1934 Jack Marvin, chair of the AHA's executive committee, warned that the association's financial outlook was "darker than at any time in the past six years." This sobering assessment was due, in part, to the progressive reduction in the National Tuberculosis Association's annual contribution to the AHA. In 1935 the gift would be only $1,000—one-tenth of their previous high.[113]

Financial pressures led the AHA leaders to reconsider their organization's mission (which some members thought was too narrowly focused) and its structure (which many members viewed as undemocratic). Their decisions were pragmatic. As membership dues became a more important source of revenue, the AHA leaders actively recruited internists and general practitioners to join their association. By 1932 they could count 1,277 members and 238 affiliated clinics. But despite a nearly threefold increase in income from dues between 1929 and 1935, total income declined from $19,513 to $12,543. The association's expenses exceeded income by $1,331.91 in 1935.[114]

Nonetheless, the AHA leaders expanded their activities to maintain their status as the sole national heart organization. The association published a detailed summary of its expanded mission in 1932. It outlined the AHA's commitment to providing public and professional education, establishing local heart associations, developing outpatient clinics and inpatient facilities for patients with acute and chronic cardiac conditions, and supporting epidemiological research. To finance this ambitious program, the AHA leaders intensified their efforts to attract donations from "individuals and foundations."[115]

They also launched a new publication. *Modern Concepts of Cardiovascular Disease,* a monthly leaflet written by academic cardiologists, first appeared in 1932. It was aimed at private practitioners, a constituency the association wanted not only to educate but also to cultivate as dues-paying members. Harvard cardiologist Samuel Levine, who edited the publication, explained that it would be "sent to as many physicians as possible," especially those practitioners "not in intimate contact with large medical centers or teaching institutions." The goal was to "keep such men better informed concerning the recent developments in the diagnosis, prognosis, and treatment of cardiovascular diseases." The first issues were devoted to brief summaries of digitalis, rheumatic fever, cardiovascular syphilis, heart disease in pregnancy, and angina pectoris.[116]

At the same time the AHA leaders sought to educate practitioners, they also looked for ways to stimulate "more widespread and cordial interest in the association and a more generous support of its work." The issues that concerned some members were governance and representation. Their rumblings induced the AHA leaders to change the bylaws "to permit of a larger national representation in the government of the association."[117] They began by enlarging the membership of various committees "to have the entire country represented more adequately in the work of the association."[118]

When tensions persisted, the AHA leaders formed a committee to address the criticisms they had received. Marvin thought prompt and deliberate action was necessary. He supported expanding the AHA board from fifteen to twenty-five doctors, with equal representation from five geographical regions. This strategy was supposed to address the growing concerns about the unchecked influence of the Northeast group. Twenty-five men were selected from different parts of the country, but virtually all of them were academic cardiologists affiliated with medical schools and university hospitals.[119]

Although practitioner cardiologists still did not have a significant voice in the organization, a few academic internists whose shared interest was peripheral vascular disease and clinical research were heard. In 1935 they successfully challenged the AHA's traditional limited view of heart disease. Between 1932 and 1936, *Modern Concepts* published forty-eight articles on diagnosis and treatment, but only two dealt with peripheral vascular disease and one with hypertension. This reflected the conscious decision of the AHA leaders to focus their efforts on the *heart* rather than on the *cardiovascular system*. Disorders of the peripheral circulation had limited interest to the public health cardiologists who founded the association and whose original focus was on rheumatic heart disease. Paul White also viewed cardiology as devoted to the heart, as reflected by his choice of the title *Heart Disease* for his 1931 textbook.[120]

Irving Wright of New York's Post-Graduate Hospital and George Brown and Edgar Allen of the Mayo Clinic were interested in the peripheral circulation, and they thought the AHA should be as well. Wright, a thirty-four-year-old Cornell graduate, took the initiative and urged his former chief, Lewis Conner, to formally affiliate "a group of workers in the peripheral vascular field" with the association.[121] Wright's medical school classmate, Irvine Page, a Rockefeller Institute scientist whose main interest was hypertension, also fought to expand the AHA's agenda. He recalled, "It seemed hard for the early cardiologists to understand that both hypertension and atherosclerosis were part of the discipline of cardiology."[122] Some practitioner cardiologists, such as Bishop, were concerned about hypertension. In 1928 Bishop stated that "the management of blood pressure has a large place in the practice of cardiology."[123]

Unlike the New York City practitioner cardiologists who formed the NYCS, Wright, Page, and their circle were academics who held appointments at teaching institutions and did research. They convinced the AHA to establish the Section for the Study of the Peripheral Circulation in 1935. Wright later recalled, "There were doubts expressed by some of the classical cardiologists regarding the adoption of this upstart, but with the encouragement and guidance of doctors Marvin, White, and others, the new and first council was admitted."[124] Wright acknowledged recently that his group was "a nuisance to the old line cardiologists, but, anyway, they finally let us in."[125]

AHA founders Lewis Conner and Haven Emerson (public health cardiologists), were nervous about this new constituency whose members had a different vision of heart . . . of *cardiovascular* disease. The executive committee minutes mention "a great deal of discussion" before they voted to establish the vascular section. Conner and Emerson worried whether "the new group [would] have any consciousness of their duties with respect to the public health aspect of the association's work." Marvin explained that these founders "expressed regret that the trend of the work of the association in recent years has been steadily away from public health and toward education of the physician, but admitted that perhaps this was inevitable and proper."[126]

The AHA's original public health orientation proved to be too narrow to appeal to an increasingly diverse membership. There was growing interest in the scientific aspects of hypertension and arteriosclerosis and their clinical sequelae of stroke and heart attack. In expanding their program to accept the peripheral vascular group, Conner and the other AHA leaders acknowledged that they were impressed by the "recent extraordinarily rapid growth of interest in the peripheral vascular disorders and their study." But the accommodation was also a strategic move to discourage the vascular specialists from forming a competing society. The AHA leaders knew Wright and his friends felt "the need of some organization and of some central outlet for their contributions." They made several concessions, including expanding the *American Heart Journal* from six to twelve issues a year to accommodate vascular papers.[127]

Wright's ascent in the AHA was dramatic. He was appointed associate editor of the journal in 1935 and elected a member at large of the AHA's board of directors the following year. Despite their small numbers (the vascular section included only twenty-three of the association's 1,141 members in 1936), Wright, Page, and Allen became influential figures in the AHA. Each eventually presided over the organization. Moreover, their vascular section was the model for the formation within the AHA of other special interest groups, called "councils."[128]

TABLE 2-2
American Heart Association Income and Expenses (1934)

INCOME	
Dues	$ 4,583.00
Grants and donations	
National Tuberculosis Association	2,500.00
Burke Foundation	2,000.00
O'Donnell Iselin	100.00
Florence Sharp	100.00
Miscellaneous	17.35
Sales ("Criteria," pamphlets, charts, films, miscellaneous)	2,618.41
Other income (interest and discount on purchases)	107.13
TOTAL INCOME	**$12,025.89**

EXPENSES	
Salaries (administrative and clerical)	$ 7,099.92
General office expense (supplies, postage, etc.)	2,190.54
General service expense (shipping, accounting, etc.)	957.74
Travel	303.51
Education expense (materials sold or distributed free)	
"Criteria for Classification and Diagnosis"	580.08
Pamphlets, charts, films, and slides	929.87
Profit on sales of "Criteria" paid to the New York Tuberculosis and Health Association	295.30
"Modern Concepts in Cardiovascular Disease"	749.26
"Bulletin of the American Heart Association"	261.28
Exhibits and meetings	320.95
Miscellaneous	62.05
TOTAL EXPENSES	**$13,750.50**

NET EXPENSES OVER INCOME (DEFICIT)	–$ 1,724.61

SOURCE: "AHA State of Income and Expense for the Year Ended December 31, 1934," Exhibit B, Minutes, AHA AM, 4 February 1934, AHA Archives.

The vascular group also set a precedent by formalizing the distinction within the AHA between the practitioners and members who were physiological or academic cardiologists. Any AHA physician could become a *member* of the new vascular section, but *fellowship* was "reserved for those particularly interested in peripheral circulation and who are *actively engaged in research in this field* [emphasis added]."[129] The distinction between self-designated cardiologists and those with some formal training was sharpened during the 1940s, when the AHA leaders played a decisive role in establishing criteria by which cardiologists would be considered eligible for board certification in the specialty.

The vascular section influenced the AHA in another important way. Deeply committed to basic and clinical investigation, they urged the association to fund scientific research, not just to encourage data collection and epidemiological studies. The academic cardiologists who led the AHA acknowledged the importance of research, but rhetoric and ambition were not enough to overcome the severe economic conditions of the depression. The association did not have enough money to achieve its main goals of educating the public and the profession about heart disease, let alone subsidize basic and clinical research (Table 2-2).[130]

By now, some of the AHA's academic cardiologists were expressing frustration about the association's traditional focus on prevention and public education. Howard Sprague, Paul White's protégé and an academic cardiologist at the Massachusetts General Hospital, told a North Carolina doctor in 1932 that although he thought the concept of periodic health examinations was "probably a good one," he was "not quite so optimistic about the amount of disease that can be prevented" by them.[131]

Sprague joined the AHA's leadership circle in 1937 when he was appointed to the ten-member executive committee and made secretary. This would be the first year that none of the influential New York public health cardiologists (Conner, Emerson, Halsey, and Wyckoff) would serve on the executive committee. During the next decade, Sprague coordinated a reform effort that culminated in the AHA's transformation into a voluntary health organization in 1948. During the late 1940s the focus of the AHA would shift from public health to science—and to fund-raising to support a greatly expanded agenda. A new generation of physiological and academic cardiologists was reshaping the AHA's agenda, which for fifteen years had reflected the interests of the public health cardiologists.

Chapter 3

<h2>Declaring War on Heart Disease</h2>

The number of practitioner cardiologists in America increased significantly between the world wars. Nearly all were self-designated partial specialists whose practice was a combination of cardiology and internal medicine. There was no standard career path for aspiring heart specialists—a source of increasing friction between doctors during the Great Depression. Shortly after the American Board of Internal Medicine (ABIM) was created in 1935, the American Heart Association (AHA) leaders lobbied to participate in the credentialing of cardiologists. This decision signaled a new role for the AHA: it would become the voice of America's growing community of heart specialists.

Despite some successes, the AHA was chronically on the verge of bankruptcy during the depression. There was no money to expand the organization's public health and educational programs, let alone support research, a major interest of many academic cardiologists. Two 1937 events—the first March of Dimes campaign to collect money for polio research and the passage of the National Cancer Institute Act— showed that the public wanted cures and was willing to pay researchers to find them. Soon, a group of ambitious physiological and academic cardiologists coordinated the AHA's transformation from a nearly insolvent professional society into a prosperous and influential voluntary health organization committed to the endowment of research.

After World War II, AHA leaders joined with a group of legislators, government officials, and concerned citizens to form the "heart lobby," which used a military metaphor to describe their goal. They told the American people and their political leaders that heart disease could be *conquered* if enough money was given to support cardiovascular research. The success of the Manhattan project to build an atomic bomb and recent medical advances such as antibiotics helped them make their case.

Paths to specialization and who patrols them

By 1940 approximately one thousand American doctors viewed themselves as heart specialists, but few had received any formal cardiology training. At the time there were 451 official residency positions in internal medicine but only four in cardiology.[1] Typically, a doctor who wanted to be a cardiologist took brief postgraduate courses on electrocardiography and heart disease after completing an internship and a year of medical residency. Some aspiring heart specialists gained additional experience by serving as an assistant to a recognized cardiologist.

A few institutions had responded to the growing interest in heart disease by sponsoring short courses for practitioners. By 1925 Paul White was offering a two-week summer course at the Massachusetts General Hospital (MGH), and the Washington University School of Medicine in St. Louis advertised an "intensive" five-day course for ten dollars. Within a decade, several institutions offered similar courses lasting from one to twelve weeks.[2] White started America's first cardiology fellowship—a year of specialized training following the completion of a medical residency—in the early 1920s. During that decade he trained fourteen cardiologists. William Stroud, an academic cardiologist who studied with Carl Wiggers, Thomas Lewis, and James Mackenzie, established a cardiology fellowship at the Pennsylvania Hospital in 1924. There were few other formal programs until after World War II, however.[3]

As the number of self-designated specialists (of all types) increased following World War I, there was growing concern about the lack of standards in training, credentialing, and practice. In 1931 a New York Academy of Medicine committee concluded that specialty training was disorganized. An aspiring specialist, it was claimed, "has to shift for himself and try to pick up whatever knowledge he requires to perfect himself in his chosen field."[4] Meanwhile, Willard Rappleye, director of a survey of medical education for the Association of American Medical Colleges, urged that postgraduate training be standardized. He predicted that "in the near future every specialist will be obliged to take adequate training to qualify him for his limited field of practice."[5]

Concerns about quality of care and economic self-interest led many practitioners to support actions that promised to formalize the process of specialization. Self-designated cardiologists competed among themselves and with general practitioners and internists for patients. Tensions increased during the Great Depression as physicians' incomes fell dramatically. In 1934 American College of Physicians (ACP) president George Piersol noted that "unbelievable changes of political, social, economic and industrial significance have taken place. Every social group, physicians along with all others, has been profoundly affected."[6]

Some observers complained that inadequately trained self-designated specialists posed a risk to patients. It was argued that the public had a right to know whether doctors claiming to be specialists and charging specialists' fees had adequate training and experience. One writer protested, "Over-specialization is unnecessary and costly to the public, particularly where self-diagnosis and selection of specialists is practiced by the patient." Acknowledging that specialization was an "essential" part of modern medicine, he demanded that the profession guarantee "that those who claim to be specialists are, in fact, experts in the field."[7]

In 1931 a nationwide survey of five thousand physicians in the United States revealed that 23 percent were full specialists, 21 percent were partial specialists, and 56 percent were general practitioners. That year a Cleveland physician protested, "The number of self-styled specialists is ridiculous." He thought laws should prohibit practitioners from claiming to be specialists unless they had received adequate training.[8] More and more doctors demanded action, but what should be done and by whom? Several organizations sensed that their constituents had a stake in the outcome, and they wanted to participate in developing and administering any process used to define specialists.

The procedures for licensing or certifying specialists could have been devised and managed by one or more organizations, including the American Medical Association (AMA) through its Council on Medical Education and Hospitals, the Association of American Medical Colleges, the American Hospital Association, the Federation of State Boards, the National Board of Medical Examiners, and the various professional societies. Although there was no obvious answer, most observers agreed that central coordination was necessary—and soon. Historian Rosemary Stevens writes, "Unless heroic measures were taken, there promised to be a rapid fragmentation into self-regulating specialist organizations."[9]

Doctors, hospitals, and medical societies considered various options for regulating the process of specialization. The organizations and coalitions that developed proposals and negotiated compromises in the 1930s had many choices. Among the issues: Who sets the criteria for defining a specialist? Should the criteria be based on training? If so, what type, with whom, where, and for how long? If examinations are judged to be necessary, who prepares, administers, and grades them? Who controls licenses or certificates signifying the attainment of specialty status? Who polices the profession to be sure doctors follow the rules, and what power do these enforcers have? During the 1930s several (but not all) of these questions were answered by groups that took responsibility for organizing the process of specialization.

The AMA had been involved in the debate about credentialing specialists for several years. James Herrick, secretary of the AMA's committee on graduate instruction in internal medicine, explained in 1921 that "certain internists specialize in restricted fields" like cardiology, infectious diseases, and gastroenterology. The committee's proposal acknowledged (and if adopted by the AMA would encourage) the growing tendency of some doctors to specialize *within* internal medicine. Internists seeking AMA certification would have had to display "mastery of at least one special field" of internal medicine in addition to having "broad general knowledge" of the entire discipline.[10]

This system was not instituted, and the AMA would not be the sole organization to determine the criteria for defining America's internists and cardiologists. It would share that responsibility with the ACP, a professional society for internists founded in New York in 1915. For a decade the ACP struggled to establish itself as a credible national organization. At first, it represented office-based internists—private practitioners excluded from the elite Association of American Physicians. According to Rosemary Stevens, the academic internists who belonged to that organization initially viewed the ACP as "pretentious, irrelevant, unnecessary, and faintly absurd."[11]

During the 1920s the ACP gained stature as academic internists began to join and assume leadership positions. They discussed how to select and classify their members as the debate about specialty certification intensified.[12] Because the ACP leaders feared that some other organization might invent (and control) a process for certifying internists if they did not act, they joined with the AMA to create the ABIM in 1935. Walter Bierring, first chair of the board, explained that it was formed "in response to a well defined movement in America to establish more definite criteria for the title of specialist."[13]

This drive to certify internists had important implications for cardiology. The ACP leaders, working through the ABIM, wanted to control the credentialing of *all types* of internists, not just general internists. A president of the college argued in 1933 that progressive specialization "threatened general medicine with disaster" because it had "torn medicine asunder, divided it up into many parts and attempted to create many separate entities."[14] An ACP governor for Massachusetts thought it would be "suicidal" if the college restricted itself to general internal medicine. He argued that physicians practicing "allied specialties" like gastroenterology and cardiology should "be discouraged from setting up their own boards."[15]

The ACP would also control the credentialing of medical "subspecialists." In 1936 college leaders decided that the ABIM would specify training guidelines and develop examinations for the "more restricted and specialized branches of internal medicine, as gastroenterology, cardiology, metabolic diseases, tuberculosis and allergic diseases."[16] This ABIM policy institutionalized a philosophy that the career path to nonsurgical fields like cardiology and other medical subspecialties would go through internal medicine. Doctors seeking certification in those fields had to be fully trained in internal medicine and to have passed the internal medicine board exam. This policy went largely unchallenged. Academic cardiologist Tinsley Harrison stated, "I don't think a man can be much of a cardiologist unless he is first of all a well rounded internist."[17]

In 1927 Louis Bishop had characterized cardiology as "the youngest child of medical evolution" and acknowledged that it had not "quite as yet come into its own as a distinct specialty."[18] Nor would it if the ACP leaders had their way. Although Bishop and Paul White viewed cardiology as a specialty, most internists (especially the academic elite) saw cardiologists as internists with supplementary training who did something in addition to general internal medicine, not instead of it. This concept was formalized when certification of internists and medical subspecialists was invented in the 1930s. Heart disease was common, and all internists saw patients with cardiac complaints. The integrity of internal medicine would be seriously threatened if cardiologists succeeded, as neurologists had decades earlier, in segregating such a large pool of patients. But there was little risk of this happening. Most internists felt capable of caring for heart patients, and most cardiologists viewed themselves as internists who focused their practice on people with cardiac disease.

The AHA founders did not envision their organization as a traditional professional society, and the ABIM leaders did not view it as one when they established criteria for granting certificates to certain groups of internists without examination. Members of the ACP, the American Gastroenterological Association, and four elite, academically oriented medical societies would be eligible for certificates via the "grandfather" method. AHA members would not be automatically granted certificates, because their society now included hundreds of general practitioners, internists, and self-designated heart specialists as a result of a successful effort to recruit more dues-paying members.[19]

Although the ABIM policy precluded the AHA leaders from establishing an independent board for cardiology, it did not prevent them from trying to influence the scheme being developed to certify heart specialists. Yale cardiologist Jack Marvin (a Harvard Medical School graduate and former cardiology fellow under Paul White who chaired the AHA executive committee) lobbied the ABIM on behalf of the association after the board announced its intention to certify subspecialists. He and other AHA leaders thought that a critical function of the cardiology board would be to assess competence in electrocardiography. This reflected their concern that many physicians who read electrocardiograms were "wholly incompetent."[20] Samuel Levine thought that electrocardiograph machines had "become so simple and comparatively inexpensive [by 1940] that there are thousands of them in use." Because "many inadequately trained physicians have assumed the responsibility of interpreting the tracings . . . there is a danger of prostituting the entire work."[21]

Quality of care was not the sole issue. The AHA leaders knew that some physicians used the electrocardiograph to affirm their self-designated status as heart specialists. Levine complained that some doctors got the "reputation" of being cardiologists by "the simple purchase of an electrocardiograph."[22] The issue concerned practitioners as well as academics. A Kansas doctor urged the AHA to "discourage all physicians (including internists) from acquiring elaborate pretentious apparatus (electrocardiograph, recording sphygmomanometer, oscillometer, etc.) which they have not had adequate training in the use of." He thought the association should "discourage all physicians from acquiring the impression that because they have given the subject [heart disease] some study that they are cardiologists."[23] Harvard cardiologist (and AHA secretary) Howard Sprague agreed: "There are far too many half baked cardiologists with all sorts of trick apparatus, who are entirely unqualified, and doing a lot of harm."[24]

In 1939 AHA leaders Irving Wright, Jack Marvin, and William Stroud (who was also treasurer of the ACP) met with ABIM chair Ernest Irons to develop a plan for certifying cardiologists. Marvin reported that Irons "was not eager to certify men in the subspecialties, but agreed to do so only because the representative bodies in each field have requested it."[25] The AHA leaders knew they had to move quickly if they were to influence the process of certifying heart specialists. They sensed a "widespread and insistent demand for some plan of certification" and worried that it would "be controlled by some other group if the American Board of Internal Medicine and the American Heart Association do not take action soon."[26] The AMA and the American Board of Medical Specialties (ABMS) approved the ABIM-AHA plan, and the first cardiovascular board examination was given in Boston in April 1941. It was an oral examination administered by White and five other academic cardiologists. That year, 223 persons were certified by the ABIM as specialists in cardiovascular disease—90 percent by virtue of their standing in the field rather than by examination.[27]

After the first examination, the AHA's board of directors demanded that the requirements for taking them "be greatly extended." Only a candidate with "undoubted qualifications of training, experience, and eagerness to advance the knowledge in his specialty" would be permitted to take the examination.[28] Tinsley Harrison urged the AHA to limit board certification to persons who had done research, except in unusual cases.[29] These policies excluded most practitioner cardiologists, because they, unlike academic or physiological cardiologists, did not perform research or write papers. A common pattern in professionalization is that an elite defines the boundaries of their discipline and attempts to exclude those who (in their opinion) do not have the proper mentors, training, experience, or credentials. In deciding who could take the cardiology boards, the AHA leaders placed great emphasis on the opinion of the candidate's "sponsor."[30] This restrictive philosophy regarding board eligibility helps explain why only 255 cardiologists were certified during the first decade the examination was offered.[31]

The development of specific training requirements for doctors seeking certification in general surgery and surgical specialties contributed to a dramatic increase in the number of residency positions between 1930 (2,028) and 1939 (4,556). The dean of Columbia University's medical faculty explained that "the various organizations of medical specialists have given great impetus to the development of long residencies with satisfactory educational content."[32] Although true for surgery, this was not the case for internal medicine and its subspecialties until after World War II. The ABIM decided not to follow the example set by the surgeons. Walter Bierring, the first chair of the ABIM, explained that rather than defining "any fixed rules," the board outlined "certain broad general principles for training." This meant that aspiring internists or cardiologists had many choices. The main criterion for board eligibility was that the candidate had worked under the "guidance of older men who bring to their clinical problems ripe knowledge and critical judgement."[33]

Unlike surgeons, whose training had to consist of a hospital-based residency, aspiring internists and cardiologists could gain their experience and become board-eligible in a variety of ways. In 1936 the ABIM explained that "graduate work" in internal medicine and its subspecialties could be carried out "in any domestic or foreign medical school, laboratory, hospital, clinic or dispensary" recognized by the AMA as having adequate facilities.[34] This liberal policy did not encourage the development of formal cardiology training programs. Most aspiring heart specialists would get their specialty training informally or by assisting a recognized cardiologist. Although academic cardiologist George Herrmann urged the AHA in 1943 to develop "standard requirements for acceptable hospital residencies in cardiovascular disease," no action was taken.[35]

Even without the development of standardized training programs, cardiology had achieved new stature as a result of the efforts of the AHA leaders. They got the ABMS and the ABIM to acknowledge that their discipline was sufficiently distinct and well developed to justify its own board examination. The ABIM did not give other medical fields, such as hematology or rheumatology, this prerogative. But cardiology would not be an independent specialty like dermatology and neurology.[36]

According to Rosemary Stevens, the timing of the ABIM's creation was critical; it allowed academic internists to gain control over the emerging medical subspecialties. By so doing, they "checked the progress of further division in [internal medicine's] related specialties."[37] By 1940 it was clear that internal medicine would not copy surgery; that field had been divided into several distinct organ-based *specialties.* Internal medicine would control cardiology and the other medical *sub-specialties.* That year, the ACP president declared that "being an internist is a state of mind. It implies a breadth of interest which inherently excludes narrow specialism."[38]

In 1940 ABIM chair Ernest Irons told Paul White that "all men applying for certification in a sub-specialty must first be good internists and be approved by the American Board of Internal Medicine."[39] White saw things differently, perhaps because he began his career as a cardiologist and never practiced general medicine. Although he favored certifying specialists, the Harvard cardiologist had misgivings about certifying general internists. He told the Harvard Medical School dean, "It is my belief that eventually the practice of medicine will be taken care of by (1) general practitioners on the front line, better trained, to be sure, than in the past and with the special ability to direct their problems straight to specialists in all fields, and by (2) the specialists of all varieties, rather than through middle men of general surgery and internal medicine." White reiterated, "I have a hunch that the internist willy nilly, and probably quite correctly, is bound to pass on, perhaps not for another generation, but the handwriting is on the wall."[40]

The AHA as a voluntary health organization

While some AHA influentials were negotiating the process of certifying cardiologists with the ABIM, others were debating their association's future. In 1939 MGH cardiologist Howard Sprague formed a "committee of activities" which sought "to collect points of view from different parts of the country, relative to the purposes and aspirations" of the AHA.[41] Despite having expanded the geographical representation in several key committees in the mid-1930s, the AHA leaders confronted new challenges. Tensions between the national organization and its affiliates were increasing. Now several local associations demanded "more information, cooperation, and leadership" from the New York–based AHA. These affiliates also wanted money to support their local programs, but the AHA was in no position to help. Marvin explained that "raising funds had proved so difficult for the national association that it was scarcely in a position to assist local groups in this important undertaking."[42]

The AHA leaders knew they could not be complacent; their national network of local associations and affiliated clinics might unravel. The creation of the New York Cardiological Society (NYCS), the cardiovascular group of the American Physiological Society (APS), and the AHA's own vascular section proved that theirs was not the only vision of American cardiology. Despite a limited budget and internal stresses, Marvin, Sprague, Wright, and their circle were ambitious. They were positioning the AHA to represent American cardiology; the association's collaboration with the ABIM was a step in this direction. As the nation entered World War II, they offered the association's "services as a cooperating body to the United States Government . . . to help in the cardiac problems of preparedness, war, or retirement from the service."[43]

By 1941 the AHA was coordinating the nation's public health campaign against heart disease through its publications and affiliated clinics, directing the certification of cardiologists, and educating doctors. That year, Sprague submitted a detailed plan for greatly expanding the AHA's agenda. He was frustrated that so little had been accomplished, but he admitted that "the situation of the association is no more static than is the country itself, and the military emergency overshadows the calmer paths of peace."[44] The war was not the main problem; the association had always been on the verge of bankruptcy. Marvin thought the AHA's agenda was "far too limited in its scope and quantity." Although the AHA was supported by "the finest men in the cardiovascular field in the country . . . its limited budget has long been a great handicap."[45]

The AHA leaders knew this did not have to be the case. Founded just five years earlier, the National Foundation for Infantile Paralysis was raising huge sums of money ($2 million in 1941) from its March of Dimes campaign. At the same time, the AHA's budget was just under $15 thousand, mainly from membership dues.[46] The National Foundation showcased celebrities like Mickey Rooney and Judy Garland to publicize their goal of conquering polio. They also had help from the White House. Polio researcher John Paul termed Franklin Roosevelt, paralyzed as a result of the disease, the "spiritual sponsor" of the foundation, which was headed by the president's former law partner

Basil O'Conner. According to Paul, "the lesson that medical scientists were supposed to learn quickly" was that if the foundation was "to succeed or even exist, a certain amount of flamboyant publicity was absolutely necessary and they must go along with it."[47]

Marvin was confident that a public fund-raising campaign would provide the AHA with enough money to support an expanded agenda. In 1942 he asked the former public relations director of the National Tuberculosis Association to draft a proposal for a national fund-raising drive. Sensing that many AHA physicians might object, Marvin assured the association's leaders that the public relations firm knew they did not want "a lot of ballyhoo and undignified publicity" and that "unjustified claims about the cure of heart disease" would not be permitted.[48]

The AHA's consultant outlined their problem: "A conservative organization of the highest integrity, with a tranquil history covering many years, now sees the opportunity to develop a more dynamic program, but lacks the budget to do so." He assured them that a national campaign would succeed for many reasons. Heart disease was the most frequent cause of death. The public was "science minded" and cardiovascular research was "fascinating." The AHA had a record of public service and was endorsed by the government and universities. More Americans than ever were giving to "worthy causes" despite the war. And AHA board members could help attract large donations from "individuals, industry and foundations" because of their personal prestige and contacts.[49]

The main obstacle was that the AHA was virtually unknown—but public relations professionals could help them overcome that problem. Marvin thought the detailed proposal was "sound, dignified, ambitious, and in general a highly desirable program for the association to adopt."[50] He was confident that the affiliated heart associations would support the plan, because if it succeeded it would help them finance the nearly one hundred clinics they represented.[51] Some AHA leaders were concerned, however. White told Marvin that he was "a little uncertain" about the wisdom of the campaign and was "fearful that we might get off with too much of a rush."[52] But Sprague and Marvin would convince White that "radical changes" were necessary if the AHA was to "break the inertia of years."[53]

When the war delayed the AHA leaders' plans to launch a major fund-raising campaign, they looked elsewhere for financial support. Marvin solicited donations from the medical directors of several large insurance companies, pointing out that premature death from heart disease reduced their profits. He told them that the AHA wanted to begin to finance basic research, which would ultimately lead to prevention, earlier diagnosis, and more effective treatment. Marvin urged the insurance company representatives to view their annual gift to the AHA as "an investment rather than a donation."[54]

The AHA's new emphasis on basic research reflected the growing influence of physiological and academic cardiologists within the organization. Most of them were deeply committed to research, and they needed funding to perform it. These scientists were interested in many types of cardiovascular disease, not just rheumatic heart disease (the traditional focus of the public health cardiologists). Marvin assured the insurance company doctors that the AHA's research program would emphasize the diseases that killed many of their company's clients— hypertension and arteriosclerosis. Statistics showed that people who purchased life insurance were more likely to suffer from hypertension, arteriosclerosis, and coronary artery disease than rheumatic heart disease. Despite the AHA's attempt to frame their campaign for corporate support in terms of a prudent investment, the results were disappointing. Insurance companies donated only $17 thousand to the AHA between 1942 and 1945.[55]

Although the physiological and academic cardiologists welcomed the AHA's plan of supporting research, the people who ran the association's affiliated clinics were more concerned with public health issues and their own financial needs. In 1943 Marvin told the board that the "central office" was receiving "an increasing number of demands that the association extend its public health activities."[56] Two years later, a frustrated and impatient Marvin told the board that there was no longer any "valid excuse for failure to expand [the AHA] in size and influence" now that the war was over. He challenged them: "As many of you know, I have several times suggested in all seriousness that the association should either expand its activities or should terminate its existence."[57]

Pressures were mounting from several directions. The authors of a 1945 book on voluntary health agencies called the "extreme disparity" between the annual incomes of the AHA ($29 thousand) and the National Foundation for Infantile Paralysis ($8.2 million) "startling" (Table 3-1).[58] Americans were growing restless; they wanted cures for diseases that threatened their livelihoods and their lives. The success of

TABLE 3-1
Income of Voluntary Health Organizations (1944)

ORGANIZATION	1944 INCOME ($)
American Heart Association	28,776
American Cancer Society	280,249
National Foundation for Infantile Paralysis	8,178,891*

*Annualized from 8 months' data.
SOURCE: S. M. Gunn and P. S. Platt, *Voluntary Health Agencies: An Interpretive Study* (New York: Ronald Press, 1945), table 5, p. 208.

the March of Dimes campaign proved that the people were willing to invest in research that promised cures. Marvin knew this: "There is an increasingly insistent demand from the public that something be done . . . toward the conquest of rheumatic fever, coronary thrombosis, hypertension, etc." He explained that the public's attention had been "focused so sharply upon the apparent value of coordinated research, as exemplified by the atomic bomb, the large contributions to cancer research, Senator Pepper's many public statements concerning the necessity for federal financing of research, and related matters, that it is beginning to clamor for some action in the field of cardiovascular research."[59]

The solution to the AHA's chronic financial problems now seemed clear: the association should follow the example of other disease foundations that were raising huge sums of money from the public for research and other purposes. But such a move would change the character of the AHA. Once transformed into a voluntary health organization, it would no longer be controlled by an academic elite. Influential laypersons would be invited to join the board, because their help with the fund-raising campaign was crucial. As the financial and programmatic implications of the proposed transformation were articulated, more AHA board members (still all doctors) embraced the reformers' goals—and their strategy.

After several meetings with "professional fund raisers, with public relations counselors, with individual members and groups," the AHA leaders had decided "to embark upon a broad expansion of activities" and had finalized their plans for a major fund-raising drive.[60] By now, even White was convinced. "We must have money to carry on what we want to do," he told Marvin. "Of course, we have in the past shrunk from all this publicity in keeping the association very scientific and conservative but obviously we have got to get away from that." White conceded, "Much as I dislike the thought of all the publicity that is coming, I believe we must undertake it."[61]

The reorganization of the AHA was catalyzed by the formation of "The Council on Heart Diseases, Inc." in 1946. This new group, which was informally linked to the powerful New York Heart Association (NYHA), alarmed Marvin and his allies. He had been warned that the new council could "eventually, by the expansion of its lay and medical boards . . . operate on a national basis, absorbing or being absorbed by the present American Heart Association."[62] Marvin complained to one of the council's founders: "A new national organization has been formed which must of necessity be in direct competition with, if not in opposition to, the American Heart Association."[63] Although Marvin learned that the council did not plan to compete with the AHA, the reformers were galvanized into action. Sprague admitted that "it is to a degree true, that the stimuli for remaking this association have come from the formation of the many other organizations, espousing the cause of heart disease, now burgeoning throughout the country."[64]

One of the "many other organizations" that worried Sprague and Marvin was the American Foundation for High Blood Pressure, formed in 1945 by Irvine Page, a physiological cardiologist at the Cleveland Clinic. He modeled his foundation after "the cancer, polio, tuberculosis and rheumatic fever associations."[65] Page, whose research interests were hypertension and arteriosclerosis, was frustrated with the AHA's continued emphasis on rheumatic heart disease. He told Marvin that the association had failed to show sufficient concern for cardiovascular disorders that were of greater "social and economic importance."

The purpose of Page's foundation was to "further research in hypertension and arteriosclerosis, problems of major importance which have failed to receive the support or attention they deserve."[66] Marvin succeeded in convincing Page to coordinate his group's fund-raising activities with those the AHA was planning. Rather than launching a public appeal, Page's foundation undertook "a quiet, personal contact approach for funds from corporations, individuals, and foundations." Four years later, Page's foundation merged with the AHA to become the Council on High Blood Pressure Research.[67]

While some AHA influentials debated what types of cardiovascular disease deserved the most support, other members addressed the balance between the association's traditional public health agenda and its new commitment to research. By now the public health cardiologists were greatly outnumbered by the association's practitioner and academic cardiologists. But numbers were not everything, and the prevention message was compelling. One AHA board member warned that "there are an awful lot of enthusiasts in public health and they sometimes like to maneuver themselves in places of power."[68]

The influence of the public health cardiologists within the AHA had waned as Conner, Emerson, Halsey, and Wyckoff were replaced by a new generation of heart specialists. Physiological and academic cardiologists were now setting the agenda. The challenge for Sprague and Marvin was to unite the AHA's diverse constituencies at this critical time. They had to deal with competing agendas and conflicting ideologies, as well as several strong egos. In 1946 Sprague told AHA president Roy Scott that the association included two camps: the "expansionists [who] favor extending the public health, public education, lay representation, federal and large scale features of the program [and] the contractionists [who] desire the emphasis upon the small, strictly scientific, professional and clinical aspects of the association."[69]

There was also disagreement about the "ideology of research," a topic that reverberated in academic circles in postwar America. Sprague explained that although some people still supported the "small investigator, the individual clinic or laboratory," they were rapidly being outnumbered by those who wanted "great central foundations" where "investigative specialists" could work "under one roof [with] our clinicians, biochemists, enzyme biologists, physicists, radiant energists, and the super-priesthood of medicine." This was already the model for the nation's program of cancer research. Meanwhile, collaborative wartime ventures, especially the Manhattan Project, demonstrated the potential of federally funded cross-disciplinary, multi-institutional research. Sprague was not enthusiastic about creating a few major centers for heart disease research. He thought that "the investigative work should be kept at the local level."[70]

Sprague worried that the expanded agenda of the AHA might be undermined by "sectionalism or local ambition." That was what was most threatening about the formation of the independent Council for Heart Diseases and the American Foundation for High Blood Pressure. The AHA reformers were alarmed at the prospect of other organizations competing with them for public funds to support cardiovascular research. Sprague appealed to Scott, "Let us by all means be, first of all, the united and dominant organization in the cardiovascular field in the country."[71]

Sprague knew they had to act quickly. In 1946 he told the AHA board about his strategy for transforming the association into a voluntary health organization. Under the new plan, the AHA would be governed by a board that included 50 percent laypersons. He promised that the fund-raising campaign would permit a dramatic expansion of the association's public health programs and make it possible to finance cardiovascular research. The directors supported the plan; the reformers had won. AHA members were told the following year that the transformation was undertaken "in order to meet the urgent need for national action in solving the medical, social, and economic problems of heart disease." The public would be told that "heart disease is our *first* national health problem."[72]

In 1946 the AHA hired Win Nathanson and Associates, a New York public relations firm, to plan their fund-raising program. The first priority was to increase public awareness of the AHA, since it was not as well known as the "organizations sponsoring campaigns to alleviate cancer, tuberculosis, polio, etc." The consultants advocated a "National Heart Week" that would be "governmentally proclaimed, nationally publicized by all major media and through all major organizations." Acknowledging the need to carefully plan this ambitious campaign, they thought 1947 "should be looked upon as a stepping stone to '48."[73]

The decision had been made to frame the fund-raising drive (and the reorganized AHA) around research. A widely circulated booklet, "One out of Three," warned potential donors that one-third of Americans died of cardiovascular disease, but it assured them that the AHA's "first objective" was to "sponsor and finance research on the causes and mechanisms of heart disease," the first step in finding cures.[74] In 1948 the "National Heart Week" strategy brought widespread attention to the AHA and its new agenda, as newspaper columnists and radio announcers championed the cause of cardiovascular research.

That year, the AHA also benefited from the "Walking Man Contest," a regular feature of the popular "Truth or Consequences" radio program. Listeners were challenged to identify a mystery guest who walked in front of a microphone while the announcer provided sketchy clues as to his or her identity. They were encouraged to send in donations for a specific charity (in this case the AHA) with their entry form. By the time (several weeks) someone correctly guessed Jack Benny, listeners had sent in $1.8 million for the AHA—compelling evidence that they supported heart research.[75]

The fund-raising drive was off to a spectacular start. Several association leaders traveled extensively to stimulate enthusiasm for the campaign among physicians and concerned citizens. AHA president Tinsley Harrison knew a lot of money was needed, because "successful research requires competent investigators who can devote all their time and energy to their work." In a Boston speech carried over the ABC radio network, he complained that many promising young researchers had been forced to abandon academic careers because there was no consistent source of funding; they were forced "to earn a livelihood in private practice." This concern led the AHA leaders to target their research support to "career" investigators willing to "devote their entire effort to research and basic problems of heart disease." Harrison saw this as the "primary objective of the American Heart Association's programs."[76]

Concern about inadequate support for research was not new; similar warnings had been voiced since the nineteenth century. In 1876 Philadelphia medical scientist Henry Chapman declared, "Everything in the long run is a question of finance." He argued that America's physiologists were not as "distinguished as those in Germany" because "they do not make their studies the business of their lives. They do not live in their laboratories, but in their carriages going from patient to patient." Most medical scientists had no choice; the government did not support medical research, and few of the nation's medical schools had any endowment.[77] Although the situation had improved significantly since Chapman protested the lack of salary support for America's medical scientists, complaints about inadequate research funding continued. In 1933 a writer on arteriosclerosis reported that there was a consensus among scientists and academic physicians that whatever research had been carried out on the subject had "been done in a scattered way without sufficient financial backing to lend that continuity over a period of years which is so essential in investigations of this kind."[78]

In 1948 the outlook for medical researchers looked brighter than at any time in the past. Isolated, underfunded scientists struggling with inadequate support staff and equipment were being replaced gradually by teams of investigators financed by grants. Initially, funding for this small but growing research enterprise came from philanthropists. Led by the Rockefeller Foundation, a number of organizations began supporting medical research during the first half of the twentieth century.[79] Now the federal government would get involved in a major way.

Alliance of Washington and the AHA in a war on heart disease

The AHA leaders looked beyond public fund-raising, corporate donations, and philanthropists to support their twin causes: cardiovascular research *and researchers*. They knew that the federal government was the most promising source for research funding. Victoria Harden has explored the origins of the National Institutes of Health, and Daniel Fox has summarized the dynamics that led the federal government to expand its research support into the area of chronic diseases during the 1930s and 1940s. Gradually, a coalition of politicians, federal officials, scientists, and academic physicians succeeded in getting the government to liberally fund research projects in private institutions. Fox characterizes their achievement as "a triumph of bureaucratic politics; of brilliant use of techniques of incrementalism, of opportunism, and of coalition-building."[80]

The government's role in financing medical research expanded dramatically after World War II. Today, the extraordinary impact of the war on medicine is largely forgotten.[81] As with all modern wars, it was a powerful stimulus for the development of technology. Although the goal of war-related research was to gain a military advantage, many medical advances, such as blood substitutes, diagnostic ultrasound, and radioisotopes for diagnosis and treatment, can be traced to wartime research programs. The Manhattan Project to develop an atomic bomb had greater implications for American medicine than any specific war-related medical advance. This program of well-funded, multi-institutional research served as a model for the nation's postwar biomedical research initiative.[82]

In 1944 Franklin Roosevelt asked Vannevar Bush, director of the Office of Scientific Research and Development, to prepare a proposal for America's postwar science program. In his report, *Science: The Endless Frontier*, Bush urged the government to assume a major role in funding research through the creation of a "National Research Foundation."[83]

Walter Palmer, chair of medicine at Columbia University, headed the medical advisory committee that Bush created as part of his comprehensive study. Palmer's committee cited the "brilliant record of medicine in World War II." Thousands of lives had been saved as a result of penicillin, better vaccines, improved transfusion techniques, and other innovations. These developments and the specialty hospital concept were credited with reducing the mortality of war-related injuries by nearly 50 percent.[84]

The issue was how to maintain the momentum in peacetime. Palmer's report concluded that more funds should be given to universities, the "chief contributors to pure science." He urged the government to support research in three ways: unrestricted institutional grants, fellowship grants to train individuals for research careers, and grants-in-aid for especially important projects. The committee recommended annual government grants of between $5 and $7 million initially, cautioning that "funds exceeding the capacity of the nation's research institutions to utilize them effectively would do harm by encouraging mediocre work and by driving away university and foundation support." Palmer's committee also recommended the creation of a new independent federal agency (the National Foundation for Medical Research) to administer the grants.[85]

Medical scientists and clinical investigators conceded that research was expensive, but they argued that the cost was justified because it produced new knowledge that would benefit humanity. Categorical, goal-directed research gained many advocates as a result of the apparent success of this approach during the war. In 1947 Everett Kinsey of Harvard appealed for the support of "laboratories investigating specific diseases." He thought they should be organized in the clinical departments of university medical schools and staffed by "well-trained, full-time workers." Kinsey acknowledged that there was "little precedent for full-time investigators in clinical specialties," but he was convinced that such a plan would promote practical discoveries and encourage medical students to become researchers.[86]

When the AHA leaders began to develop a plan for winning government support for cardiovascular research, they knew they were competing with other groups lobbying on behalf of *their* diseases—especially cancer. A coalition of scientists, politicians, and citizens had succeeded in getting Congress to pass the National Cancer Institute Act in 1937. The cancer research program was a model for the activists who hoped to achieve similar success for heart disease. As they formulated their strategy, AHA leaders worked with businesswoman Mary Lasker and several politicians, including Senators Claude Pepper and Lister Hill and Congressmen Frank Keefe and John Fogarty.

Mary Lasker's husband Albert, a wealthy advertising executive, had created a foundation in the mid-1930s to fund research into the "causes, nature, prevention, and cure of degenerative diseases" such as cancer and disorders of the heart and kidneys.[87] Mary Lasker became interested in the cause of chronic diseases shortly after she married him in 1940. That year, New York public health cardiologist Ernst Boas characterized chronic illness as "a great, destructive force in society."[88] Concern about the socioeconomic consequences of chronic or "degenerative" diseases was gradually increasing. As Daniel Fox notes, Boas and Alfred Cohn were among the first to emphasize their significance.[89]

Lasker was especially concerned about cancer, heart disease, and arthritis. James Patterson characterizes her as a "key figure" in the transformation (in the mid-1940s) of the American Society for the Control of Cancer from an association run by a "medical elite" into the American Cancer Society, a voluntary health organization controlled by a coalition of physicians, scientists, and influential laypersons.[90] With the help of politicians and several disease-specific foundations, Lasker got "government involved in medical research in a big way," according to historian Stephen Strickland.[91]

In 1944 Lasker and her friend Florence Mahoney, the wife of an influential newspaper publisher, persuaded Senator Pepper to focus his health care hearings on the future of medical research. The testimony (and Lasker's persistent lobbying) led Pepper to conclude that the amount of medical research carried out in America should not be "limited by lack of money."[92] While several disease lobbies urged concerned citizens and the government to support their cause, the case for heart disease was especially compelling. In 1948 Pepper told his Senate colleagues that heart disease was a "killer more deadly than cancer." He also expressed concern that there were few trained cardiovascular specialists and "hardly any facilities where research was being carried on in this field."[93]

Meanwhile, the House of Representatives was considering several bills relating to the establishment of a "National Institute for the Study of Heart Disease." Wisconsin Republican Frank Keefe claimed that "every member of Congress is thoroughly aware of the tremendous inroads that diseases of the heart are making upon the American people." He urged the creation of a "heart control program" patterned after the government-sponsored cancer program. One aspect of the proposal had tremendous implications for cardiology. The heart control program would not only support research; it would also subsidize the training of heart specialists. Keefe argued that new knowledge was of little value to the American people unless there were highly trained "clinicians and doctors" to translate research breakthroughs into patient care. He assured the politicians that they had nothing to fear from their constituents if they funded the heart program. Citing the public's response to the Walking Man Contest, Keefe claimed, "the American people are way ahead of Congress."[94]

Surgeon General Leonard Scheele supported the establishment of a National Heart Institute (NHI) and a National Heart Council to help coordinate cardiovascular research across the country. This would "pave the way for a full-scale, comprehensive attack on the nation's number one killer—heart disease." Portraying existing facilities for cardiovascular research as "pitifully inadequate," Scheele protested that "funds and facilities in heart disease research have lagged far behind the resources and money which have been made available for other illnesses, some of which are less prevalent and less deadly." He also advocated federal support for clinical cardiology training and urged the government to coordinate its efforts with those of the AHA, "which had been performing such a valuable function in this field."[95]

The AHA was formally represented on Capitol Hill by president Tinsley Harrison and medical director Charles Connor. They pledged full cooperation with the government and urged Congress to support "extramural" research at sites other than the National Institutes of Health (NIH), a critical issue for the nation's academic physicians. Stephen Strickland has shown that there was broad support for a program of extramural grants to supplement the monies spent in Bethesda.[96] The heart lobby knew this. They also knew that cardiovascular disease had touched almost every American, at least indirectly. Mary Lasker told members of Congress that her parents had died of cardiovascular disease: "I am sure you have all felt equal losses." Contrasting the $2 billion spent to produce the atomic bomb with less than $3 million of private and government funds targeted for cardiovascular research, she complained that the total expenditures for the latter amounted to just $3.98 per death.[97]

But research funding was not enough; there had to be money to train both investigators *and* clinical specialists. Lasker insisted that it was crucial to increase the "present meager force of physicians specializing in diseases of the heart and circulation." The number of cardiologists, "about 638 out of a total effective force of 135,000 doctors," was wholly inadequate. She challenged the politicians: "Leadership in the fight at this moment rests with Congress. The American people fervently await your action."[98]

Congress passed the National Heart Act "to support research and training in diseases of the heart and circulation," and Harry Truman signed it into law on 16 June 1948. The act established the NHI as a division of the NIH and the National Advisory Heart Council (NAHC). The NAHC was charged with reviewing grant requests for research projects and training programs. It dispensed grants-in-aid to individual researchers at the NHI and elsewhere and allocated funds to public and private institutions for research and training and for the construction of laboratory and clinical facilities.[99]

The NAHC was a powerful group because it controlled the funds that academic medical centers could use to develop or expand cardiology research and training programs. It included four ex-officio government representatives and twelve "leaders in the fields of fundamental sciences, medical sciences, education, and public affairs," of which six were "leading medical or scientific authorities . . . outstanding in the study, diagnosis, or treatment of heart diseases." Paul White, Tinsley Harrison, Duckett Jones, Irvine Page, and Mary Lasker were among those present at the first meeting, chaired by Surgeon General Leonard Scheele in September 1948.[100]

Cardiovascular research: The AHA's new "primary purpose"

The AHA now had a wealthy ally—the federal government—in its campaign to endow heart research. In 1948 the association formed a research committee chaired by physiological cardiologist Louis Katz of Chicago. He thought the "primary purpose" of the AHA reorganization was to "increase the amount of money available for cardiovascular research." Although Katz conceded that the AHA's public health activities were worthwhile, they were "not so important as advancing knowledge by research."[101] The public health cardiologists saw things differently, but their influence was limited; physiological and academic cardiologists now controlled the association.

In 1950 the AHA board voted to devote half of the association's budget to research. Edgar Allen of the Mayo Clinic reassured Sprague (who had presided over the turbulent meeting) that he had "no regrets about the insistence that 50 per cent of the funds of the AHA be devoted to research." Allen closed his letter, "It is unfortunate that considerable bitterness was expressed, but I presume that all wounds will heal."[102] Sprague responded, "I certainly hope that the matters discussed so heatedly in California will be viewed by all of us in the proper perspective." The next challenge was to convince people across the country to donate money to support research in urban academic medical centers rather than to fund heart clinics in their own area. Sprague knew it would be "terribly difficult to get this over in smaller communities from which, perhaps, much of our funds must come."[103] Association leaders knew they needed the support of their local affiliates. Their fund-raising goal for 1949 was $5 million, an ambitious target for an organization whose budget was less than $30 thousand five years earlier.[104]

Katz's research committee included twelve members representing arteriosclerosis, hypertension, rheumatic fever, vascular disease and vascular surgery, physiology, other basic sciences, public health, and practitioners. As they debated how to allocate the AHA's research budget (almost $1 million in 1949–1950), the committee had to decide whether basic research or clinical investigation deserved more support; whether the focus should be on arteriosclerosis or rheumatic heart disease; whether grants should go to institutions or individuals; and what should be the amount and duration of each grant.[105]

Several institutional models for research had evolved during the twentieth century: university-based programs, private foundations (like the Rockefeller Institute in New York), hospital-based research programs (like Katz's at Michael Reese Hospital in Chicago), and multi-institutional networks (like the one Cornell cardiologist Irving Wright developed to study anticoagulation). Katz rejected the large institute model, embodied in New York's Sloan-Kettering Institute, which historian Harry Marks characterizes as "the public's symbol of cancer research."[106] In 1949 a writer in *Time* stated that Sloan-Kettering possessed "the world's most impressive array of cancer-fighting weapons." In addition to vast laboratories, experimental equipment, and animals, it housed "scholarly chemists, physicists, biologists, clinicians all working in unison to defeat the common enemy: cancer."[107]

A few days after the *Time* essay appeared, Katz told Sprague that creating "huge institutes to which investigators are brought is, in my opinion, the wrong approach in the cardiovascular field." He thought their size stifled "that competitive instinct and originality which is as prevalent in our society in research as it is in industry and which has proven so fruitful." Katz favored smaller institution-based centers (like his own) because they were "built to permit a leader in the field to develop to his full capacity." The "primary need" in cardiology was to "develop more first class leaders of research and to have them widely disseminated." This view was consistent with the proposal Walter Palmer's committee had submitted to Vannevar Bush four years earlier.[108]

Reflecting this philosophy, Katz's committee decided to provide financial support to "established investigators" in 1949. They purposely chose to support *investigators* with a record of accomplishment rather than specific short-term *projects*.[109] The AHA's "career investigator program" was designed to provide a few outstanding scientists with long-term financial support so they could devote themselves almost exclusively to cardiovascular research. The AHA leaders chose to link the number of career investigator awards to the association's annual income—a strategy that encouraged academicians to support the AHA's fund-raising activities.[110]

This ambitious research program required money, and the AHA's public relations consultants pledged to help raise it. They proposed the "fullest development of press coverage in newspapers and magazines . . . network and local radio stations." The Advertising Council would be approached "to secure higher priorities and allocations of radio time. . . . The newspaper wire services and syndicates will be heavily cultivated." This media blitz would coincide with the distribution of 10 million fund-raising pamphlets and 100 thousand plastic hearts to collect pocket change from concerned citizens.[111]

The intense campaign heightened the public's awareness of (and concern about) heart disease. Readers of *Business Week* were told, "A bad heart is bad business." Applauding the AHA's reorganization, the writer decried how little was spent on cardiovascular research: "In comparable years heart research grants for the entire U.S. were 17 cents per death while those of polio $5.02 per death." Heart disease not only cost lives, it hurt the nation's economy. Disability due to cardiovascular disease resulted in a loss of $1.2 billion annually, making it "the greatest drain on America's human resources."[112]

Ed Sullivan told readers of his syndicated column, "One person dies every minute from diseases of the heart, which is No. 1 killer in all age brackets."[113] The subtitle of a 1950 *Fortune* article "Why Executives Drop Dead" explained "It's from cardiovascular diseases." The writer declared, "Reading the obituaries on a bad morning, one might easily get the impression that business is a hazardous occupation. The number of executives nipped in mid-career seems to be rising, and the frequency with which 'heart failure' is cited almost gives this the status of an occupational disease."[114]

Despite the success of their fund-raising drive, some AHA leaders were impatient. In 1950 Andrew Robertson, chair of the AHA board (and of Westinghouse), complained, "There are still many people in the world who apparently have no intention of giving money to the association!" One problem was that "cardiovascular diseases are difficult to dramatize." He thought more funds would be raised "if we could put a man suffering from a heart attack in a public window."[115] Fund-raisers knew that compelling images stimulated donations. One writer explained, "The picture of the suffering child takes priority over any appeal concerning adults. . . . Men at a luncheon club are stirred into giving by the sight of a crippled child."[116]

Robertson admitted that "such antics are inappropriate," but he thought the AHA should publish "cumulative lists of famous men who died of heart attacks" to impress the public with the impact of cardiac disease. His goal was "to put our work so vividly before the public that it will be discussed over the lunch tables, in the board rooms of corporations, at social gatherings generally, not to mention the smoking rooms and the lounge cars, to the end that everyone not only knows that there is a disease called heart disease, but is interested in the dramatic contest that is being waged to find a cure."[117]

The AHA had been working to increase public awareness of the risks of heart disease for nearly a quarter of a century when they began sending official representatives to Capitol Hill in 1948. But they now carried a powerful new message: research can *cure* heart disease. The AHA's media consultant told them that the public was becoming desensitized to "startling statistics." His advice: "Stop talking about America's #1 killer and begin to show how the American Heart Association is using public funds to arrest this killer." Katz and other AHA scientists who wanted the association to support basic research recognized the need to reinforce the message that cures ultimately depended on the work they and their peers were doing in laboratories scattered across the country.[118]

Paul White, who had long been influential in the AHA, was appointed executive director of the NAHC and chief medical advisor to the NHI. He first appeared before Congress in February 1949. White, Lasker, Wright, and other members of the "heart lobby" stated and restated their simple message. If the nation invested in academic medical centers—facilities, researchers, and equipment were needed—practical discoveries were inevitable. Wartime programs proved that systematic support of categorical research produced results. In the case of heart disease, the goals were prevention, earlier diagnosis, better treatments, and *cures.* Individuals would be helped, but the nation would be the true beneficiary. Lower mortality and morbidity from heart disease would result in a healthier and more productive workforce.

All it took was money, and a lot of it. Mary Lasker put it bluntly: "No funds are sufficient until a large and successful attack has been made."[119] The heart lobby worked tirelessly to ensure continuous (and generous) government support of the nation's few cardiovascular research and training programs. Heeding their consultants' advice, they stressed what research had already accomplished in the fight against cardiac disease. White often brought recovered patients to the hearings "as concrete evidence of the benefit that previous funds had procured for the citizens of the United States."[120]

Irving Wright (now deeply involved in an AHA-sponsored study of the value of anticoagulants in treating acute myocardial infarction) knew how crucial Mary Lasker was to the effort to endow cardiovascular research. In 1950 he sent her several of his recent publications with the assurance, "I wanted you to know that the funds which you have given during the past have been put to good use and have resulted in the addition of new and important knowledge in the field of heart and blood vessel diseases for the benefit of mankind."[121] Wright and the other members of the heart lobby believed deeply that research was the way to improve the nation's health. He still held this view four decades later: "What is needed is new knowledge if you're going to really improve the care of the patients."[122]

The First National Congress on Cardiovascular Diseases, jointly sponsored by the AHA and the NHI, was held in Washington in 1950. Irvine Page considered the three-day conference "the first formal indication that cardiovascular disease was to become both big business and politically significant in Washington."[123] The AHA told tens of thousands of people through their widely circulated publication *American Heart* that "196 experts from 32 states" attended the conference. These "professional and lay leaders" participated in three separate sections: research, professional education, and community service.[124]

Heart disease at mid-century: Practices and promises

Several recent medical advances helped the heart lobby make their case to America's citizens and their political leaders. In the decade following World War II, new drugs dramatically changed the way doctors cared for patients with cardiovascular disease. Antibiotics, oral diuretics, and effective antihypertensive medications were all introduced at this time. The significance of these and other advances is underscored by the case of Franklin Roosevelt. Crippled by polio, the president died from complications of malignant hypertension just before effective antihypertensive drugs were developed.

Doctors (and their patients) sensed they were entering a new era in the diagnosis and treatment of cardiovascular disease. In his popular 1949 book on heart disease, New York cardiologist Charles Friedberg emphasized the "swift pace of recent advances."[125] This was not hyperbole. Many things *had* changed since Paul White published his unintentionally dreary assessment of the treatment of heart disease in 1931. The first truly dramatic therapeutic advances—ones that offered heart patients the possibility of cure—were in the emerging field of cardiovascular surgery. Although a few surgeons had tried to repair diseased cardiac valves earlier in the century, they abandoned the approach because nearly all the patients died.[126] There was renewed interest in cardiovascular surgery after Boston surgeon Robert Gross successfully ligated a patent ductus arteriosus in 1938, and Swedish surgeon Clarence Crafoord successfully repaired a coarctation of the aorta six years later. These operations for congenital defects of the great vessels attracted worldwide attention.

Meanwhile, a powerful new diagnostic technique—cardiac catheterization—was being developed. Although it was only available in a few academic centers in the late 1940s, cardiac catheterization signaled a new era in the diagnosis of heart disease. Just as the electrocardiograph made it possible to study cardiac electrophysiology in living humans, the cardiac catheter allowed doctors to evaluate the heart's structure and function. German surgeon Werner Forssmann had performed the first human cardiac catheterization in 1929—on himself. His goal was not to advance cardiac diagnosis, but to improve on a standard therapeutic procedure used in some cases of cardiac arrest. He hoped to find a safer way than direct cardiac puncture to deliver medicines like epinephrine into the central circulation following cardiac arrest. Forssmann introduced a flexible ureteral catheter into his basilic arm vein and pushed it toward his heart. After it reached its goal (he followed its progress with a fluoroscope), Forssmann walked to the x-ray department, where he documented his experiment on film.[127]

Twelve years later, André Cournand, Dickinson Richards, and their colleagues at Bellevue Hospital in New York reported the results of the first series of heart catheterizations in humans. These researchers showed that cardiac output and intracardiac pressures could be measured in humans, but they were interested in cardiopulmonary physiology, not cardiac diagnosis. By 1945 the catheter was being used to study human cardiac physiology in Boston (Lewis Dexter), Atlanta (James Warren and Eugene Stead), London (John McMichael and Edward Sharpey-Schaefer), and Paris (Pierre Maurice and Jean Lenègre).[128]

One surgeon's desire for more accurate preoperative diagnosis catalyzed the transformation of cardiac catheterization from a research technique into a clinical diagnostic tool. In 1944 Johns Hopkins surgeon Alfred Blalock performed an operation that inaugurated a new era in the treatment of cardiovascular disease: the "blue-baby operation" for tetralogy of Fallot (the most common form of cyanotic congenital heart disease), which he had developed in collaboration with pediatric heart specialist Helen Taussig.

Taussig conceived how such an operation might help counter the serious physiological consequences of this heart defect. Blalock, working with his African-American laboratory technician Vivien Thomas, perfected the surgical technique. The operation was designed to correct the hypoxemia and cyanosis, caused by severe pulmonary stenosis in association with a ventricular septal defect, by connecting the left subclavian artery to the pulmonary artery, thereby supplying blood to the lungs. This extracardiac operation created a shunt that increased blood flow through the lungs and transformed cyanotic, frail children with severely limited exercise tolerance into pink, active youngsters. The change in the patient's color was immediate and visible. Following recovery, the improvement in their exercise tolerance was dramatic and sustained.[129]

Houston heart surgeon Denton Cooley was a surgical intern when he assisted Blalock with the first blue-baby operation. Cooley recalled recently that during that operation he sensed that he "was really at the dawn of a new era. And it turned out to be just that."[130] A contemporary writer proclaimed the "revolutionary" operation a "God-send to the blue baby."[131] The Blalock-Taussig operation electrified the medical community, and scores of surgeons visited Baltimore to observe and to learn to perform it. André Cournand told Blalock, "Watching you operate Saturday will stand out in my mind as a most impressive manifestation of mastery, one to be compared to a work of art."[132] Harris Shumacker Jr., who worked under Blalock from 1937 to 1941, claimed recently that after the blue-baby operation was reported, "Physicians altered their attitude and started to think of cardiac surgery as an essential component in the therapeutic armamentarium for disorders of the heart."[133]

Once surgeons began performing heart operations that were both life-saving and life-threatening, the limitations of standard cardiac diagnostic techniques (history, physical examination, auscultation, electrocardiography, x-ray, and fluoroscopy) became more apparent. By June 1945, less than a year after he performed the first blue-baby operation, Blalock was operating on several children with tetralogy of Fallot each week. After one child died during surgery, Blalock's resident William Longmire Jr. noted in his diary that the child "was found to have transposition of the great vessels rather than tetralogy as had been diagnosed before operation."[134] This incident emphasized the limitations of routine diagnostic approaches. Even Helen Taussig, whose skill in cardiac diagnosis (despite a hearing impairment) was legendary, was not infallible.

Blalock knew that accurate diagnosis was crucial, and he thought the new technique of cardiac catheterization could provide useful physiological information as part of the routine preoperative evaluation of his heart patients. In 1945 he hired Richard Bing to organize the world's first *diagnostic* cardiac catheterization laboratory at Johns Hopkins. Bing had fled Nazi Germany in 1933 along with many other prominent or promising scientists and clinicians. He had worked as a clinical scientist at the Rockefeller Institute, Columbia University, and New York University, where he learned to use catheter techniques while investigating renal function with physiologist Homer Smith. Bing recalled recently that Blalock's desire for more preoperative information transformed cardiac catheterization from a "physiological tool" into a "diagnostic thing."[135]

In 1945 Samuel Levine encouraged Lewis Dexter to develop Boston's first diagnostic cardiac catheterization program at the Peter Bent Brigham Hospital. The following year, Dexter published a paper that emphasized the value of catheterization in the evaluation of children with congenital heart disease. Once catheterization was shown to be clinically useful, physiologists and physiological cardiologists introduced several innovations that enhanced the value of the cardiac catheter as a diagnostic tool. These included technical advances (such as improved pressure gauges and instruments to measure oxygen saturation) and new approaches (such as injecting dyes into the circulation to document intracardiac shunts).[136]

Like Bing, Dexter feels that surgeons were initially more interested in cardiac catheterization than were cardiologists or pediatricians. He explained recently, "Now they could have a diagnosis and know what they were dealing with." At first, cardiac catheterization grew slowly. According to Dexter, the technique was received "with great hesitation. I mean sticking tubes down into people's hearts was not a very comforting thought. Because the heart was always such a sacred organ in people's minds."[137]

But recent wartime surgical experience had proved that the heart was not such a fragile organ after all. Several innovations during World War II contributed to the development of cardiovascular surgery, but one was especially significant. Boston surgeon Dwight Harken adopted an aggressive approach for removing shell fragments that had lodged in and around the heart and great vessels. Harken explained recently, "I don't think the technical trick of pulling the shell fragment out was the important thing." He thought his main contribution was proving that this amount of manipulation of the heart was both feasible and safe. The "big step" was getting beyond the belief that operating on the heart "was 'verboten'." Following the war, Harken resumed studies on the surgical treatment of mitral valve obstruction (stenosis) that Boston surgeon Eliot Cutler had abandoned two decades earlier.[138]

Mitral stenosis, a serious long-term complication of rheumatic fever, usually led to progressive shortness of breath, congestive heart failure, and eventually death. In June 1948 Harken in Boston and Charles Bailey in Philadelphia independently performed successful operations on patients with mitral stenosis. Harken relieved the obstruction by splitting the fused valve leaflets with his finger, while Bailey used a special scalpel blade attached to his finger. Although several of their first patients died, they persisted and proved that such an operation could help some people with mitral stenosis. Blalock was impressed. After watching him operate, he told Bailey, "You are certainly to be congratulated on your pioneering work and I wish you continued success."[139]

During these procedures, the surgeon inserted a finger through an incision in the left atrial appendage while the heart was full of blood and beating. There was still no way to temporarily interrupt the circulation, although machines to accomplish this goal were under development. Willem Kolff's recent invention of an "artificial kidney" led Philadelphia surgeon John Gibbon Jr. to conclude that his twelve-year project to invent a machine to oxygenate the blood (permitting temporary arrest of the circulation) might soon come to fruition.

In 1949 Gibbon updated Blalock on the status of his heart-lung machine, designed to "take over, temporarily, a part of the cardiorespiratory functions." Gibbon made it sound simple: "It is only necessary to heparinize a patient, withdraw blood from a vein, introduce oxygen and allow carbon dioxide to escape, and then inject the blood into a peripheral artery." Although he had yet to invent a "suitable apparatus" for a clinical trial, Gibbon was optimistic and thought the difficulties would be overcome in the "not too distant future." He had already performed the procedure in animals and could "see no reason why it cannot ultimately be done in patients." Gibbon knew that a reliable heart-lung machine would revolutionize cardiac surgery. He told Blalock, "It would permit, of course, operations within the heart under direct vision."[140]

Gibbon's 1949 prediction that intracardiac surgery under direct vision would be possible using a heart–lung machine came true in five years. It was an exciting time for surgeons and for patients they treated. Working alone or in collaboration with engineers and scientists, several surgeons were busy trying to develop operations to treat a variety of congenital and acquired cardiovascular diseases. The dramatic advances in cardiovascular surgery during the next several decades depended not only on innovative and technically adept surgeons; they relied on literally thousands of developments in science, technology, pharmacology, and medicine. For example, open-heart surgery required some way to prevent blood from clotting, which was only possible after heparin was introduced into clinical practice in the late 1930s.[141]

"Miracle drugs" and the transformation of medical practice

At the same time as Blalock and Taussig's operation signaled a new era in the surgical treatment of heart disease, the introduction of penicillin into civilian medical practice seemed to herald an age in which people would no longer die from infections. In 1950 academic internist Paul Beeson was impressed that antibiotics were transforming the lives of patients and doctors alike. Their advent had resulted in "striking changes in medical practice."[142] Sulfonamides had been introduced before World War II, but they proved less effective and more toxic than penicillin, an antibiotic first used in 1940. Six years later, penicillin's discoverer, Alexander Fleming, declared: "It seems likely that in the next few years a combination of antibiotics with different antibacterial spectra will furnish a 'cribrum therapeuticum' from which fewer and fewer infecting bacteria will escape."[143]

The introduction of antibiotics is one of the most significant advances in the history of medicine. During the war, the public had heard that penicillin had resulted in dramatic cures and lower mortality rates. When it became available to civilians at the end of the war, the antibiotic had many champions: cured patients, elated families, relieved doctors, and the media—often prone to sensationalism. Reminding doctors that penicillin was not a cure-all, Fleming cautioned: "Press publicity in the last few years has given many people the idea that penicillin is a panacea."[144]

Penicillin changed cardiology because it was effective in treating (and preventing recurrent) streptococcal infections, which had become recognized as the underlying cause of acute rheumatic fever. As the incidence of rheumatic fever declined, so did the dreaded cardiac complications. Penicillin also transformed bacterial endocarditis from a disease with a "hopeless prognosis" (Paul White, 1931) into "the most frequent curable cardiac disease" (Charles Friedberg, 1949).[145] There were other medical advances that had important implications for patients with heart disease. By 1950 it was clear that anticoagulants (intravenous heparin and oral dicoumarol) were useful in the prevention and treatment of some forms of cardiovascular disease.

America's cardiologists sensed that they were entering a new era in the diagnosis and treatment of heart disease. It seemed likely that antibiotics would eliminate cardiovascular syphilis and rheumatic heart disease. Some surgeons predicted that the dramatic cardiovascular operations introduced during the 1940s were just the beginning. They anticipated an increasing role for their emerging specialty in the care and *cure* of heart patients. This would be a welcome new focus for thoracic surgeons, who soon found that they were performing fewer operations for pulmonary tuberculosis as a result of the introduction of antibiotics.[146]

Doctors and patients were hopeful, and their mood was elevated further as postwar euphoria swept the nation. The AHA leaders were also optimistic, with good reason. Their specialty seemed poised for unprecedented growth, and they had established the AHA as *the* national organization representing heart disease and heart doctors. The academicians who led the association influenced every aspect of cardiovascular medicine. They controlled a (suddenly prosperous) voluntary health organization. They were key members of the heart lobby that convinced Congress to endow cardiovascular research and training programs. They played a dominant role in the cardiology boards. And they and their protégés held positions in America's leading medical schools that were targeted for government support. But the AHA's successes also set the stage for unexpected new tensions between some of the nation's academic and practitioner cardiologists.

∿∿∿∿∿

CHAPTER 4

Doctors with a Different Vision: The American College of Cardiology

Many American Heart Association (AHA) members (all of them physicians or medical scientists) were unhappy when their society was transformed into a voluntary health organization in 1948. Although the AHA leaders did not realize it initially, certain aspects of the plan alienated their largest constituency: the practitioner cardiologists, internists, and general practitioners who cared for heart patients in their offices and in community hospitals across the nation. Some of these doctors thought that the AHA leaders—busy debating the proper balance between their organization's traditional public health mission and its new emphasis on research—were ignoring their concerns. Eager to learn about the new approaches to diagnose and treat heart disease, practitioner cardiologists wanted more educational programs.

Franz Groedel, a German heart specialist who had emigrated to the United States fifteen years earlier, could see that many acknowledged and aspiring practitioner cardiologists were frustrated with the reorganized AHA. He took advantage of their discontent to create the American College of Cardiology (ACC) in 1949. By focusing on continuing medical education, Groedel's new professional society promised to address issues that concerned practitioners whose primary interest was patient care rather than public health or research. When the ACC began to recruit members in 1951, the AHA leaders feared the worst. They worried that the college would compete with them for members and, more importantly, for public funds. This chapter describes the complex dynamics that led to the creation of the ACC and the AHA's hostile reaction to it.

Groedel was largely responsible for inventing the ACC. His passionate struggle to develop the college, despite a series of setbacks and an intense campaign by AHA leaders to undermine his recruiting effort, can be understood only if one appreciates the challenges Groedel and other immigrant physicians faced when they arrived in the United States in the 1930s and 1940s. Meanwhile, other stresses affected native-born physicians. Groedel took advantage of the growing strain between America's expanding community of academic physicians and medical scientists and the much larger (but less influential) body of practitioners. His new organization offered practitioner cardiologists and internists an alternative to the AHA, which an increasing number of them viewed as elitist and indifferent to their needs.

The AHA Scientific Council: Its creation and consequences

The tensions among the various physician groups that made up the AHA increased during the 1940s. They peaked late in the decade after a Scientific Council was established within the organization. Association leaders had considered creating a membership hierarchy for several years. In 1940 AHA secretary Howard Sprague told executive committee chair Jack Marvin that he favored dividing the association into "a relatively small group of fellows, and a much larger group of members."[1] Although the concept reflected the elitist tendencies of some AHA leaders, there was a more pragmatic issue. Sprague had received complaints that some "unqualified practitioners" were using their AHA membership to "pose as heart specialists."[2]

Marvin embraced the concept of selecting a small group of "fellows." Physiological cardiologist and AHA influential Louis Katz also supported the idea and suggested limiting fellowships to people chosen "by virtue of their meritorious scientific, teaching, public health, or medical activities."[3] The designations had practical implications: fellows would have special privileges. Under the proposed scheme, they alone could present papers at the annual meeting, hold offices, or serve on committees. Ordinary members (most practitioners would be in this category) could not.[4]

Although this membership hierarchy scheme was similar to that employed in other medical societies, it contributed to the strain between practitioners and academicians, who were much more likely to qualify for fellowship based on the AHA criteria. Physiologist Harold Rice acknowledged in 1947, "The general practitioner in medicine knows little of the aims and objectives and ideals of the academic man, and he calls his work impractical and of little use. On the other hand, the academic group tends to scorn the practitioner as an ignoramus and empiricist." Another medical scientist thought "academic snobbishness" was part of the problem.[5]

The AHA leaders did not implement a hierarchy system until their association became a voluntary health organization in 1948. That change promised to greatly increase the AHA's budget, but it carried risks, which the AHA leaders underestimated. From the start, the association had been a society *of* physicians run *by* physicians. The reorganization changed this. Under the new plan, the AHA welcomed nurses, social workers, and interested citizens as members. More importantly, it would be governed by a board that included 50 percent laypersons.

Some of the AHA's influential academic and physiological cardiologists worried that the new agenda and revised governance structure might result in an overemphasis on public health activities at the expense of supporting scientific research.[6] Physicians and medical scientists interested in cancer had raised similar concerns when their American Society for the Control of Cancer was transformed into the American Cancer Society (a voluntary health organization) a few months earlier. Historian James Patterson concludes that the society's "doctors and scientists, in danger of losing control, reacted with predictable alarm and outrage" to the "invasion of business people" intent on a massive publicity and fund-raising campaign.[7]

The voices of the AHA's academic and physiological cardiologists were heard. To reassure this influential constituency that their interests would be served, the reformers decided to create a Scientific Council within the AHA.[8] Sprague characterized the council as the AHA's "nucleus" and urged that membership in it be limited to "scientifically qualified individuals who will be primarily interested in furthering knowledge of cardiovascular disease." The council would be an powerful body responsible for the *American Heart Journal* (the AHA's official journal until *Circulation* was launched in 1950), the annual scientific meeting, the allocation of research funds, and other professional activities. AHA members who were board certified in cardiovascular disease would automatically become council members. Other professionals could be nominated and elected to membership, "particularly internists, pediatricians, and thoracic surgeons [who] have made major contributions to the knowledge of cardiovascular diseases" and scientists "who have made contributions to cardiovascular research."[9] In May 1948 AHA president Arlie Barnes of the Mayo Clinic invited 676 people to join the "founder's group" of the Scientific Council. Shortly thereafter, a final list of 548 founding members was circulated.[10]

Although the council had broad geographical representation and included board certified practitioners in addition to academic cardiologists and medical scientists, many of the association's doctors felt disenfranchised. Fewer than one-fifth of the AHA's 2,351 physician members were invited to join. This was because few of them had published articles and only a small fraction of them were board certified; there were only 338 board certified cardiologists in the country at the time.[11]

A social scientist hired to help plan the transition to a voluntary health organization warned the AHA leaders that by limiting membership in the council and making it "self-electing," they had formed a group "considerably more aristocratic than the American Heart Association previously was."[12] An AHA executive director described the response: "Almost immediately, the structure and restrictions on the membership [in the Scientific Council] caused dissatisfaction."[13] The council held its first formal meeting in 1948 in Chicago during the InterAmerican Cardiological Congress. Franz Groedel, an AHA member, attended the congress, but he was not invited to join the council despite a bibliography of more than 300 publications, mainly on the heart.[14]

Franz Groedel: An immigrant physician who created the ACC

Once a prominent physician and clinical scientist, today Franz Groedel is virtually unknown. It is important to summarize his career in order to understand why he created the ACC and why the AHA leaders responded to it as they did. The son of a physician, Groedel was born in 1881 in Bad Nauheim, Germany.[15] In 1904 he received his medical degree from the University of Leipzig, home of the world's leading physiological institute during the second half of the nineteenth century.[16]

Groedel then served as assistant to Friedrich von Müller in his renowned medical clinic in Munich. Müller was a role model for several first-generation clinical scientists (including Lewellys Barker of Johns Hopkins and Rufus Cole of the Rockefeller Institute Hospital). In 1912 one American educational reformer portrayed Müller as an example of "the best type of teacher of modern scientific medicine."[17]

Cardiac diagnosis was entering a new era when Groedel joined his father in practice at Bad Nauheim around 1906. A proponent of physiological pathology, young Groedel appreciated the value of pulse tracings, fluoroscopy, and later electrocardiography as clinical and research tools. In 1909 he invented the first machine for taking serial x-rays; his *Fallkasettenapparat* exposed twenty-five film cassettes in five seconds. A few years later, Groedel published a study of cardiac motion in which he combined electrocardiography with x-ray cinematography. He also invented an improved orthodiagraph, an x-ray apparatus that facilitated the accurate measurement of heart size. After his book on x-ray examination of the heart was published in 1912, he was viewed as a world authority on cardiovascular radiology.[18]

Groedel was among the first clinical scientists to write extensively about electrocardiography. He helped establish the value of recording the electrocardiogram from different sites on the chest wall using "precordial" leads. In 1934 Groedel summarized two decades of research in a book that included his controversial theory that each cardiac ventricle generated an independent or "partial" electrocardiogram. Frank Wilson criticized Groedel's theory of partial electrocardiograms and resented the fact that he ignored the role Americans (especially his own group) had played in inventing precordial leads.[19]

Another of Groedel's main interests, hydrotherapy or balneology, was also controversial. Long a popular health resort because of its hot mineral springs, Bad Nauheim had become a world center for the treatment of cardiac patients by the turn of the century. Like his father and other Nauheim physicians, Groedel advocated hydrotherapy as an adjunctive treatment for cardiovascular disease and actively promoted it in a series of publications.[20] There was no consensus on the value of hydrotherapy in the treatment of heart disease during the first decades of the century. In 1905 William Osler, the English-speaking world's leading internist, advocated the Schott treatment (a combination of warm saline baths and special exercises developed by a family of Nauheim physicians) in cases of "myocardial weakness from whatever cause" and in cases of "neurotic heart."[21]

The following year, Harvard physician Joseph Pratt protested the lack of interest among American physicians in hydrotherapy. He argued that "modern hydrotherapy" was "founded on the solid rock of physiological and pathological knowledge" and challenged medical schools to provide instruction on the subject. Pratt knew that hydrotherapy was "still looked upon with suspicion by our best physicians" because it had "received such scant attention by the medical leaders, and had been accorded such extravagant praise by irregular practitioners."[22] British physician James Mackenzie, whose opinions regarding heart disease carried great weight, was very skeptical of hydrotherapy as a method of treating cardiac patients. Despite mixed reviews, patients flocked to Bad Nauheim: more than 425,000 baths were given to 30,000 people in 1908.[23]

Groedel succeeded his father as head of a popular private hospital and spa at Nauheim after World War I. As the nation recovered and tensions eased, the facility once again became a magnet for wealthy and socially prominent patients from America, Great Britain, and the Continent. Groedel's main link to the United States was his reputation as a pioneer in the study of the physiological aspects of hydrotherapy. During the 1920s, Bernard Baruch, a wealthy financier and philanthropist, became Groedel's most vocal advocate in America. Baruch's father, Simon, was a physician, an expert on hydrotherapy, and a strong proponent of Nauheim baths for heart patients.[24]

Bernard Baruch chaired a state commission to explore the possibility of developing a German-style spa, an "American Nauheim," at Saratoga Springs, New York. The commission arranged for New York Heart Association (NYHA) president John Wyckoff and three other physicians to visit Nauheim and other European spas in 1930. Wyckoff's group concluded, "Although in the past the reputation of the average spa physician has not always been of the highest," after the war "many very able clinicians have taken up work at the health resorts." Especially impressed by Franz Groedel, Wyckoff's group encouraged the New York legislature to create a Nauheim-like spa at Saratoga Springs.[25]

Baruch's commission continued to ask Groedel for advice because this "leading balneologist" gave them the "best testimony" on their questions about scientific hydrotherapy. He came to America several times during the late 1920s and early 1930s to deliver lectures on hydrotherapy, cardiac radiology, and other topics. In 1931 he was formally appointed consultant to the Saratoga Springs Commission. The following year, the AHA's *Bulletin* characterized Groedel as an individual who "has made valuable contributions" to the investigation of the cardiovascular effects of hydrotherapy.[26] Baruch told New York governor Franklin Roosevelt (a proponent of spa therapy) that a dinner honoring the German physician "was attended by many members of the medical profession and some members of the legislature who are evincing real interest in the matter."[27]

Despite the worldwide depression, things seemed to be going well for Groedel. In 1929 a former patient, Los Angeles industrialist William Kerckhoff, left $4 million to create a research facility at Nauheim for the scientific study of hydrotherapy. Groedel (designated lifetime director of the Kerckhoff Institute) spared no expense in designing and equipping the facility. Irish physician P. T. O'Farrell had nothing but praise for it after a 1932 visit. It included clinical and research units, as well as departments of experimental pathology, statistics, and education. O'Farrell was especially impressed by Groedel's x-ray cinematography unit, his electrocardiograph-phonocardiograph machines, and the animal research laboratory. He concluded, "Bad Nauheim has good reason to be proud of her institutes of cardiac research . . . [and her] zealous staff of workers who are advancing the study of cardiology with a thoroughness characteristic of the German people."[28]

By 1932 Groedel had published nearly 300 papers, held an academic appointment as full professor at the University of Frankfurt, had a thriving cardiology practice at Nauheim, and was director of a world-class cardiovascular research institute that was unmatched by anything in the United States. But suddenly everything changed for Groedel because one of his parents was Jewish.

Adolf Hitler's election as chancellor of Germany in 1933 led to laws that institutionalized anti-Semitism and severely restricted opportunities for "non-Aryans." A writer in the *Journal of the American Medical Association* (*JAMA*) explained that Jews, defined by the Nazis as "anyone who had one parent or one grandparent of Jewish race," would be dismissed from committees and boards of German medical societies. Jews could no longer matriculate at German universities.[29] David Krasner points out that the Nazis' "legal devices rendered the study, teaching, and practice of medicine by Jews almost impossible" in Germany.[30] This was Groedel's new reality.

Immigrant physicians and their encounter
with a troubled profession

Many Jews tried to leave Germany as the Nazis fanned the flames of anti-Semitism and severely limited their social and professional opportunities. Tens of thousands of Jewish doctors, scientists, writers, musicians, lawyers, bankers, architects, and others fled Germany if they could. Between 1933 and 1942, about 5,600 refugee physicians arrived in the United States, three-quarters of them Jewish. Almost half of the immigrant physicians were still in New York City by 1942.[31] They could not have come at a worse time. The nation's citizens and their institutions were struggling as a result of the Great Depression, which spared no one. Doctors, hospitals, and medical schools were all affected. In her study of immigrant intellectuals, Laura Fermi observes that "the mere size of the [physician] group constituted an obstacle to its smooth resettlement, for it was inevitable that this inundation of foreigners, in a time of economic crisis when some doctors charged only fifty cents a visit, should alarm the American medical profession."[32]

New York neurologist Bernard Sachs formed an "Emergency Committee in Aid of Displaced Foreign Physicians" in 1933. In a letter published in *JAMA*, the committee's secretary reassured the nation's doctors that its members recognized "the plight in which so many American physicians find themselves at present because of the economic depression." He vowed that the committee would not encourage foreign physicians to emigrate to the United States "for the purpose of engaging in medical practice."[33] But many of the nation's doctors remained skeptical; they feared *any* competition as their incomes fell during the depression.

Leaders of organized medicine heard the concerns, and they responded. American Medical Association (AMA) president Dean Lewis, a Johns Hopkins surgeon, argued that overproduction and improper distribution of doctors justified restricting the number of immigrant physicians.[34] In 1934 Lewis's successor Walter Bierring, an Iowa internist who would chair the American Board of Internal Medicine (ABIM) when it was created two years later, protested, "In many urban communities, there are two doctors for every call and many can barely earn a decent living." Bierring described the physician surplus as "a distinct social economic menace that requires the most earnest consideration on the part of organized medicine."[35] Alfred Cohn, a member of the emergency committee, admitted that "practitioners have all but demanded . . . that newcomers shall not be set up in competition with them."[36]

The AMA intensified its campaign to protect its members from the influx of European doctors. In 1935 its delegates demanded legislative action "to stop entirely the 'selective injustice to the American physician' resulting from the immigration into the United States of foreign physicians." The AMA board of trustees was advised "that it seems practicable to exclude immigrant physicians . . . by making them a selected group against which restrictive legislation would have to be directed."[37]

Physicians were not the only group of refugees challenged by anxious Americans. Some people tried to stem the tide of anti-immigrant feeling and rhetoric. In 1939 theologian Henry Leiper protested the "great hue and cry . . . about the number of German refugees reputedly displacing American workers." Admitting that some people had lost their jobs to immigrants, Leiper rejected the "generalizations as to thousands of Americans displaced by refugee workmen." He thought "rumors about the competition exerted against American professional men by refugees are almost as far-fetched" and noted that the "most common story deals with the German refugee doctor. But one also hears of the dentist, the lawyer and other professionals."[38]

Many institutions were overwhelmed by requests from European doctors and scientists hoping to resume their careers in America. Even if they were willing to hire refugees (and most were not), few institutions had the resources to do so. In 1933 Cohn informed a Nauheim doctor, "The Depression has affected the universities so that their resources are much reduced. They are themselves dismissing their staffs and taking on no new assistants." He explained that most institutions were receiving "numerous applications like yours."[39] In 1933 James Means, chief of medicine at the Massachusetts General Hospital, told the director of the division of medical sciences of the Rockefeller Foundation, "I don't suppose at the present time any hospital or even any university could see its way clear to taking on regular salary an exiled German Jew." Money was a critical factor. If the Rockefeller Foundation could fund such a person as a fellow, Means thought it "might be splendid for all concerned."[40]

When they arrived in the United States, refugee physicians (especially those who had held academic posts in Germany) found that

America's system of social stratification was very different from what they were used to. Their former status as members of an intellectual elite was not automatically transferrable to their new country. Stresses related to this cultural transition were intensified because some Americans were quick to identify personality traits that conformed to stereotypes of German immigrants. In 1937 Cohn learned that several refugees were practicing medicine in Kansas City, but one was having trouble getting a license, despite "much political pressure and influence." Cohn's informant thought this was because "the first few exiles who appeared on the Missouri scene made themselves obnoxious by an attitude of superiority and an I-know-more-than-thou complex."[41] Cohn responded, "What you say about the overbearingness of German physicians, and the refugees are no exception to the rule, is I fear only too true."[42]

Challenging the stereotype, David Edsall, former Harvard Medical School dean and chair of the Boston Committee on Medical Emigrés, claimed that "on the whole" the refugee physicians "are not aggressive or self-assertive. . . . they are generally earnest people, cultured, possess a good command of English and give promise of ready adaptability to the American environment."[43] Economic conditions, a perceived oversupply of doctors, inherent prejudices, and stereotyping contributed to the hostile response many refugee physicians confronted when they arrived in America during the 1930s and 1940s.

Discrimination of all sorts was widespread and generally tolerated at the time. In 1933 former New York governor Alfred Smith editorialized that as America "has become older and wealthier, as bigotry and snobbishness have raised their ugly heads among us, we have tended to forget that this country was built up by immigrants." He urged citizens to welcome the European refugees, many of whom were "people of superior education and great ability."[44] Although immigrant doctors heard and read rhetoric like this, they experienced a very different reality. Most experienced discrimination and were marginalized. A few years later, Harvard bacteriologist Hans Zinsser declared, "To pretend that we do not discriminate against Jews in this country is mere self-deception. Let us be honest. We discriminate in our colleges, in our clubs, and in our hotels."[45] The same was true of medical schools and hospitals.

Franz Groedel was part of the flood of immigrants. His life and career changed suddenly and forever when Hitler's regime instituted restrictive laws targeting non-Aryans early in 1933. Although he had converted to Christianity two decades earlier, that was irrelevant; in Hitler's Germany, Groedel was Jewish. Historian William Coleman describes the plight of physicians like Groedel after Hitler came to power: They "found themselves disastrously placed in the political and social warfare launched in the name of the state by the Nazis."[46] Groedel seized the opportunity provided by his New York contacts to start a new life and rebuild his career in America. Bernard Baruch and Louis Bishop, who had known him since before World War I, were influential patrons. Groedel was among the first German physicians to gain refuge in the United States. Fluent in English, wealthy, and well-connected, he got a medical license and opened an office as a "consulting cardiologist" on Park Avenue in New York in 1934.

Groedel could claim many accomplishments by this time. Possessing a superior education, he had a track record of successes as a clinician, medical scientist, and administrator. Many people, including several American doctors, thought highly of him. In 1934 Alfred Cohn maintained that Groedel "enjoys an excellent reputation both as a physician and as a man."[47] At the same time, John Wyckoff, dean of New York University Medical College and president-elect of the NYHA, characterized him as "one of the great authorities of balneology" and "an investigator of note."[48]

But some New York physicians thought otherwise, especially after Groedel arrived in their city as an immigrant. The occasional visitor was now a refugee practitioner—a competitor. Groedel was no longer viewed as a knowledgeable consultant to the Saratoga Springs Commission who was trying to rationalize hydrotherapy and place it on a solid scientific footing. He was no longer characterized as a pioneer of cardiac radiology who ran a world-class cardiovascular research institute. Several members of the New York medical elite came to view (and to portray) Groedel as an arrogant refugee physician who had made his name as a spa doctor, gaining wealth and influence by pampering the elite of European and American society. Groedel's scientific accomplishments were belittled: balneology was portrayed as inherently unscientific, and his concept of isolating the electrocardiogram from the right and left ventricles was considered false (which it was).[49]

Groedel's friend Louis Bishop Jr. recalled, "The American medical profession which had always been most cordial to the visiting professor from the Continent was not quite so cordial when they discovered that he had finally come here to stay and to set up a practice of his own."[50] Groedel was unable to rebuild the academic and research aspects of his career. Excluded from New York's elite medical institutions, he joined the staff of the Beth David Hospital, a 154-bed institution on West 90th Street. Albert Hyman, the hospital's cardiologist and a founder of the New York Cardiological Society (NYCS), respected Groedel's scientific work and got him the position.[51]

Immigrant physicians lucky enough to obtain medical licenses were unable (with very few exceptions) to get privileges in New York's major teaching hospitals (except for Mt. Sinai), regardless of their former experience, reputation, or academic rank. In 1934 the New York-based Emergency Committee in Aid of Displaced Foreign Physicians compiled a list of refugee doctors with jobs as interns, residents, or outpatient physicians in American hospitals. Of the ninety physicians listed, sixty-nine were placed in New York hospitals, including Mt. Sinai (thirty-five), The Hospital for Joint Diseases (eleven), Beth Israel (eight), Montefiore (six), Brooklyn Jewish (six), Israel Zion (two), and Babies Hospital (one). The remaining doctors got positions in various Jewish hospitals around the nation, including Michael Reese in Chicago, Cedars of Lebanon in Los Angeles, and Jewish Hospital in St. Louis.[52]

Initially, Groedel tried to associate with America's and New York's leading cardiologists. He and Louis Bishop Sr. were among the thirteen physicians present at the 1935 annual AHA business meeting. But the association's leaders (influenced by some prominent members of the NYHA) did not accept Groedel into their circle. A few years later, Jack Marvin admitted that the AHA board, consisting of fifteen members in the early 1930s, "was self-perpetuating. . . . It was a closed body, without the slightest pretense of democracy."[53]

Groedel was frustrated that he was excluded from New York's medical elite. In Europe he had been a prominent member of several medical societies. He was president of the Deutsche Röntgen-Gesellschaft (German Radiological Society) in 1922 and was a founder and executive committee member of the prestigious Deutsche Gesellschaft für Kreislaufforschung (German Society for Cardiovascular Research) six years later.[54] Once in America, Groedel, like most refugee physicians, was marginalized to secondary institutions. Understandably, he became cynical about the attitudes of American doctors—especially the academics with whom he initially identified—toward immigrants.

In 1943 Groedel told a refugee doctor who was having trouble getting a paper published, "You have had the same unfortunate experience we all more or less have, namely, that the American scientific societies as well as the scientific journals are reserved rather for a certain clique of men. . . . This has nothing to do with the merits of your manuscript."[55] The same year Groedel complained to the president of the Medical Society of the County of New York about a derogatory editorial on refugee physicians published in the society's journal.[56] In 1945 Groedel presided over the Rudolf Virchow Medical Society, a half-century-old organization whose members were mainly German immigrants. He told its members, "We are a minority and . . . are not welcome nor accepted by the majority or, even if temporarily accepted . . . may be dropped someday."[57]

Groedel's blunt assessment of the plight of refugee doctors annoyed some members of the establishment. His assertiveness conformed to—and may have fostered—the stereotype of German immigrant physicians (most of whom were Jewish) as arrogant and aggressive. The fact that Groedel had converted to Christianity a quarter-century earlier was irrelevant. The stereotype prevailed. Speaking of the period, sociologist Charles Stember explained that most Americans viewed the terms "refugee" and "Jewish refugee" as "almost synonymous." Summarizing five national public opinion surveys conducted between 1938 and 1940, he found that "about three-fifths of the population consistently thought Jews as a group had objectionable traits." They were perceived as "domineering, aggressive, [and] obstinate."[58]

Although some Americans actively condemned the anti-Semitism that pervaded their society in this era, most were silent. Paul White told Supreme Court Justice Felix Frankfurter in 1940, "I shall certainly do all I can to combat the anti-Semitic feeling which has been rising in the country."[59] But White, like many native-born Americans, was irritated by some of the character traits attributed to the refugee physicians. After telling Alfred Cohn that aggressiveness was sometimes reasonable, he protested, "when carried to the Nth power as on occasion it is, it can be extremely annoying. Examples: two or three recent refugee physicians, names not given."[60]

Groedel's exclusion from the NYHA and AHA elite is partially explained in a letter Paul White wrote in 1955 to Bruno Kisch,

Groedel's long-time friend, fellow immigrant, and ACC cofounder. One problem was White's perception—shared by Howard Sprague and other AHA leaders—of Groedel as a clinician and investigator. White told Kisch, "He did not impress a good many of us in the U.S.A. as being a very scientific worker." But there was more. The Harvard cardiologist explained:

> One other early experience antagonized a good many of the doctors in this country including those in New York whom later on he met when he came there. It was his custom on several summers, I think in the late twenties or early thirties, to send printed cards saying that he would be coming to various parts of the U.S.A. and would be in the vicinity of various cities on certain dates. He announced that he would be able to see our patients in consultation with us. Unhappily, but quite naturally, this irritated most of the physicians who received the announcement since the notices seemed patronizing and in poor taste. I'm sure that such experiences with him constituted one of the most important reasons why, when he came to this country, he was not received with open arms right there in New York. I suspect that that early experience of Groedel's in New York City may have embittered him and stimulated him to establish an organization of his own in competition with the local heart association there in New York and with the mother group, the American Heart Association. At least that is the way the beginning of the American College of Cardiology was viewed by I think almost all of us who did some of the pioneering in the field over here.[61]

Groedel and the New York Cardiological Society: Progenitor of the American College of Cardiology

The attitudes and actions of the leaders of the NYHA and the AHA reflected those of society at large. Although the public health programs of these organizations evidenced the social conscience of their leaders, the physicians who ran them in the 1930s and 1940s shared the biases of other successful professionals of that era. That Groedel and virtually all other recent immigrant physicians were excluded from New York's medical elite and from positions of influence in the NYHA or the AHA (both based in New York) fits with historian Marcia Synnott's view that between the world wars America was characterized by "pervasive social snobbery and professional exclusiveness."[62]

During the 1940s Groedel became active in the NYCS, the city's organization for practitioner cardiologists. After becoming NYCS president in 1949, he convinced several members of the small society to help him create a new national organization for cardiologists. Referring to the AHA's recent transformation into a voluntary health organization, Groedel told them that there was no "representative national cardiological society at present, which restricts its membership to physicians only, who are interested in the advancement of the study of the heart and circulation." He characterized the AHA as "primarily a lay organization with a few interested physicians participating, interested in obtaining public support in building up funds for cooperative research." He complained that the AHA meetings were too crowded "because of the tremendous numbers of interested lay members who pack the auditorium, the halls, the balcony, and even the many rooms which are wired for reception."[63]

Another stimulus for inventing a new national organization was Groedel's desire to publish a cardiology journal. This would allow him and other refugees such as Kisch to publish their research papers in an American periodical devoted to cardiovascular disease. During the 1940s most of Groedel's several dozen clinical and research papers had appeared in *Experimental Medicine and Surgery,* founded in 1943 by Kisch. A prolific medical scientist, Kisch escaped Germany in 1938 with the help of Groedel and Bernard Baruch. He shared Groedel's view that most American medical editors routinely rejected papers written by immigrants. Kisch characterized his new journal as something akin to an "Art Salon des Refusés" where artists whose paintings were shunned by major galleries could display their work.[64]

Groedel thought the NYCS might take over the *American Heart Journal* in 1950 when it was scheduled to be dropped by the AHA. Association leaders had decided to end their half-century relationship with the C. V. Mosby Company because they were frustrated by their inability to influence the journal's editorial policies. They would have complete editorial control over (and would own) *Circulation,* their new official journal.[65] But Groedel's plan was stymied when Mosby was unwilling to turn over the *American Heart Journal* to the NYCS because he wanted a national rather than a local society to sponsor the publication.[66]

But Groedel's ambitions were not limited to gaining control of an American cardiology journal; he wanted to form a new national organization. Several members of the NYCS supported the idea. Albert Hyman, who had coordinated the formation of the NYCS two decades earlier, suggested they form an "American Cardiological Society."[67] Walter Bensel, who had presided over the NYCS for the previous eight years, moved that "the society shall be changed from local to national, with an appropriate change of name to indicate the wider scope of activity. To take effect immediately." The motion passed unanimously, and Groedel appointed committees to select a name and draft a constitution for their new organization. He thanked the members who "had refused to accept the status quo and elected by unanimous vote to meet the future not merely by dreams, but by concerted action, by proper aggressiveness and by inextinguishable enthusiasm."[68]

On 28 November 1949, an organizational meeting of the "American College of Cardiologists" was held in Groedel's Park Avenue office. As president pro tem of the proposed college, he chaired the meeting, during which a draft constitution was presented, revised, and signed by fourteen physicians. The founders next hired a lawyer to "secure the name American College of Cardiologists in the District of Columbia." But Bensel was becoming concerned about the local implications of transforming the NYCS into a national organization. The seventy-nine-year-old physician had helped organize that society two decades earlier and was one of its most loyal and active members. In a move designed to ensure Bensel's continued cooperation, Groedel withdrew his name after being nominated for college president. Thereafter, Bensel was unanimously elected president of the new American College of Cardiologists.[69]

The scheme did not work; Bensel's ambivalence turned into procrastination, which delayed the process of incorporation. Groedel's patience was exhausted. According to Philip Reichert, his confidant and colleague at Beth David Hospital, Groedel decided to act independently, "bypassing the society's lawyer." Groedel hired his own attorney and paid the necessary fees to complete the process of incorporation. The college's charter was granted on 2 December 1949 in Washington, D.C.[70]

Ironically, neither Bensel or Groedel was the first official president of the new college: that position was held by Max Miller, Groedel's lawyer. Miller's son Melvin (also a lawyer) was elected secretary-treasurer. Presumably, lawyers were chosen to head the college during its developmental stage—before the founders could recruit members or hold formal meetings—because legal rather than medical skills were necessary to launch it. Before Groedel could inaugurate a membership campaign, the college had to be established as a legal entity, and the lawyer-president was charged with drafting and filing "such papers as may be required to qualify this corporation to do business in the states of Delaware, Illinois, Ohio, New Jersey, Pennsylvania, Texas, California, Minnesota and Massachusetts." In addition to the lawyers Miller, three German-American physicians (Groedel's friends George Kaufer, Julius Ottenheimer, and Paul Borchardt) made up the original five-member board of trustees.[71]

Four days after the "American College of Cardiology" was incorporated in Washington, the "American College of Cardiologists, Inc." was chartered in Delaware. The legal documents for that organization were signed by eight NYCS members—but not by Bensel, Groedel, or Reichert. Groedel's lawyer later explained that this dual incorporation was designed to block another group with a similar name from getting a charter.[72] Despite the conspicuous absence of Groedel's name on the official documents, he was working behind the scenes in all three societies—the NYCS and the new colleges.

Officially, the two colleges were inactive for a year, until 2 December 1950, when the board of the American College of Cardiology met in New York. During the year, Groedel had met three times with "Dr. X" (an unofficial representative of the AHA) in an attempt to win the association's support. The discussions were unproductive, and Groedel concluded that "the Heart Association does not want to cooperate with us."[73] By this time, the official founding trustees (the Millers, Kaufer, Ottenheimer, and Borchardt) had resigned, and Groedel, Reichert, and Dr. Max Miller (Groedel's assistant, not to be confused with his lawyer of the same name) had replaced them on the board. Groedel was elected president and Reichert secretary of the American College of Cardiology "for the ensuing year." At the same meeting, Groedel announced that he had also succeeded Bensel as president of the Delaware-incorporated American College of Cardiologists, Inc.[74]

Finally, Groedel had orchestrated a merger of his two colleges. The result of these complex legal maneuverings was a single organization whose officers and board of trustees were designated the official founders of the American College of Cardiology.[75] The next step was to recruit members and organize the first formal scientific meeting.

Setting sail into stormy seas: Groedel launches the college

Marginalized by the elite of New York and American cardiology since his arrival in the United States in 1933, Groedel had become increasingly resentful. Although they were diminishing, tensions persisted between native-born and refugee physicians. In 1948 an official of the New York state licensing board characterized immigrant physicians as having an attitude "of arrogance and superiority." He claimed, "The majority has shown no friendliness or thankfulness to be allowed to come to this free and democratic country."[76]

At the same time, the actions of the AHA leaders following World War II caused many American-born cardiologists to feel disenfranchised. When the Scientific Council was created to reassure academic and physiological cardiologists that their needs would be met, many of the nation's heart specialists were excluded. Groedel took advantage of the discontent resonating through the practitioner community as he planned and launched the ACC. In December 1950 the college's newly constituted board authorized the officers "to invite those physicians known to be interested in cardiology and residing in the United States and its possessions, Canada, Central America and South America, to become members of the American College of Cardiology."[77]

Groedel wasted no time. When the first issue of the *American College of Cardiology Bulletin* appeared the following month, he explained that the society was "formed by a group of doctors, specializing in cardiology and angiology, who felt that there was a need for a college in this field whose membership was limited to physicians and scientists interested in the advancement of cardiology and angiology." Groedel told readers that the ACC founders renounced elitism and rejected the concept of limited membership; they wanted a "College" not a "Royal Club, restricted to a small fixed number of 'the chosen'."

But the ACC would not be confined to practitioners. Groedel wanted a college of teachers and scholars: "Each can learn from the other: the practicing physician from the research man, the research man from the practitioner."[78] Groedel, Reichert, Miller, and Kisch (rather than the entire board) formulated the college's policies and outlined its program (Table 4-1). This ambitious agenda emphasized education and included no mention of public health programs.

In January 1951 Groedel sent a letter explaining the college's purpose and a membership application to eighteen hundred doctors

---

TABLE 4-1

Objectives of the American College of Cardiology (1951)

To promote and advance the science of cardiology and angiology

To cooperate with other organizations of practitioners and scientists dealing with the same or related specialties

To arrange for mutual meetings of cardiologists and angiologists with scientists interested in cardiovascular physiology, anatomy, pathology, pharmacology, and allied sciences

To make available free postgraduate training in cardiology and angiology

To create cardiological centers for clinical treatment and research in cardiovascular diseases

To edit and publish a journal, articles, and pamphlets pertaining to cardiology and angiology.

SOURCE: *Am. Coll. Cardiol. Bull.* (February 1951): 1–2.

---

who had indicated in the AMA directory that they had a special interest in heart disease. Reichert recalled that Groedel "started a whirlwind letter-writing project" targeting practitioners. Self-designated cardiologists ("every M.D. in the United States who put a 'C' after his name in the national directory") were invited to apply for membership. Reichert explained that "those who were recognized cardiologists, either by hospital appointment or as diplomats of the national board, were to be admitted as 'Fellows' with the right to use F.A.C.C. after their names."[79]

The AHA leaders were startled by the sudden flurry of activity from the ACC, which had been dormant throughout 1950. Groedel's meetings with Dr. X were unofficial, and there is no mention of the ACC in the AHA minutes or the preserved correspondence of Howard Sprague or Paul White until 1951. Once the college announced its agenda and launched its membership campaign, Sprague, White, Marvin, and other AHA leaders reacted intensely. Just as they had feared competition from the Council for Heart Disease, Inc., five years earlier, they now worried that the ACC would confuse the profession and the public. Most of all, Sprague (now AHA president) and his circle thought it would harm their fund-raising campaign, the engine that drove their ambitious new agenda. The association's leaders worried that their bold initiative would be harmed if the profession did not support local fund-raising programs, a vital source of income. The tension was heightened because they knew many practitioner cardiologists were ambivalent about the AHA's new orientation.

Several AHA leaders were furious when they received Groedel's letter—and they let him know it. Duckett Jones, chair of the AHA's Council on Rheumatic Fever, responded that he was "distressed to hear of the incorporation of your organization for reasons that must be obvious to you." Jones closed with a theme the AHA leaders adopted as they tried to suppress the college: "I personally feel that to develop competing scientific organizations will serve no useful purpose and probably do little good, if not actual harm, to cardiovascular disease knowledge."[80]

But Jones missed the point. Groedel and his circle (along with most of America's practitioner cardiologists) had been excluded from the Scientific Council, and they resented the elitism it symbolized. Moreover, Groedel did not plan to duplicate the AHA's broad mission, which was geared to supporting public health activities and academic research programs. Although the college's agenda was ambitious, its centerpiece was professional education. The AHA mission also included education, but many doctors thought their programs of public education were excessive whereas those for physicians were inadequate. Physiologist Maurice Visscher complained to the AHA executive director in 1950, "We all know that the prime essential in connection with the application of new knowledge in medicine is the education of the physicians." He warned, "the AHA cannot under any circumstances expect to have the support of the medical profession if it tells patients that lay instruction is the primary method by which use can be made of medical advances."[81]

Groedel's response to Jones was polite but firm. Explaining that the AHA's transformation into a voluntary health organization had triggered the college's creation, Groedel declared, "since every specialty has its college, a purely scientific organization of physicians and scientists, we need the college for cardiology in addition to and complementing the Heart Association." Groedel (still an AHA member) reassured Jones, "we have no desire to compete with such a meritorious organization."[82]

In a second letter, Jones reiterated the AHA's main concern—competition: "We cannot afford to dissipate the voluntary efforts, interests and abilities of any individuals, multiple organizations can only be competing."[83] Groedel persisted, no doubt reinforcing the stereotype of German immigrants as overly aggressive. He told Jones he could see no reason for doctors and scientists "to limit themselves rigidly to membership in a single society if they feel that 'multiple organizations' are needed for the furtherance of various facets of their interests."[84]

When the AHA leaders realized they could not dissuade Groedel from recruiting members for his new organization, they tried to discourage Scientific Council members—cardiology's elite—from joining. Jack Marvin, chair of the council, informed its members, "In our best judgment, this new association duplicates the purpose of our own Scientific Council."[85] But the doctors most likely to join the college were *not* the academic and physiological cardiologists; they were the two thousand practitioner cardiologists and internists who belonged to the AHA but were excluded from the council. Groedel told one AHA influential that he formed his organization "only because of the request of a great number of cardiologists who told me that there is a real need for such a college." He closed with a claim that must have worried the AHA leaders: "This need seems to be well substantiated by the number of membership applications we have received."[86]

Expanding his propaganda effort to suppress the ACC, Sprague informed *all* AHA physician members that it was the organization's "considered opinion that the establishment of competing scientific associations serves no useful purpose." He included a copy of the Scientific Council's rules and regulations and urged the doctors "to review article three on membership."[87] But Sprague was out of touch with ordinary practitioners, some of whom were offended by his letter. The pamphlet's wording reinforced their concern that the AHA cared mainly about academicians. It stated that "all who have made significant contributions to the knowledge of cardiovascular diseases are eligible for membership in the Scientific Council, provided they are or become members of the American Heart Association." The doctors attracted to the ACC were practitioners who wanted to learn about and use new knowledge; they were not the researchers who created it.[88]

For Sprague, Groedel and the other founders were not the only problem; America's doctors were partly to blame. He told a New York internist, "It is pretty hard to stem the tide of new societies when there are a lot of men who are willing to pay twenty-five dollars to get some sort of a certificate that they can frame for their offices. It results in a great deal of confusion and the possibility of racketeering."[89] The AHA president protested to one of his former residents that membership in the college "purports to confer some authoritative status on the holder." In Sprague's opinion, the college was "merely offering a lot of

L.M.D.'s, heavily sprinkled with refugees, the privilege of putting up a certificate in their offices to impress the public with the idea that they are heart specialists."[90]

As the college succeeded in attracting members, the AHA leaders became increasingly frustrated—and desperate. Sprague informed a Toledo cardiologist that the ACC was "merely the attempt of a few individuals who have apparently been unable to make the adjustment between the American scene and their refugee status."[91] Sprague's statement reveals his failure to fully comprehend the discontent of many AHA members. It also reflects a stereotype that emerged about the ACC founders, a majority of whom were foreign-born. Sprague's insensitive characterization of them (which became part of an oral tradition among AHA leaders in the 1950s and 1960s) was not entirely groundless. College founder Philip Reichert (American-born and Cornell-trained) told Louis Bishop Jr. in 1960, "The college started under a cloud. Groedel had an arrogant German manner and the founding board was not representative of American cardiology."[92]

Sprague was especially annoyed when some prominent scientists and one of his own trainees joined the college. Groedel had written to 350 medical scientists selected by Kisch. Sprague was shocked when David Bruce Dill (president of the American Physiological Society) and Carl Schmidt (president of the American Society for Pharmacology and Experimental Therapeutics) accepted Groedel's invitation to become vice presidents of the college. In addition, physiological cardiologists Carl Wiggers and Frank Wilson and renowned vascular surgeon Rudolph Matas accepted honorary fellowships. Sprague warned Louis Katz, "You can see that this outfit has hooked in some good men and we cannot disregard it."[93]

Ashton Graybiel, one of White's and Sprague's former residents, also accepted Groedel's offer to become one of the society's three vice presidents. Sprague complained to him, "I note with a good deal of disappointment that you have consented to be a vice president of the American College of Cardiology." The Harvard cardiologist continued, "I wonder if you know how questionable the antecedents of this organization are. . . . The founder of this organization has not been held in the highest repute." He claimed that both Wiggers and Wilson now regretted accepting honorary fellowships in the organization and that Paul White "was steered away from it just in time." Claiming that "some other friends of mine have discovered that they were tying up with a bunch of second and third raters [and] have resigned," Sprague warned, "Frankly, Ash, I think this is [a] racket and you ought not to get burned."[94]

Graybiel told Sprague that while reading his letter indicating that "the college did not have the blessing of the American Heart Association . . . the possibility came to mind that you might not be in the position of an unprejudiced judge or observer."[95] Sprague's terse reply reveals the important role that some NYHA members played in shaping the opinions of the AHA leaders about Groedel and his circle. Obviously annoyed, he told Graybiel, "I can only add that my friends in New York recognizing the College of Cardiology is an outgrowth of the New York Cardiological Society wouldn't touch it with a 10 foot pole."[96]

Louis Katz, AHA president-elect in 1951, was intensely opposed to the ACC. Katz claimed that Irving Wright (a recent NYHA president set to succeed him as AHA president) was his source for information about the college. Wright, an ambitious academic vascular specialist and longtime AHA influential, had told Sprague two years earlier, "As you know, I have a deep sense of loyalty to the American Heart Association."[97] Louis Bishop Jr. later recalled, "My friends in the New York Heart Association and the American Heart Association did not hesitate to tell me to have nothing to do with [the ACC]."[98] Wright was surely one voice that Bishop heard. According to Wright, they were "very, very close friends."[99] Initially Bishop decided not to join the ACC, but he changed his mind two years later.

Long-standing tensions in the New York medical community set the tone for the AHA's response to the college. In 1946 a sociologist studying the American medical profession interviewed a Catholic Italian-American surgeon who practiced in New York. He thought that "medicine in this city is a clique affair. A big part of the clique is a set of old doctors who caught on during the last war." The surgeon described "plenty of discrimination against" Italian and Jewish physicians. Based on his study, the author concluded that a "group of Yankee, East Side specialists occupies a position of pivotal importance." This elite, who "belong to the democracy of first names . . . can designate the appointees" to hospital positions, and by "continually recruiting young men to their offices they maintain the stability of their group through time." He identified "an inner fraternity within the medical profession, a specially segregated group, homogeneous with respect to ethnic and religious affiliations, involved in the lucrative specialized fields of medicine, occupying the dominant hospital posts, and having preferred claims on the good paying clienteles of the city." Wright was part of this elite. The ACC founders, most of whom were foreign-born Jews or Italian Catholics, were not.[100]

Katz denounced the formation of the college and denigrated its founders. This physiological cardiologist had fought hard to convince the AHA's leaders to embark on an ambitious program of research funding. Too much was at stake; the AHA budget (and many academic careers) depended on the support of the medical profession and the patronage of the public and their government. There was no room for a new national organization that might compete for doctors *and* dollars. Speaking of the college, Katz told Sprague that "any move that the American Heart Association can take to accelerate its dissolution would be beneficial."[101]

The fact that Katz was Jewish suggests that the lingering impression (based on an oral tradition) that anti-Semitism was the sole explanation for the hostile response of some AHA and NYHA leaders to the formation of the college is an oversimplification. This is not to say it was not a factor. As I pointed out earlier, anti-Semitism was prevalent in America until after World War II, when it began to diminish. It is safe to assume that the AHA and NYHA leaders reflected the cultural attitudes of their time with respect to issues of religion, race, and gender. During the 1940s American medicine (especially academic medicine) was dominated by white, Anglo-Saxon, Protestant males.[102] When it was created in 1948, the AHA Scientific Council included a few Jewish immigrants such as Richard Bing, Harry Gold, Richard Langendorf, and David Scherf. But they, unlike the ACC founders, were viewed as *scientists*.[103] The NYHA also appointed or elected Jewish physicians such as Ernst Boas, Irving Roth, and Robert Levy to leadership positions in this era.

Philip Reichert's widow, who knew all of the ACC founders, provides an interesting perspective: "As I see it, neither anti-Semitism nor anti-immigrants [*sic*] was the basis for the AHA initial antagonism [toward the ACC]. It was the natural reaction of a prestigious group to thirteen unknowns, men without national reputation who dared to invade the established AHA territory, and with such an academic title. Had those same men been American Protestants, their announcement of an ACC would still have shocked and disturbed the AHA."[104]

When it became apparent to Sprague that the AHA could not suppress the ACC, he devised a new strategy. The association would compete with the college by offering practitioners an alternative to it within the AHA framework. In the spring of 1951 Sprague told the Scientific Council executive committee that many association members had complained about the council's "restricted membership."[105] To counter the "dissatisfaction" among "physicians throughout the country," he suggested that the council be opened to *all* AHA doctors. The committee agreed and changed the bylaws.[106]

Discussing the radical change in philosophy, Sprague admitted that "the immediate burr under the saddle was the American College of Cardiology."[107] As a result of these discussions, the "Section on Clinical Cardiology" was formally established by the AHA board of directors on 5 June 1952. The section's official mission was to "facilitate and encourage investigation, prevention, treatment and education in the field of clinical cardiology." Its unstated objectives were to arrest the growth and limit the impact of the ACC.[108]

Groedel resented the AHA leaders' campaign to ruin his fledgling organization. He told a friend that they "became active sending letters around, mentioning my name, giving up their aristocratic snobbishness and inviting God and the world to join the scientific council of the American Heart Association." Although practitioner cardiologists responded to Groedel's invitation to join the college, his and Kisch's efforts to attract academic and physiological cardiologists were largely unsuccessful. Kisch, a productive scientist in Europe, hoped to attract teachers and researchers to the college. In addition to recruiting practitioners, he appealed to "scientists (anatomists, physiologists, pharmacologists, pathologists) with adequate experience in cardiovascular research" to consider joining.[109]

Two months after 350 applications had been sent to medical scientists, only a dozen had responded. Groedel even offered special incentives to recruit researchers, but to no avail. He had "approached several scientists to become trustees but so far without success."[110] Groedel knew the AHA campaign had been effective in keeping academic physicians and researchers from joining the college: "This propaganda frightens . . . many who hope to get a little bit of the milk from the cow (populace) the American Heart Assn. is milking so cleverly for some years."[111]

As he recruited members, Groedel knew that the tensions resulting from the AHA's transformation into a voluntary health organization were helping his cause. A practitioner cardiologist from Youngstown, Ohio, told Sprague he disliked the new AHA, "a lay organization with some doctors as members." Previously, "every doctor felt he was a part of the association and there was a good 'esprit-de-corps' in the group." This physician also resented the Scientific Council, "composed of a self-chosen, a self-perpetuating few members who dominate, control the organization, and dispense the funds as they see fit. The rest of us are merely on the level of the lay members except for the dues which are $15.50 for physicians and $2.50 for lay members."[112]

Fund-raising was another problem for this doctor and for many AHA members. He complained, "Since the advent of social workers, paid secretaries, and innumerable personnel attending the meetings and others working in many cities over the country, it would appear that the association has become an advertising medium and collecting organization." His local colleagues agreed with him that the AHA's fund-raising campaign was a "racket" like those for polio and cancer. "Perhaps," he told Sprague, "this new organization known as the American College has sensed the situation and wishes to get away from a mixed group. Perhaps many members resent the social organization with butterflies flitting hither and thither; doctors and lay men shouting from the roster of luncheon clubs; newspaper stories about saving a life, and various other misrepresentations of the facts concerning research workers and the profession at large."[113]

These were the main reasons that many doctors were unhappy with the AHA, which they had perceived as *their* organization until its transformation. While Sprague was writing an essay, "What the Heart Association does for the practicing physician," to reassure practitioners the new AHA was relevant to them, Groedel seized the opportunity to achieve his personal goal of inventing a new cardiology organization.[114]

Groedel surely had the courage of his convictions. Academic internist William Bean complained to him, "I can see no useful purpose in the incessant and endless multiplication of such groups [like the ACC], particularly when there are admirable ones in being. I can see no very promising future other than that of a mutual admiration society." Groedel responded sarcastically, "Being a physician you should know how dangerous it is to make a prognosis. Nevertheless, mutual admiration . . . is better than mutual hate and mutual fights about money."[115]

Practitioner cardiologists join the ACC

The AHA's attempts to discourage doctors from joining the ACC were only partially successful. In just a few weeks, hundreds of them joined the college. These practitioners—and nearly all were practitioners—decided to join for different reasons, but there were common themes. The ACC promised them additional opportunities for continuing medical education at a time when they were struggling to keep up with new knowledge, approaches, and procedures. It also offered them the chance to be part of a *professional* society that limited its membership to physicians and medical scientists.

Despite the AHA's campaign to discredit the college and its founders, many doctors saw the new organization as a way to validate their status as self-designated heart specialists. Traditionally, doctors displayed diplomas and certificates indicating their educational attainments to impress (or at least reassure) their patients. A New Jersey practitioner told Groedel, "The certificate of the American Board of Internal Medicine is so attractive and very desirable in the office that I wondered . . . if the men would not also receive some pride of having an attractive certificate for the American College of Cardiology reside on the walls of their offices."[116] Groedel and the ACC founders decided to issue certificates to fellows and associate fellows.

The majority of practitioners who joined the college were designated fellows, and even members could claim to belong to a *college* of *cardiologists*. In addition to a certificate, fellows received a gold key and could use the initials F.A.C.C. For many practitioners, this designation implied achievement and status, like fellowship in the American College of Physicians (F.A.C.P.) or the American College of Surgeons (F.A.C.S.). Some doctors thought the title F.A.C.C. would pay dividends by helping to distinguish them from general practitioners, internists, and other self-designated heart specialists who did not possess the credential.

The AHA leaders were irritated by the college's decision to issue certificates. After all, *they* had cooperated with the ABIM for more than a decade in deciding who was eligible for certification as a cardiovascular specialist, and *they* ultimately determined who achieved this distinction. But certification was beyond the reach of most practitioner cardiologists, since their training and accomplishments did not meet the standards set by the ABIM and AHA. Sprague and other AHA leaders feared that the ACC certificate might undermine the signifi-cance of formal board certification. The relative "value" of board certi-fication and fellowship in a professional society was debated at the time, especially by surgeons, whose hospital privileges might be deter-mined by these credentials.

Each professional society set its own standards for selecting fellows. Initially, the ACC leaders chose not to require board certification in cardiology as a prerequisite for election to fellowship.[117] Johns Hopkins cardiologist Cowles Andrus, one of the AHA elite and an influential member of the National Heart Advisory Council, told Paul White that the college "supplies what some physicians need, or think they need, namely, a formal recognition of the fact they are 'specialists'."[118]

Becoming a fellow of the college did affect the way practitioner cardiologists were perceived by patients and other doctors in their communities. Frank Gouze, the Marshfield Clinic's first formally trained cardiologist, had practiced there for a decade before becoming an F.A.C.C. in 1959. Until he got that credential, Gouze found it somewhat difficult to get consults. Although his cardiology practice was already growing, it increased dramatically after the local newspaper reported his election to fellowship in the college. The fellowship desig-nation "helped a lot to get cases, not only from my own colleagues, but from people who came to the clinic who thought they had heart trouble and wanted to see the cardiologist. . . . Suddenly, I was over-whelmed with a whole bunch of patients." This practitioner cardiolo-gist valued his ACC fellowship because it signaled his colleagues that he was "qualified to take care of the cardiac problems of the day."[119]

Many practitioners joined the ACC because it focused on continu-ing medical education. The postwar era was a dynamic time for many specialties, especially for cardiology and the new field of cardiovascular surgery. Doctors and patients alike were impressed by recent innova-tions in the diagnosis and treatment of heart disease. Cardiac catheter-ization and dramatic new surgical approaches to treat stenotic mitral valves and some forms of congenital heart disease proved there was more to cardiology than electrocardiography. In this context, postgrad-uate courses held special appeal for physicians—internists and general practitioners as well as cardiologists—who cared for patients with heart disease. Even if they did not intend to perform any of the new proce-dures such as cardiac catheterization, doctors were urged to learn about them so they would know when (and where) to refer their patients.

For example, a reviewer recommended André Cournand's 1949 book on cardiac catheterization "to all internists, pediatricians, and cardiologists with interest in congenital heart disease in order that they might become more closely acquainted with a procedure they are or will be advising their patients to undergo."[120]

The ACC held its first scientific meeting in New York on 6 October 1951. Groedel, too ill to participate, died a week later. Bruno Kisch opened the meeting with a brief overview of the history of cardiology and his interpretation of the college's agenda. Two hundred seventy-five doctors attended the Saturday meeting, which was devoted to the pathophysiology, diagnosis, and treatment of coronary artery disease and its complications. Charles Connor, the AHA's medical director, attended the conference and told Sprague that the papers were "well presented and excellent." He was impressed that many of the attendees were from outside New York City, including one from Hawaii and "many" from the Midwest. Connor reported that there was no specific mention of the AHA, "but on several occasions it was emphasized that the college was a physician's organization, made up of physicians, run by physicians, and for physicians." He informed Sprague that the college hoped to recruit "full-time teachers or research men" as fellows "so that they may join with the clinicians and discuss common problems."[121]

Although he had been seriously ill for several weeks, Groedel's death devastated the ACC trustees, especially Kisch and Reichert, with whom he had worked so closely to invent and launch the college. Kisch, who succeeded Groedel as college president, portrayed the death of his "best and most trusted friend" as a tremendous loss that jeopardized the future of the young organization.[122] But Kisch, Reichert, and other founders were determined to proceed. Max Miller, who now chaired the ACC board of trustees, told a California member that "our group will go ahead with the development of the college as outlined by the late Dr. Groedel. The opinions of local, state, or national societies who may oppose us will not enter into our decisions."[123]

The ACC not only survived Groedel's death, it grew rapidly. Meeting certain needs perceived by practitioner cardiologists and internists, the college achieved (in just a few months) the momentum necessary to endure the loss of its ambitious and determined founder. At the first annual meeting in June 1952, Reichert reported that 739 people had joined: 442 fellows, 156 associate fellows, and 141 members.[124] These statistics show that the published requirement that fellows must "have had at least five years of training in the specialty of cardiovascular diseases or angiology" was not enforced. The ACC founders interpreted the term "training" liberally, crediting practice experience if the doctor focused on the care of heart patients. This was similar to the philosophy that the leaders of the American College of Physicians (ACP) adopted in the 1930s when they decided that internists could become board eligible and achieve fellowship status in several ways and in diverse settings.

During the 1940s and early 1950s, many aspiring heart specialists got much of their training while serving as assistants to recognized cardiologists in private offices, clinics, and hospitals following completion of a rotating internship and a one- to three-year internal medicine residency. In 1952 there were only twenty-seven ABIM-approved cardiology training programs, which offered just thirty-six first-year and twenty-five second-year positions. Five years of formal training was simply not an option.[125] Many practitioner cardiologists entered practice as internists and became (partial or full) heart specialists as they concentrated their practice on patients with cardiovascular disease, just as Louis Bishop had done half a century earlier.

Because there were so few formal training programs, the ACC leaders granted fellowship status to an individual who was "regarded as a cardiologist" as a result of "his training and his practice." In June 1951 Jerome Bodlander, president of the college's California chapter, spent several hours discussing ACC policies with Groedel. He learned from the founder that the college would be "very lenient" in enforcing membership requirements "at least until we had an organization which was functional."[126] The membership committee placed emphasis on the candidate's local reputation as a consultant. Successful candidates for fellowship had to be viewed as cardiologists by their peers and "present the highest standards of ethics and dignity."[127]

For years, the college, like many other specialty societies, struggled with its membership criteria. If the requirements were too strict, the society would be small, perhaps so small that the critical mass necessary to sustain it would not be maintained. Lenient fellowship criteria would prompt criticism from other organizations like the AHA, as happened almost immediately. It might also discourage some cardiologists from joining. Bodlander warned Groedel, "a good number of cardiologists are sitting by and watching to see who we accept."[128]

At the beginning, the officers were pragmatic. Reichert explained that Groedel and the trustees agreed that although "examinations and diplomas are important in considering the qualifications of a man for our fellowship, the really important thing is what has he accomplished, and what does he accomplish in his day-to-day practice for his colleagues in the place where he does practice."[129] Reichert's choice of words, implying that men alone were considered for fellowship, reflected contemporary conventions of expression. Although only 5 percent of American physicians were women in 1951, Groedel made it clear that they were welcome to join the college. He told the president of the New York Academy of Medicine that fellowship was open to "professional men and women actively engaged in practice or research relating to diseases of the heart and circulation."[130]

The ACC was off to a good start. It consisted almost exclusively of practitioner cardiologists and internists, however; the AHA leaders had succeeded in discouraging academicians from joining. Much of the college's early success resulted from its members' desire to keep up with the rapidly changing field of cardiology and its leaders' commitment to sponsoring continuing medical education meetings that emphasized clinically relevant topics.

In a 1950 summary of recent innovations in the cardiovascular field, AHA president Tinsley Harrison emphasized the need for innovative approaches to facilitate the prompt transfer of new knowledge from academicians to practitioners. He thought this required "some plan which brings medical research and medical education closer to the profession."[131] Ironically, this was exactly the role Groedel, Kisch, and Reichert envisioned for the ACC. As a result of the creation and rapid expansion of cardiology training programs during the 1950s and 1960s, more heart specialists entered practice—and joined the college. The AHA leaders discovered that their fears that the ACC would harm their fund-raising campaign were exaggerated. The association's income rose steadily from $4 million in 1950 to $24 million in 1959.[132]

At mid-century America's heart specialists sensed that their field was poised for growth. One specialty organization was not enough; academic and practitioner cardiologists had distinct but complementary needs. A reinvented and suddenly wealthy AHA would address the concerns of academics who wanted to create new (or enlarge existing) research and training programs in order to generate knowledge and produce heart specialists. The fledgling ACC would focus on transferring new concepts and innovations in diagnosis and treatment to practitioners. During the second half of the century, there would be much more knowledge and many more cardiologists as the federal government pumped millions of dollars into academic cardiology programs.

CHAPTER 5

Cardiology and the Federal Funding of Academic Medicine

The federal government inaugurated an ambitious campaign of research funding after World War II that energized academic medicine in the United States. This resulted in discoveries and inventions that transformed medicine in general and cardiology in particular.[1] Specialty training also changed dramatically when the government began subsidizing research programs in university medical centers. After the war, dozens of cardiology training programs were created, resulting in a national network of academic units poised to produce new knowledge and heart specialists. Structured subspecialty fellowships replaced informal advanced residencies and apprenticeships. This chapter describes the creation of this academic infrastructure and three innovations that stimulated demand for cardiologists: heart surgery, cardiac catheterization, and the coronary care unit.

American physicians entered the second half of the twentieth century with confidence and optimism. They (and their patients) marveled at what seemed to be an endless series of medical "breakthroughs." Like many other fields, cardiology was changing rapidly. Antibiotics were revolutionizing patient care, and it appeared that syphilitic and rheumatic heart disease might be eliminated.[2] Meanwhile, innovative surgical procedures offered the hope of cure for some types of congenital and acquired heart disease. The introduction of cortisone (which seemed to alter the natural history of rheumatoid arthritis and acute rheumatic fever) signaled "a new era in medical research and practice," according to Surgeon General Leonard Scheele.[3] Antidepressants and antipsychotic drugs promised to reform the treatment and improve the prognosis of the mentally ill. The Salk polio vaccine seemed capable of preventing a disabling and deadly disease.

Some social instruments for delivering care (e.g., tuberculosis sanatoria and rheumatic fever wards) disappeared as a result of these and other innovations. Several therapeutic technologies (e.g., iron lungs) and procedures (e.g., psychosurgery and tuberculosis surgery) became obsolete as well. In the United States, the death rate from infectious diseases continued to decline as a result of improvements in sanitation and nutrition and the advent of antibiotics. This contributed to the growing concern about "degenerative" conditions like heart disease, cancer, stroke, and kidney failure, which caused enormous disability and were responsible for the majority of deaths of Americans over the age of forty-five.[4]

Historian Daniel Fox identifies Alfred Cohn as "the leading advocate" for promoting a "higher priority for chronic illness in health policy" between the world wars. A public-minded scientist concerned about the socioeconomic consequences of chronic (especially cardiac) diseases, he mounted a campaign to "challenge the priorities of medical research." Cohn and others who shared his views (e.g., Surgeon General Thomas Parran and his successor Leonard Scheele) succeeded in drawing the government's attention to chronic illness. Rather than emphasizing public health measures, the reformers embraced the ideology of research. This coalition of academics, influential citizens, and government officials lobbied successfully for federal funding of academic research programs that targeted chronic diseases.[5]

Federal support of collaborative research during World War II accelerated the application "of a large backlog of scientific data accumulated through careful research in the years prior to the war," according to academic internist and government consultant Walter Palmer. Most government-supported wartime medical research would be classified as "applied" rather than "basic."[6] After the war, programs and policies were designed to distribute millions of dollars for medical research though the National Institutes of Health (NIH). Historian Stephen Strickland points out that medical scientists and clinical investigators eagerly applied for these grants because they were "brimming with ideas" but had been chronically underfunded.[7]

Spending on biomedical research grew at a remarkable rate after the war. Between 1945 and 1949, the NIH budget for extramural research increased one hundredfold to $10 million. Institute officials coordinated the process with the help of academic scientists and physicians who formed "study sections" to evaluate research programs and grant requests.[8] The pace of discovery and the practical application of new knowledge accelerated as Washington pumped tens (and later hundreds) of millions of dollars into academic medicine and biomedical research.[9]

Cardiology was only one of several specialties that benefited from the government's decision to endow research and the production of investigators. Most medical schools took advantage of federal grants to augment their research programs, expand their full-time faculty, and train more fellows. They created subspecialty divisions to enhance their ability to attract disease- or organ-specific research funds. Two academics whose careers spanned half a century were amazed at how generous government funding transformed their fields. The NIH had "an enormous influence on the growth and development of research in hematology," according to Maxwell Wintrobe.[10] Joseph Kirsner thinks that the "impact of the NIH on gastroenterology . . . by supporting an increasing number of categorical research projects and postdoctoral training programs via federal funds was . . . profound."[11]

The creation of academic cardiology by Congress

The heart lobby, like the cancer lobby, promised Congress and the American people that liberal research funding would lead to practical advances that would improve productivity and save lives.[12] Beginning in 1947, a succession of American Heart Association (AHA) leaders and National Heart Institute (NHI) directors (with the help of Mary Lasker and several influential politicians) urged Congress to subsidize academic cardiology programs in order to unravel the mysteries of heart disease and train specialists to translate discoveries into better patient care. The politicians listened. By endowing academic cardiology, they created a national resource poised to produce a steady stream of practitioner cardiologists when demand for them rose as a result of innovations in cardiac diagnosis and treatment (e.g., coronary angiography and the coronary care unit), the expansion of hospital insurance, and the invention of a reimbursement program (Medicare) that rewarded doctors who performed procedures.

The nation's small but growing community of academic cardiologists and their institutions benefited from the creation of the NHI in 1948 and its program of extramural grants for researchers, facilities, equipment, and staff. Many medical school deans, hospital administrators, and academic cardiologists became convinced that federal funds for heart research were theirs for the asking. Institute officials traveled extensively to "talk up the grants," according to Franklin Yeager, who headed the Heart Grants Section from 1952 to 1965.[13] By 1949 the NHI's newly created National Advisory Heart Council (NAHC) had received proposals totaling more than $36 million. Within two years, more than two-thirds of the nation's seventy-nine medical schools would apply for or express interest in an NHI construction grant to help them develop a cardiovascular research center.[14] Many institutions requested funds to establish a cardiac catheterization laboratory where physiological cardiologists could study the heart's function for clinical and research purposes.[15]

The NHI offered several other types of grants: "research training grants" for directors of programs that trained investigators; "research fellowships" for postdoctoral students seeking research training; "clinical training grants" for faculty members who trained "people who will utilize the results of research in the form of diagnosis, therapy, and preventive medicine, particularly as academicians"; and "clinical traineeship awards" for individuals seeking this type of specialized cardiology training.[16] In 1949 the NHI awarded nearly $11 million in grants to medical schools, teaching hospitals, and research institutes in 32 states (Table 5-1).

Paul White was executive director of the NAHC from 1948 to 1957. Chaired by NHI director Cassius Van Slyke, the council set the policies and distributed the money that created modern academic cardiology in America. White and Mary Lasker knew that the NAHC was empowered by the huge research and training grants it controlled; the council was shaping academic cardiology.[17] In 1954 they urged former AHA president Irving Wright to accept Surgeon General Scheele's invitation to join the council. Concerned when he hesitated, Lasker cabled, "Implore you to go on heart council as it is largest single fund for heart research and training. Your wisdom and influence vital and can effect faster reduction of death rate." Wright agreed to serve.[18]

In addition to shaping the character of academic cardiology programs, the NAHC indirectly influenced the geographical distribution of practitioner cardiologists, many of whom eventually practiced in or near the cities where they trained. The council decided to support many academic institutions. Members rejected the notion of setting an arbitrary limit on the number of cardiovascular research centers they

TABLE 5-1
National Heart Institute Grants Awarded (1949)

TYPE OF GRANT	$ AMOUNT	NO. GRANTS	NO. INSTITUTIONS	NO. STATES
Research	3,864,307	326	86	32
Construction	6,000,395	24	24	16
Teaching	649,088	46	46	28
Research fellow	184,700	53	53	22
Traineeship	215,000	61	52	26

SOURCE: *National Heart Institute Circular* no. 2 (November 1949): 1–4, Rutstein Papers.

would help create in the nation as a whole or in a single large city like New York, Chicago, or Boston. Although the NAHC funded academic medical centers across the country, it favored institutions with productive research programs, such as those run by physiological cardiologist Louis Katz at Michael Reese Hospital in Chicago. This policy reflected the overall NIH strategy of preferentially supporting successful research institutions. NHI grants, capped at $1 million per institution, would go to those places "where we know the ablest researchers already work and teach."[19]

Research funding was the main concern of the physiological and academic cardiologists who had helped transform the AHA into a voluntary health organization. Most of them supported the heart lobby's efforts to convince Congress that money was the key to conquering cardiovascular disease. Many original members of the AHA's elite Scientific Council were researchers, and several of them now applied to the association and the NHI to fund their investigations. Joseph Wearn, dean at Western Reserve, expressed "hearty approval" for Wiggers's plan to request NHI funding for twelve positions in his cardiovascular research training program. Both men were founding members of the Scientific Council.[20]

In 1948 David Barr, chief of medicine at New York Hospital, urged Irving Wright to apply for federal funds to form a cardiovascular division. Wright told Barr that "large amounts of money are now becoming available for research and training in this field from numerous sources," including the NHI, the AHA, the New York Heart Association (NYHA), and private foundations. He was confident that funds would be "allocated to medical schools throughout the country which are in a position to offer definite plans for the development of research in this field." Wright knew that government grants would also be available to finance construction and help train clinical cardiologists.[21]

Reflecting the broad scope of the National Heart Act, the NHI also awarded grants to encourage medical schools to enhance instruction in cardiovascular disease. By 1949 it had received thirty-seven requests totaling $1.4 million to support teaching activities. Within five years, almost every medical school had identified a "program director" in order to receive a teaching grant. This was an important innovation; each school now had a cardiology representative at the national level. It also created a new network of academic cardiologists. In 1953 eighty-six persons were invited to attend the first annual program directors' meeting which would be chaired by AHA president-elect Cowles Andrus, who also headed the NIH cardiovascular study section charged with reviewing grant requests.[22]

Reflecting the government's commitment to laboratory and clinical investigation, NAHC members often discussed the problem of keeping "well trained and extremely able men interested in research." Their early experience was encouraging. By 1952 the NHI had supported 121 research fellows, three-quarters of whom were still devoting all or part of their time to research.[23] The number of academic cardiologists grew steadily as federal grants created opportunities for them in the nation's medical schools and teaching hospitals. This was part of a larger trend: federal money fueled a dramatic increase in the number of full-time clinical faculty positions in many specialties.

The chairs of departments of medicine in the nation's medical schools were especially eager to recruit cardiologists. In 1952 they were asked to project the number of full-time medical subspecialists they thought their departments would need eighteen years later. The anticipated need for full-time academic cardiologists was impressive; of eighteen types of medical subspecialists, only general internists were in greater demand.[24] The results of the survey accurately predicted the growth of academic cardiology divisions.

At Yale, the number of full-time faculty members in the department of medicine exploded from twelve in 1952 to sixty-five in 1965. Paul Beeson, who chaired the department during those years, attributed this extraordinary increase to the "huge sums of money [that] became available for biomedical research and training after World

TABLE 5-2
American Academic Medicine and Research Grants (1950–1975)

YEAR	MEDICAL SCHOOLS[a]	MEDICAL STUDENTS[a]	FULL-TIME CLINICAL FACULTY[b]	TOTAL NIH GRANTS[c] ($MILLION)	TOTAL NHI BUDGET[d] ($MILLION)
1950	79	26,000	2,000	42	16
1960	86	30,000	7,000	328	62
1970	103	40,000	18,000	873	171
1975	114	56,000	29,000	1,880	328

SOURCES: Adapted from [a]W. G. Rothstein, *American Medical Schools and the Practice of Medicine, a History* (New York: Oxford Univ. Press, 1987), table 11.2, p. 225; [b]ibid., table 11.3, p. 226 (1975 faculty data are actually for 1976); [c]E. Ginzberg and A. B. Dutka, *The Financing of Biomedical Research* (Baltimore: Johns Hopkins Univ. Press, 1989), table 2.2, p. 12; [d]*National Heart, Lung, and Blood Institute Fact Book. Fiscal Year 1993* (Bethesda, Md.: NHLBI, 1994), p. 63.

War II." The "largesse available to academic medicine seemed almost unlimited," according to Beeson, who recalls thinking, "What *else* should I be asking for?"[25] Similarly, the number of full-time physicians in the department of medicine at the University of Rochester increased from eight to one hundred between 1939 and 1974.[26]

These experiences were typical of many research-oriented academic medical centers. According to James Shannon (NIH director from 1955 to 1968), the federal government's annual support of biomedical research increased a thousandfold from $3 million to $3 billion between 1940 and 1975.[27] Between 1950 and 1975, NIH grants increased more than fortyfold, from $42 million to $1,880 million, and the total NHI budget increased by more than twentyfold, from $16 million to $328 million (Table 5-2).

The money disbursed by the AHA and the NHI after 1948 fueled a dramatic expansion in cardiovascular research activity in America. In the inaugural issue of the AHA's new journal *Circulation* (1950), association president Jack Marvin stressed the recent "remarkable" increase in research studies related to circulatory physiology.[28] Three years later, the AHA launched *Circulation Research* to accommodate the continued "acceleration of cardiovascular research."[29] The NHI extramural grant program was successful in stimulating the creation or expansion of academic cardiology programs—a key component of the government's strategy for increasing the nation's research capacity. Many academic medical centers established formal cardiology (and other subspecialty) divisions within their medical departments in order to take advantage of categorical NIH grants.[30]

The politicians who passed the National Heart Act wanted to be sure that their constituents benefited from the discoveries that academicians promised would result from the endowment of research. They thought this goal could best be achieved by producing more and better-trained practitioner cardiologists. The act charged the NHI with providing grants to train clinicians "in the institute and elsewhere in matters relating to the diagnosis, prevention, and treatment of heart diseases."[31] The NAHC discussed various strategies for increasing the number of well-trained cardiologists in 1948. Paul White favored subsidies that would encourage more academic centers to create structured cardiology fellowships. One proposal was to distribute $1 million to "train about 300 men at a salary of $3,000 for unmarried and $3,600 for married men per year." Reflecting the NHI's main agenda—research— in the end, only $75 thousand was appropriated in 1949 to train clinical fellows. Fifty-one heart traineeship grants were awarded in 1950, bringing the total expenditure for this program to a quarter-million dollars.[32] The number of formally trained practitioner cardiologists increased steadily during the 1950s in large part because many trainees supported by "research fellowships" eventually entered practice.

Hans Hecht, an academic cardiologist at the University of Utah, described a typical cardiology training program in 1954. After completing a medical internship and a year of residency (which included some instruction in electrocardiography), the trainee became a cardiology fellow. Much of that year was spent in the catheterization laboratory "as an active member of the team." Following a year of fellowship, the aspiring heart specialist was "a useful member of the unit" and would probably be asked to "try his hand in active independent investigative pursuits." This experience would "test him as a future clinical research worker."[33]

Hecht acknowledged that most cardiology fellows did not pursue academic careers but completed "another year of medical residency" and then took "the 'plunge' into practice." His summary reflects the emphasis cardiology training programs placed on teaching fellows to perform catheterization. Hecht's comments also reveal the tensions between the full-time academic faculty and part-time practitioners. He argued that full-time academic cardiologists were able to teach the "art of medicine" and "bedside diagnostic techniques" as well as or better than the "overburdened and hurried practicing physician."[34]

Other tensions became evident as the government endowed academic medicine. Although there was broad public support for federal
research funding, there was debate about the policies and practices
used to distribute grants. Politicians, scientists, educators, and others
observed (and reacted to) the government's programs of research support.[35] In 1948 Clarence Mills, professor of experimental medicine at
the University of Cincinnati, complained that academic medical centers
in the Northeast got a disproportionate amount of federal funds. He
attributed this in part to the fact that 80 percent of the National
Research Council members (who awarded the grants) were from that
region. Mills argued that "equity and wisdom in the distribution of
federal research funds" would be "of paramount importance in the
years ahead," because the amount of money the NIH planned to
disburse would "dwarf into insignificance previous distributions for
research."[36]

A detailed study of almost thirteen thousand government and
private grants awarded from 1946 through 1951 documented regional
variations in disease-specific research funding. The "Middle East" states
(Delaware, District of Columbia, Maryland, New Jersey, New York,
Pennsylvania, and West Virginia) received more funding than other
regions for most major disease categories. This region included large
cities with research-oriented medical schools like Johns Hopkins and
the University of Pennsylvania. During this five-year period, the leading categories in total medical research funding were cancer ($26 mil-
lion), infectious diseases ($24 million), and cardiovascular diseases
($12 million). By 1951, however, the gap between cardiovascular dis-
eases and the leaders had narrowed considerably as a result of the
reinvention of the AHA and the creation of the NHI.[37]

Sensitive to these concerns, some NAHC members argued that NHI
grants should be distributed geographically in a manner calculated to
prevent criticism. This policy helped create academic cardiology programs focused on research in many medical centers throughout the
country. Other controversies regarding government funding of research concerned principles rather than processes. According to James
Shannon, most "senior academicians in medicine" worried about federal interference with their research programs in the "immediate postwar period."[38] In addition, some scientists resented the trend toward
funding programs and centers instead of individual researchers. The
AHA's career investigator awards attempted to address the concern.[39]

Surgeon General Leonard Scheele raised another issue in a 1951 paper in which he summarized the government's expanding role in medical research and research training. Although he supported those initiatives, Scheele worried that too much emphasis on research might harm teaching activities, "the major function of medical schools." Medical schools were changing rapidly as a result of liberal federal funding. Only a few years earlier, according to Scheele, "the establishment of modest research opportunities for faculty members was a major problem." Now many deans hoped to maintain a teaching program "of reasonable quality in the presence of a large and growing research structure."[40]

This rhetoric reflected the growing realization that a choice had been made. The main business of elite academic medical centers would be the creation of new knowledge. Abundant federal research funding reinforced this vision of academic medicine; dollars drove the agenda. By endowing the full-time clinical faculty system, the NIH embraced a strategy articulated a generation earlier by a small but influential group of academicians who sought to enthrone medical research.[41] In the quarter-century following World War II, James Shannon watched the "elements of education specifically related to the production of physicians become only a small part of the complex activities" of academic medical centers, which came to offer the "whole range of research, education, and service."[42] Most of the new full-time faculty members were subspecialists who defined their careers by their research activities.

Increasingly, medical students on clinical rotations, interns, and residents were taught by these full-time research-oriented subspecialists. Despite growing emphasis on research in academic medical centers, the great majority of students who entered medical school (even research-oriented institutions like Harvard and Johns Hopkins) eventually became practitioners—usually specialists and subspecialists like their mentors. For a generation, most observers believed this served the national interest. The politicians who passed the National Heart Act that created the NHI had been convinced that the nation needed more and better-trained heart specialists.

Today, when 2,633 doctors are enrolled in the nation's 210 cardiology fellowship programs, it is hard to comprehend how few structured training programs existed before the passage of the National Heart Act a half-century ago. In 1947 there were just seven American Medical

Association (AMA)-approved cardiology training programs that offered just fifteen positions. Continuing a pattern that had emerged decades earlier, most aspiring heart specialists gained practical experience by assisting a recognized cardiologist after completing a residency in one of the nation's 318 internal medicine programs.[43] Although internal medicine residents cared for many cardiac patients and may have been exposed to practitioner cardiologists, most of them did not receive focused, intense training in the diagnosis and treatment of heart disease. This would change rapidly after World War II.

The creation of the NHI (and the government funds it disbursed) had an immediate impact: the number of cardiology training programs and fellowship positions quadrupled in just five years. By 1952 twenty-seven training programs were offering sixty-one positions.[44] NHI director Van Slyke, who had survived a heart attack five years earlier, told senators that the clinical training grants were designed to "increase the number of physicians in this country competent to handle the specialized work that the patient with heart disease presents."[45] In 1952 he told House members that there were barely "600 people in this country qualified as heart specialists. . . . if we are going to do the kind of job we should be doing in heart disease, applying what we already know, we just do not have enough people competent in the field."[46]

Year after year, NHI officials urged Congress to appropriate more money for their intramural and extramural programs; the heart lobby was always on hand to reinforce the message. The case for supporting cardiovascular research was compelling. In 1953 Van Slyke told Congress that heart disease was the leading cause of death, claiming more than 750 thousand lives annually. Arguing that almost ten million Americans suffered from cardiovascular diseases, he declared, "Its price is equally staggering in social and economic terms." Choosing his words carefully, Van Slyke told the politicians, "Heart disease exacts an enormous economic cost in medical and institutional care, in military manpower, and in industrial production." What could they do about diseases that cost America 150 million work days each year? Appropriate more funds for research and for the production of more formally trained heart specialists![47]

Van Slyke thought the NHI clinical traineeship program was of "marked benefit to the community . . . because many of the young physicians thus trained go out to assist in teaching capacities in hospitals and medical schools as well as to general or specialized medical practice."[48] Between 1949 and 1952 the NHI funded 148 clinical train-eeships to begin supplying the country with better-trained practitioner cardiologists.[49] This transfer of specialized skills and knowledge from academic centers to community hospitals was part of an organizing principle in health care delivery the Public Health Service described as a "coordinated hospital system." Daniel Fox terms the concept "hierar-chial regionalism."[50]

In addition to sponsoring education and research programs, aca-demic medical centers delivered patient care. Clinical investigation required more than researchers, facilities, equipment, and support staff; patients were a vital part of the equation of discovery and applica-tion. Academic cardiologists knew that most heart patients got their care from general practitioners in the nation's small towns and from internists in larger cities. Although they never envisioned a time when *every* heart patient would be cared for by a cardiologist, they did want local doctors and their patients to think that the most advanced cardiac care was available only at academic medical centers. This would ensure a referral base—a critical source of patients for teaching and research.[51]

In 1949 AHA president Tinsley Harrison told the association's med-ical director, "There can be no first rate patient care without first rate education in intimate association." Moreover, "there can be no first rate education without research."[52] This argument, reflecting an opinion shared by many academic physicians, placed the university medical center in a unique position. It meant that patients could get state-of-the-art care only in academic medical centers. The corollary was that these institutions deserved special financial support for the research and educational activities that were vital to their unique brand of patient care. This interpretation was compatible with the government's new philosophy. The government endowed academic medicine be-cause Congress had been convinced it was the best way to improve the health of Americans. This philosophy went largely unchallenged for a generation.

Liberal government funding of academic medical centers beginning in the late 1940s led to an extraordinary expansion of the nation's capacity for biomedical research. And the funds kept coming. In 1957, less than a decade after the creation of the NHI, the institute's budget exceeded $33 million.[53] That year the AHA budget was $20 million, half of it targeted to support research.[54] The money was having the desired effect: it had already resulted in more investigators, more research, and more well-trained cardiologists. Academic physicians had a powerful incentive to focus their effort on research once promotion and salary decisions came to be based primarily on research productivity, as measured by numbers of publications.[55]

Academic cardiology programs began producing a flood of new knowledge and technology. They also created a sophisticated new type of clinician, one whose outlook and practice reflected the growing influence of the physiological cardiologist tradition. Beginning in the 1950s, most cardiology fellows participated in some research during their training. When they entered practice—as most if them did—their focus shifted to patient care. But they took with them an appreciation of what research was and what it promised in terms of patient care. Although most new cardiological knowledge came from academic centers, significant advances, such as the coronary care unit concept and selective coronary angiography, were introduced by practitioner cardiologists working in other settings. As more nonuniversity hospitals established research and training programs, more institutions and individuals participated in clinical investigation and education.

A growing arsenal to combat heart disease

The way doctors cared for patients changed dramatically in the years following World War II. The era of the general practitioner who cared for the whole family and made house calls was coming rapidly to a close. Norman Rockwell's portrayal of a white-haired, old-time doctor evoked nostalgia, but American medicine was now being framed in terms of science and technology. Empathy was all right, but action was better. Patients wanted cures, and more than ever it seemed that medicine—modern scientific medicine—could deliver them. This transformation took place over decades, but the pace accelerated greatly during the second half of the twentieth century. Doctors could not have anticipated how quickly their profession would change.[56]

A Texas internist declared in 1950, "The contents of the doctor's bag continue to be a most important facet of medical practice." His essay provides an interesting perspective on the physician's armamentarium in this transitional era. The list of "essential" drugs the doctor should carry reflects the frequency of cardiac disease and the number of medicines available to treat acute heart problems in this era. Of the seventeen medications that belonged in every bag, almost half were cardiac drugs.[57] This doctor could not have known how soon the black bag, the "everyday symbol of the medical profession," would be shelved. Increasingly, patients traveled to doctors' offices, clinics, or hospitals, where their complaints were evaluated with an ever-increasing array of sophisticated laboratory tests and technological tools. Continuing a trend that began half a century earlier, diagnosis and treatment of all but the simplest conditions became a complex process requiring a team of professionals and technical assistants.

Between the world wars, many pharmaceutical firms began collaborating with universities, hoping to improve their chances of developing effective and marketable drugs. In addition to cardiac drugs, these joint research programs led to the synthesis of insulin, numerous antibiotics, several cancer chemotherapy agents, and many other medicines.[58] Before World War II, doctors had few effective drugs for treating cardiovascular diseases. For example, there was no safe and effective medical therapy for high blood pressure. Shortly after starting an internal medicine fellowship in 1949, one Mayo Clinic physician was struck by the sudden "explosion in antihypertensive pharmacotherapy." At clinical conferences, he "began to hear names of strange drugs such as veriloid, veratrum viride, hexamethonium, dibenzyline, rauwolfia serpentina, and 1-hydrazinophthalazine."[59] Within fifteen years, several effective antihypertensive drugs were on the market.[60]

Unlike hypertension, "the silent killer," congestive heart failure was a serious condition accompanied by disabling symptoms, notably shortness of breath and limited exercise tolerance. Digitalis, rest, and salt restriction were the mainstay of treatment for congestive heart failure until such effective oral diuretics as chlorothiazide and spironolactone were introduced in the late 1950s. Although mercurial diuretics were available, they were potentially toxic and had to be administered by injection to obtain a significant diuresis. When furosemide was introduced in 1964, practitioners finally had a powerful drug that could be given orally and intravenously to treat severe congestive heart failure.[61]

These new drugs and other innovations had implications for the organization of cardiac care. Most advances fell into one of two major categories, depending on whether any doctor or just a selected few could use them. Any licensed physician could prescribe new medicines, no matter how powerful or potentially dangerous (such as dicoumarol to prevent blood clots, procaine amide to treat cardiac rhythm disturbances, and reserpine to treat hypertension).[62] Likewise, any mid-twentieth-century American doctor who chose to buy laboratory equipment for examining body fluids, an electrocardiograph, or a fluoroscope was free to do so. But most doctors would not have access to new, hospital-based technologies and procedures such as cardiac catheterization and angiography. They had to send their sickest heart patients to cardiologists or other specialists in referral centers for these and other complex diagnostic procedures.[63]

Heart surgery: Helplessness transformed to hopefulness

The introduction of antibiotics, anticoagulants, effective antihypertensive agents, and powerful diuretics affected millions of Americans. But in the minds of many, these advances were overshadowed by the invention of operations for various types of congenital and acquired heart defects during the middle third of the twentieth century. Although risky, especially during the developmental stages, these surgical procedures offered patients the hope of dramatic symptomatic improvement, a longer life, and even *cure*.

In 1937 Vanderbilt surgeon Alfred Blalock presented a paper on the surgical treatment of heart disease he had written with physiological cardiologist Tinsley Harrison. But the operations he described did not involve cutting into the organ itself; such procedures were still a decade away. Blalock focused on surgical removal of the heart's outer covering (pericardiectomy) for constrictive pericarditis.[64] William Witt, professor of clinical medicine at Vanderbilt, was impressed by this curative procedure: "Blalock's paper primarily serves to call our attention to the fact that not all heart cases are merely calls for rest, sedatives, and digitalis." Witt emphasized that some heart patients' symptoms were caused by "purely mechanical situations," and they required "purely, or largely, mechanical means [surgery] for their betterment."[65]

The evolution of cardiovascular surgery is beyond the scope of this book, but it is important to discuss a few innovations that directly stimulated the growth of cardiology. Surgeons had developed operations to treat a few cardiovascular conditions before 1950: patent ductus arteriosus (1939), coarctation of the aorta (1945), tetralogy of Fallot (1945), pulmonic stenosis (1948), and mitral stenosis (1948).[66] Although some surgeons had devised operations to attempt to treat angina pectoris, their procedures did not involve the coronary arteries and they were controversial.[67]

The surgeons who developed these and other heart operations were experimentalists: they were physiological surgeons.[68] As discussed in Chapter 1, physicians began to frame disease in terms of pathological physiology, rather than pathological anatomy, during the late nineteenth century. Surgeons took part in this paradigm shift, especially after asepsis, endotracheal anesthesia, and other technical innovations allowed them to operate in the chest, the cavity containing the body's most dynamic organs. The authors of a 1955 review of the history of thoracic surgery concluded that "the most important reason for the continued advance of surgery during the past fifty years has been the incorporation of physiological thinking and knowledge into surgical practice."[69] Many of the heart operations devised between 1945 and 1955 were performed to correct abnormal physiology by augmenting or restricting blood flow.

American surgeons who made important contributions to the early development of heart surgery included Alfred Blalock (Vanderbilt and Johns Hopkins), John Gibbon Jr. (Jefferson), Charles Bailey (Hahnemann), Dwight Harken (Harvard), John Kirklin (the Mayo Clinic), and Walton Lillehei (Minnesota), among others. Like the physiological cardiologists, they were interested in applied cardiovascular physiology. They used physiology's main experimental approach—vivisection—to develop and test operations for congenital and acquired cardiovascular diseases before trying them in humans.

The surgeons who created heart surgery collaborated with physiologists and physiological cardiologists as they invented operative techniques, surgical equipment, and implantable devices such as artificial heart valves.[70] Speaking of his institution, surgeon Owen Wangensteen wrote, "The intimate cooperation of surgeons and physiologists since the mid-1930s at the University of Minnesota paid off handsomely in the 1950s . . . in lending great impetus to the development of intracardiac surgery."[71] The Mayo Clinic cardiac surgery team of the mid-1950s (responsible for many innovations) included specialists in thoracic surgery, cardiology, pediatric cardiology, physiology, biomedical engineering, and anesthesiology.[72]

The media shared the medical profession's excitement as reports of new operations for heart defects were published and presented at professional society meetings during the 1940s and 1950s. Popular writers knew there was a story in heart surgery—a dramatic new field where heroic doctors worked wonders to save the lives of helpless cardiac patients, many of them children. The media blitz began almost immediately after Alfred Blalock and Helen Taussig reported their "blue-baby operation" for tetralogy of Fallot in 1945, and it caused some problems. Blalock told Taussig that an officer of the American Surgical Association had criticized him "because of the newspaper and magazine publicity in connection with our work." The representative "considered it bad for you and for me and for American medicine." But Blalock thought he and Taussig had "made an honest effort to avoid publicity" and were "the victims of circumstances."[73]

Doctors also wanted to meet Blalock and Taussig and learn about their dramatic new operation. When they were invited to speak at the New York Academy of Medicine in 1946, Blalock initially declined. Taussig urged Blalock to reconsider, because the academy planned to invite Harvard surgeon Robert Gross if he would not participate. She explained, "Bob Gross knows nothing about tetralogies and that is mainly what they want to hear." Taussig predicted a large audience, a "good group of about 500 surgeons and internists." The Johns Hopkins surgeon changed his mind and joined Taussig for the New York program.[74]

Although risky, the Blalock-Taussig operation for tetralogy of Fallot and the Bailey and Harken procedures for mitral stenosis were dramatic and often effective. Physiological surgeons interested in the heart knew that other cardiac defects were potentially correctable, but they faced major obstacles. They needed to see what they were doing inside the heart and have time to do it—no small feat in a beating, blood-filled organ. After a series of animal experiments, John Lewis and Mansur Taufic of the University of Minnesota successfully closed an atrial septal defect in a five-year-old girl in 1952.[75] They had achieved a bloodless field for five and one-half minutes by temporarily blocking the return of blood to the heart. The brain and other vital organs were partially protected from lack of oxygen during this period by moderate total body hypothermia at 79°F.

Although this was the first successful "open-heart" operation (the right atrial wall of the empty heart was incised so the surgeon could see the defect while repairing it), the method used was impractical because circulatory arrest led to brain damage in just a few minutes, even in hypothermic patients. Two years later, the Minnesota group summarized the problem: "The curative surgical attack on a number of intracardiac lesions has been stymied by the lack of a safe and satisfactory method for operating in a leisurely fashion under direct vision within the open chambers of the heart."[76] Even the most adept surgeon faced the absolute obstacle of time.

Several ingenious methods were devised to allow surgeons to operate in a bloodless intracardiac field for a few minutes, but this time was totally inadequate for all but the simplest defects. The solution was obvious: a mechanical substitute for the heart and lungs that would deliver oxygen to the body while the heart was open and empty. Researchers working on the problem faced many complex physiological and technological problems, however. Several groups were developing mechanical oxygenators or "heart-lung machines" at the time, but none were ready for human use. One contemporary observer remarked, "Physiologists and clinical investigators are rivaling the searches of Diogenes for an honest heart-lung machine."[77]

In 1954 Lillehei's group at the University of Minnesota introduced the innovative (and controversial) "controlled cross-circulation" technique in which a human "donor" served as the oxygenator for the patient undergoing open-heart surgery. Reflecting his group's focus on congenital heart disease, the first patients were children and the typical donor was a parent with compatible blood. Lillehei's first patient was a one-year-old boy hospitalized for nine months with heart failure due to a large hole between the heart's two main pumping chambers, a ventricular septal defect. Although the cross-circulation technique gave surgeons more time to operate in a dry field and was hailed as a major advance, it was impractical for widespread use because suitable donors were not always available.[78]

Meanwhile, a few other physiological surgeons started operating on patients using heart-lung machines they were developing. In 1953 John Gibbon Jr. performed the first successful open-heart operation using a heart-lung machine. in which he closed an atrial septal defect in an eighteen-year-old girl. That year, John Kirklin and his associates at the Mayo Clinic began using a Gibbon-type heart-lung machine they had built. In 1955 his team reported the results of eight operations (performed to correct atrial and ventricular septal defects, tetralogy of Fallot, and persistent atrioventricular canal) that proved the feasibility of the approach. Because half of the patients died, some doctors argued against using the heart-lung machine in clinical practice. Kirklin persisted, because there was no alternative if intracardiac repairs were to be attempted, and an initial 50 percent mortality rate was not unusual in this era for new cardiac surgical procedures.[79] As the equipment and techniques were refined, the operative results improved and the skeptics were silenced. The heart lobby could point with pride to these achievements, many of which represented the application of knowledge gained through basic research that was sponsored, at least in part, by the NHI.

Although these new heart operations were risky, many patients (or their parents) chose them because they offered the only hope of a cure. For many, the alternative was certain death. Symptomatic patients with some forms of congenital heart disease or advanced valvular heart disease had a very poor prognosis. In 1955 Dwight Harken reported that 88 percent of thirty-four patients with severe aortic stenosis died within six months after refusing aortic commissurotomy (a procedure for reducing the obstruction to blood flow by separating the fused valve leaflets).[80]

Despite many challenges, cardiovascular surgery was a growing field. Hospital administrators and professional staff members of academic medical centers wanted referring physicians and their patients to view their institution as *the* place to go for state-of-the-art diagnosis and treatment. Intellectual and competitive forces led most academic medical centers (and many other large urban hospitals) to establish heart surgery programs during the 1950s. St. Michael's, a 400-bed hospital in Newark, New Jersey, did so in 1952 because of the "large number of patients looking for relief" at a time when "the few pioneers in the field of cardiovascular surgery were swamped with cases."[81]

There were indeed many patients with rheumatic heart disease. It was estimated that there were 1.5 million Americans with mitral stenosis, half of whom were "severely incapacitated" at the time.[82] In 1953 surgeons at New York's Montefiore Hospital discussed the impact of the recent introduction of operations for this disabling condition. "At the present time, cardiac centers everywhere are under great pressure from physicians and patients alike to offer this type of surgery." Patients with advanced symptoms (usually profound shortness of breath) "ardently want surgery. After years in which their sphere of activity has progressively shrunk, they seize upon this as their last hope."[83] Within a decade, mitral commissurotomy evolved from an experimental operation "performed with hesitancy and reticence" into "a routine procedure," according to one Philadelphia surgical team.[84] Mitral stenosis surgery offered hope, and experience and technical innovations had reduced the operative mortality to less than 10 percent by 1953.[85]

Cardiologists were also optimistic. That year, University of Pennsylvania cardiologist Francis Wood declared that there was a "ten to one chance" that the "surgical treatment of heart disease will be revolutionized" within five years. After recounting the heart operations already being performed in some centers, Wood predicted that by that time "a few surgeons will be regularly *opening* the heart and will be able to do a careful plastic repair on abnormal valves, or even close congenital defects between two sides of the heart *under direct vision.*"[86]

More surgeons began operating on the heart as demand increased. Most of the doctors who organized the nation's first cardiac surgery programs were originally general and thoracic surgeons who had little or no formal training in heart surgery. Their main thoracic surgery experience had come from operating on patients with lung disease, especially tuberculosis.[87] Lillehei warned that "the transition from extracardiac to intracardiac techniques requires not only broad operative experience in thoracic surgery but a dedicated interest [in] . . . the physiology of respiration and circulation, not to mention cardiology." Still, he reassured those "surgeons beset with early failure" who exhibited "traces of doubt" to persist, since "this lack of courage upon their part to carry through can be expected to pass."[88]

Blalock, Lillehei, and other physiological surgeons worked in teaching institutions where they trained academic and practitioner surgeons in addition to performing research and operations. Like their medical colleagues, these academic surgeons benefited from the government's endowment of research and the full-time faculty system after World War II. Much of the research that led to the invention of modern heart surgery was supported (at least partially) by NIH grants. By the mid-1950s several of the nation's academic medical centers were producing (or prepared to produce) cardiac surgeons.

The excitement in this new surgical specialty was evident at the International Symposium on Cardiovascular Surgery held in Detroit in 1955. Sixty participants, including many of the world's heart surgery pioneers, presented papers to an audience of almost five hundred doctors from thirty-five states and twenty-two foreign countries.[89] In an atmosphere charged with self-congratulation and anticipation, London surgeon Russell Brock boasted, "There are several immortals in the field of cardiac surgery here tonight." He thought they deserved credit for stimulating cardiologists to invent new diagnostic techniques; the advent of heart surgery had "caused a true Renaissance in cardiology," which "had seemed to be progressing slowly."[90]

The new field of cardiac surgery was perceived (and portrayed) as glamorous, action-filled, and life-saving. In 1957 *Harper's Magazine* described the heart surgeon as "the Prince of the operating room, the man the big league hospital can't afford to be without."[91] Academic surgeons were training practitioner cardiac surgeons to help meet the growing demand. Two years later Lillehei boasted, "The field of intra-cardiac surgery is a burgeoning specialty."[92]

Cardiologists shared their surgical colleagues' excitement at the advent and promise of open-heart surgery. In 1956 Paul White tried to give an audience of doctors "a little idea of the thrills that have been vouchsafed to those of us who began to practice medicine in the dark days before any success had attended the primitive attempts at the surgical correction of cardiovascular lesions." He reminded them that until recently surgeons never dreamed that it would be possible to "work on the heart itself." White discussed sixteen heart conditions, "almost all of which are now amenable to amelioration if not indeed to complete cure at the hands of the expert surgeon."[93]

Surgeons knew that most patients who underwent heart surgery were improved rather than "cured." Speaking of operations for mitral stenosis in 1955, Charles Bailey admitted "we often merely convert seriously ill or incapacitated cardiac patients into less handicapped cardiac patients." Medical and surgical cardiologists were collaborators rather than competitors. Cardiologists would not lose patients to cardiac surgeons, according to Bailey, because people who had undergone corrective surgery required "careful medical supervision indefinitely."[94]

The earliest cardiac operations were performed on children with relatively simple congenital heart defects and on middle-aged adults with rheumatic mitral stenosis. Before long, however, several physiological surgeons were developing procedures and inventing devices to treat other heart problems. In 1958 the *Saturday Evening Post* told readers that an artificial heart valve designed and implanted in humans by Georgetown University surgeon Charles Hufnagel promised to help "thousands whose lives are restricted by 'aortic insufficiency'—leakage in the body's most vital artery." Pictures showed Hufnagel sewing his plastic ball valve into the descending thoracic aorta. After surgery the patient proclaimed that he was "expecting to live to a ripe old age." The writer, who had watched Hufnagel operate, was impressed by his technique and by ongoing research that promised to produce "not only artificial valves but also whole hearts."[95]

Cardiac catheterization: "A relatively safe procedure"

Cardiac surgery was the stimulus that transformed cardiac catheterization from a physiologist's research tool into a clinician's diagnostic technique. Once surgeons could cure some heart patients, there was a compelling reason to invent and diffuse new diagnostic techniques such as catheterization and angiocardiography. These procedures helped cardiologists and surgeons classify heart defects, quantitate their severity, and plan treatment.[96] They were already spreading from academic medical centers to larger community hospitals in 1949, when two academic radiologists observed that "the development and widespread application of surgical methods for the treatment of congenital heart disease has taken the problem of diagnosis in this condition out of the hands of the academic few and placed it into the hands of the medical profession at large."[97]

Cardiac catheterization and angiocardiography became part of the routine preoperative workup of patients scheduled to undergo heart operations during the 1950s.[98] Initially, cardiac catheterization and angiocardiography were independent procedures. Generally, cardiologists did the cardiac catheterizations and radiologists did the angiocardiograms. In some centers, surgeons actually performed (or helped to perform) these techniques during the 1940s and 1950s. The tests were rarely combined until the late 1950s when cardiologists began to become involved in angiocardiography.[99] As more cardiologists were trained to perform catheterization (and angiocardiography), they assumed primary responsibility for performing these procedures in most institutions. This work pattern conformed to the traditional division of labor, where nonsurgeons focused on diagnosis and medical treatment and surgeons performed operations. The physiological information provided by cardiac catheterization was greatly extended during the 1950s as a result of many technical innovations, including the invention of techniques to catheterize the left side of the heart.[100]

With the advent of diagnostic cardiac catheterization in the mid-1940s (and its widespread diffusion during the next quarter-century), the boundaries between clinical cardiologists and physiological cardiologists became increasingly indistinct. In 1954 pediatric cardiologist William Rashkind declared that "the alert cardiovascular clinician uses continuously the advances and techniques developed by physiologists. Indeed, though both may resent the designation, the cardiologist is a physiologist and has as much to contribute to the basic knowledge of cardiovascular physiology as the physiologist has to contribute to clinical progress."[101]

In 1950 a University of Washington cardiologist described cardiac catheterization as "a relatively safe procedure usually performed on a relatively unsafe patient."[102] Recognizing the inherent risks and expanding use of these new "invasive" diagnostic techniques, the AHA created a cardiac catheterization and angiocardiography committee in 1952. It included physiologists André Cournand (chair) and Earl Wood; physiological cardiologists Richard Bing, Lewis Dexter, Louis Katz, and James Warren; and radiologist Charles Dotter. They thought that cardiac catheterization and angiocardiography could best be performed "in the large centers, using specially trained medical and technical personnel."[103] Despite this advice, competitive forces and patient demand led many hospitals to construct cardiac catheterization laboratories and angiography suites.

Very few cardiac patients were referred to heart specialists before the advent of cardiac surgery; most were cared for by their general practitioner or internist. This was still true in the 1950s, when a review of population studies revealed that 26 percent of people with heart disease or hypertension saw a physician, 2.6 percent were hospitalized, 0.4 percent were referred to another physician, and 0.2 percent were referred to a university medical center for those problems in any given year.[104]

Referrals to heart specialists increased as cardiac patients and their family doctors learned about catheterization and heart surgery, as cardiologists and surgeons introduced these procedures into more hospitals, and as more Americans were covered by hospital insurance. By 1960 the nation had 86 medical schools, almost 7,000 hospitals of all types, 1,307 internal medicine residency programs, 72 cardiology training programs (most partially supported by the NHI), and 110 thoracic surgery residency programs. The American Board of Internal Medicine (ABIM) had certified a total of 653 cardiovascular specialists (some deceased or retired), and the American College of Cardiology (ACC) had 1,987 members (Fig. A4). Total personal health care expenditures

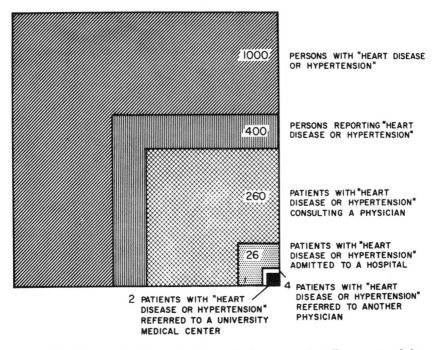

1000 — PERSONS WITH "HEART DISEASE OR HYPERTENSION"

400 — PERSONS REPORTING "HEART DISEASE OR HYPERTENSION"

260 — PATIENTS WITH "HEART DISEASE OR HYPERTENSION" CONSULTING A PHYSICIAN

26 — PATIENTS WITH "HEART DISEASE OR HYPERTENSION" ADMITTED TO A HOSPITAL

4 PATIENTS WITH "HEART DISEASE OR HYPERTENSION" REFERRED TO ANOTHER PHYSICIAN

2 PATIENTS WITH "HEART DISEASE OR HYPERTENSION" REFERRED TO A UNIVERSITY MEDICAL CENTER

Annual distribution of cardiovascular disease in the community (all persons) and the roles of physicians, hospitals, and university medical centers in relation to the overall problems.
SOURCE: K. L. White and M. A. Ibrahim, "The distribution of cardiovascular disease in the community," *Ann. Intern. Med.* 58 (1963): 627–636, fig. 2, p. 634. Reproduced with permission.

were $23.9 billion, and approximately two-thirds of Americans had hospital insurance.[105]

A survey of almost 7,000 American hospitals published in 1961 documented the rapid diffusion of cardiac catheterization and heart surgery from academic medical centers to community hospitals. There were 513 cardiac catheterization laboratories, 649 angiocardiography suites, 327 open-heart surgery programs, and 777 closed-heart surgery programs. There were 303 "fully equipped centers" offering all four procedures—six times the number expected from informal discussions with government and AHA representatives. That year, 30,654 catheterizations, 18,095 angiocardiograms, 8,792 open-heart operations, and 8,448 closed-heart operations were performed. Sixty percent of the diagnostic procedures and 69 percent of the open-heart operations were for congenital heart disease.[106] These statistics underscore how

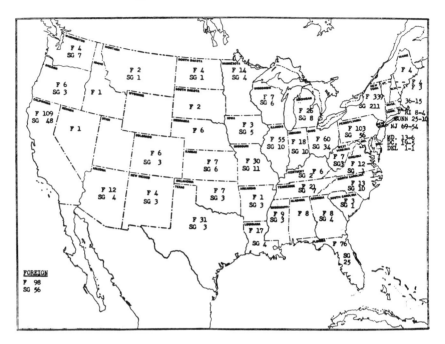

Location of ACC members (1960). F = fellows, SG = subordinate grades.
SOURCE: L. F. Bishop, "President's column," *Am. J. Cardiol.* 6 (1960): 1000–1001, fig. 1, p. 1000.
Reprinted with permission from the *American Journal of Cardiology.*

much cardiology and cardiac surgery would change when two new techniques—selective coronary angiography and saphenous vein coronary artery bypass graft surgery—were introduced shortly after the survey was completed.

During the 1960s the focus of cardiology and cardiac surgery research and practice shifted from congenital and rheumatic heart disease to coronary artery disease. This trend was greatly accelerated by three innovations: selective coronary angiography, the coronary care unit, and coronary artery bypass graft surgery. Coronary angiography had the greatest impact on cardiology practice. Beginning in 1945, a few radiologists and physiological cardiologists attempted to develop techniques to visualize the coronary circulation by injecting contrast material into the proximal aorta. Although a number of ingenious "nonselective" techniques were devised, they did not consistently provide adequate images of the coronary arteries, because most of the contrast material flowed down the aorta rather than into the coronary vessels.[107]

Mason Sones Jr., a cardiologist at the Cleveland Clinic, invented "selective" coronary angiography, a technique essential to contemporary cardiology practice, in 1958. He had been hired eight years earlier to start a cardiac catheterization laboratory at the institution, having learned the technique at the Henry Ford Hospital in Detroit. After arriving in Cleveland, Sones became interested in visualizing the coronary arteries. He accidentally invented selective coronary angiography while performing an angiogram in a twenty-six-year-old man with rheumatic heart disease. The tip of a cardiac catheter (placed just above the aortic valve in preparation for injecting contrast to assess the severity of the patient's aortic insufficiency) migrated inadvertently, and contrast was injected directly into the right coronary artery. Sones was relieved when the patient suffered no ill effects; he expected him to have a cardiac arrest as a result of so much contrast entering the artery.[108]

Sones realized he had discovered a technique for obtaining clear and detailed pictures of the entire coronary circulation. He described the procedure at the 1959 annual meeting of the ACC.[109] Before this, almost no radiologists or cardiologists were interested in coronary arteriography, and those who were used indirect techniques. Radiologist Charles Dotter remarked two years later, "Considering the importance of coronary disease, it is surprising to discover that of the countless thousands of scientific articles published during the last quarter century, little more than three dozen . . . deal with man's attempts to visualize the coronary arteries during life."[110]

Although Sones's oral presentations stimulated some interest in coronary arteriography, few persons attempted it until 1962, when he published a brief paper on his selective technique in the AHA's widely circulated educational leaflet *Modern Concepts of Cardiovascular Disease.* He summarized the technique, the indications for performing it, and the complications observed in more than 1,020 procedures. The most common problem was occlusion of the brachial artery at the site of catheter insertion. The death rate in his series was 0.29 percent.[111] Although concerns about the safety of Sones's technique led one author to declare it unsuitable "for widespread application," some radiologists and many cardiologists began using it in the early 1960s.[112] This technique and other innovations in patient care were placing coronary artery disease at the center of cardiology research and practice. The trend accelerated when the coronary care unit concept was introduced almost simultaneously.

The coronary care unit: Saving "hearts too good to die"

The most feared complication of coronary artery disease was (and is) acute myocardial infarction with its associated risk of sudden death. The coronary care unit was an innovation in heart care designed to reduce this risk. Experience during World War II convinced some doctors that special care units were efficient and saved lives. Surgeons created the first intensive care environment, the postoperative recovery room, during the 1940s.[113] These innovations reflected a conviction that grouping patients with special needs in a place where technological and human resources could be united enhanced efficiency and improved outcomes.

In 1953 the director of the Peter Bent Brigham Hospital (where heart surgeon Dwight Harken worked) explained, "The modern trend is to group related subjects for the convenience of both patients and doctors." He described his hospital's new "custom-built cardiovascular unit for research and treatment." The eight-bed unit and associated cardiac catheterization laboratory cost $343 thousand, 70 percent of which was paid for by an NHI grant. Harken's postoperative cardiac patients were cared for in the unit; it was not created for heart attack patients.[114]

"Special care units" were not only convenient, they saved "lives, nurses and money" according to a surgeon and hospital administrator at the Mary Hitchcock Hospital in Hanover, New Hampshire. Their unit, opened in 1955 for acutely ill medical and surgical patients, was "an unqualified success in its fundamental purpose: better care." Nurses played a key role in assuring a good outcome; they became "expert in the care of acutely ill patients, recognizing complications and changes in condition at their inception, thus permitting rapid treatment." The special care unit had implications for staff morale as well as patient care. It was "a godsend to the harassed staff nurses on duty in the remainder of the hospital."[115]

The advent of specialized patient care technologies such as mechanical respirators, artificial kidneys, and cardiac monitors also encouraged the development and diffusion of intensive care units. An "intensive treatment center" was created at St. Joseph Hospital in Burbank, California, in the late 1950s "for the purpose of bringing together modern methods of applied physiology for the clinical management of patients with renal failure, electrolyte problems, cardio-

vascular failure, and failure of the respiration." The physician who headed this unit declared, "the diagnostic and therapeutic procedures of applied physiology are here to stay" and predicted that patient demand would "call for the establishment of similar units in most leading hospitals."[116]

Innovations in the detection and treatment of disorders of the heartbeat (arrhythmias) introduced into clinical medicine during the 1950s set the stage for the invention of the coronary care unit concept a few years later. Two new technologies gave doctors the power to control some life-threatening arrhythmias. The electric defibrillator, which delivered a shock to the heart, was useful for treating ventricular tachycardia (a serious form of rapid heartbeat) and ventricular fibrillation (a common cause of sudden death). The electronic pacemaker which sped up the heart, was used to treat severe bradycardia (slow heartbeat), which might cause fainting, shock, and death.[117]

Doctors and medical scientists had first attempted to use electricity to treat cardiac arrhythmias in the nineteenth century. During the middle of the twentieth century, several teams of researchers (which often included electrical engineers, physiological cardiologists, physiologists, and surgeons) made discoveries and invented devices that resulted in the clinical introduction of the defibrillator and the pacemaker. Claude Beck, a heart surgeon at Western Reserve University, reported the first successful human resuscitation using a defibrillator in 1947. He delivered the electric shock directly to the patient's heart after opening the chest to compress the organ (direct cardiac massage). Beck's report stimulated great interest in defibrillation as an adjunct to the drug treatment of cardiac arrest.[118]

Surgeons, who had only recently begun operating on the heart, were enthusiastic about the technique, which promised to help save the lives of some patients who suffered cardiac arrest during surgery. This catastrophe occurred during the induction of anesthesia and with many types of operations, not just during cardiac procedures. Anesthesiologists and surgeons viewed cardiac arrest differently from cardiologists. Surgeons saw it as a surgical problem, because 85 percent of cardiac arrests in hospitalized patients occurred in the operating room and treatment required an operative procedure (immediate thoracotomy to expose the heart so it could be manually compressed and defibrillated). Surgical teams rehearsed this dramatic emergency procedure so they could carry it out "with firedrill precision."[119]

Meanwhile, cardiologists (and other nonsurgeons) saw cardiac arrest as a sudden catastrophe that took the lives of many heart attack patients. The first reports of successful resuscitation following acute myocardial infarction were published in 1956. Claude Beck thought heart attack patients could be resuscitated if they suffered cardiac arrest in a hospital and if "supplies and personnel trained in resuscitation methods are available as soon as the patient dies."[120] But even if a doctor was present when the arrest occurred (and they rarely were), few of them were trained to open a patient's chest to perform direct cardiac massage. Most physicians were powerless to treat cardiac arrest until resuscitation techniques that did not require opening the chest were invented.

In 1956 Boston cardiologist Paul Zoll reported that ventricular fibrillation in humans could be terminated by a shock delivered through the chest wall. His transthoracic (closed-chest) defibrillator was a major advance in the treatment of this lethal arrhythmia.[121] Because irreversible brain damage occurs within five minutes following cardiac arrest, immediate treatment is necessary. Zoll knew this and advocated using a "practical monitoring device" in patients thought to be at risk for cardiac arrest "to signal immediately the cessation of circulation" so resuscitation attempts could begin at once.[122]

In 1960 Boston cardiologist Harold Levine speculated that these approaches might be useful outside the operating room. He noted that there were a few reports of successful resuscitations following acute myocardial infarction using emergency thoracotomy and open cardiac massage. Although Levine condemned "indiscriminate thoracotomy in patients who have just died of acute myocardial infarction," he thought that "bloodless efforts at reviving such patients with the external pacemaker or defibrillator" might be practical.[123]

Electrical engineer William Kouwenhoven and his colleagues at Johns Hopkins reported their nonoperative method for treating cardiac arrest in 1960. It consisted of closed-chest cardiac massage, mouth-to-mouth artificial respiration, and transthoracic defibrillation. The following year they reported a success rate of 33 percent when their combined technique was used to resuscitate patients who had suffered a cardiac arrest while convalescing at the Johns Hopkins Hospital following a heart attack.[124] Their innovation almost immediately changed the way doctors treated patients with cardiac arrest. The closed-chest method replaced the "ghastly ritual" of open cardiac mas-

sage and demystified the technique of cardiopulmonary resuscitation. No longer would resuscitation be limited to surgeons and those few nonsurgeons bold enough to wield a scalpel to open a cardiac arrest patient's chest. Eventually, all physicians, and even many laypersons, would be encouraged to learn how to resuscitate people.[125]

Meanwhile, other researchers had developed practical methods for accelerating the heartbeat. Physiologists began using electricity to stimulate the heart in the nineteenth century. New York practitioner cardiologist Albert Hyman invented an "artificial cardiac pacemaker" for clinical use in the early 1930s, but it was impractical because its power supply lasted only a few minutes.[126] In 1950 Canadian surgeons Wilfred Bigelow and John Callaghan reported their research on electrical stimulation of the heart. Zoll extended their studies and two years later described how he had used a transthoracic pacemaker to stimulate the heart of a patient who had developed asystole (cardiac standstill).[127] Later in the decade, other researchers—most notably Lillehei's group in Minneapolis, Seymour Furman's in New York, and Åke Senning's in Sweden—developed reliable permanent cardiac pacemakers for clinical use. These devices revolutionized the treatment of symptomatic bradyarrhythmias.

These inventions led a few doctors to devise new strategies for delivering care to heart attack patients. Some physicians began using a cathode ray oscilloscope or other techniques to monitor the heartbeat continuously once they had tools (the defibrillator, pacemaker, and antiarrhythmic drugs) to treat the arrhythmias these machines detected.[128] In 1961 academic cardiologist Desmond Julian of Edinburgh and practitioner cardiologist Hughes Day of Kansas City, Kansas, independently developed a team approach for promptly resuscitating patients who had a cardiac arrest while hospitalized after a myocardial infarction.[129] The innovation was to group vulnerable patients in a specific hospital setting—an intensive coronary care unit—equipped with cardiology's new electronic tools and staffed with nurses trained to use them (together with mouth-to-mouth respiration and closed-chest cardiac massage).[130]

Julian learned of Kouwenhoven's technique in 1960 from a forty-year-old former Johns Hopkins physician who had a cardiac arrest at Edinburgh's Royal Infirmary following a heart attack. After being resuscitated with open cardiac massage and internal defibrillation, the doctor-patient told Julian about the less invasive closed-chest cardio-

pulmonary resuscitation technique recently developed at Johns Hopkins. In addition to adopting Kouwenhoven's approach, Julian began to monitor heart attack patients in order to recognize life-threatening arrhythmias. In 1961 he reported his experience with continuous electrocardiographic monitoring and closed-chest cardiopulmonary resuscitaton in five heart attack patients who suffered cardiac arrest. Although only one patient survived, Julian thought the survival rate would increase with more experience. He urged hospitals to create "special intensive-care units" equipped with cardiac monitors and a defibrillator, and staffed with nurses trained in the new cardiopulmonary resuscitation techniques.[131]

Hughes Day published the first comprehensive description of the cardiac arrest team concept the following year. He too was impressed with Kouwenhoven's cardiopulmonary resuscitation technique and formed a "code blue emergency" team of trained staff who responded immediately to any cardiac arrest in his hospital. Day created a "crash cart," a large mobile cabinet that included a defibrillator, thoracotomy instruments, intubation and tracheostomy equipment, a temporary pacemaker, and several cardiac drugs (e.g., epinephrine, calcium chloride, quinidine gluconate, procaine amide, and digitoxin). His hospital was creating an "intensive coronary care area" where patients with acute cardiac conditions would be continuously monitored with an "Electrodyne scope-pacemaker." Day closed his article claiming that recent advances made it "imperative that all hospitals should establish programs of cardiac resuscitation."[132]

In 1963 Day reported that his coronary care unit staff treated thirty-two heart attack patients during the first five months the unit was open. All seven patients who had cardiac arrest (during 8,567 hours of monitoring) survived: five responded to the "external automatic pacemaker" and two to external cardiac massage. Day was convinced that the staff rather than the structure of the facility was what mattered. Nurses were taught cardiopulmonary resuscitation and empowered to initiate the procedure. He thought the "greatest impact in an acute coronary care area comes from its constant nursing attention." Day's detailed description of the facility, equipment, staff, procedures, and philosophy provided a model for other institutions seeking to establish a coronary care unit.[133]

Day's comprehensive coronary care unit strategy was revolutionary, but most physicians were unaware of it and others were initially

unimpressed. He published his first two papers on the coronary care unit concept in the *Journal-Lancet,* an obscure American medical periodical, "for the simple reason that I could not get any national journal to publish them."[134] Academic cardiologist Thomas Killip, an early participant in the coronary care unit movement, recalls that "many of us in academic medicine had trouble recognizing the importance of what Hughes Day did." The coronary care unit movement gained momentum once other groups published their experiences with the approach in 1963 and 1964.[135]

Doctors were impressed, if not overwhelmed, by the explosion of new knowledge and innovations in the diagnosis and treatment of heart disease fuelled by federal funding following World War II. As they struggled to keep up, many practitioner cardiologists turned to the ACC for help. The college responded by adapting standard educational techniques and inventing new ones. Although the AHA would play a role in transmitting new knowledge to practitioners, it would focus on funding the research efforts of academicians. Both organizations grew during the 1950s and 1960s as cardiology continued to expand.

CHAPTER 6

~~~~~~~~~~

Continuing Medical Education: A Link between Academics and Practitioners

After the federal government endowed research and the full-time faculty system following World War II, America's scientists and clinical investigators began to produce new knowledge and invent diagnostic techniques and therapeutic strategies at an unprecedented rate. Doctors needed to learn about these innovations if they hoped to incorporate them into their practices. Medical educator Willard Rappleye challenged the profession: "No physician should ever be satisfied with his present knowledge."[1]

Concern about staying current was not new. Harvard's poet-anatomist Oliver Wendell Holmes said in 1878, "We must have the latest thought in its latest expression. . . . Our specialists, more particularly, depend on the month's product, on the yearly crop of new facts, new suggestions, new contrivances, as much as the farmer on the annual yield of his new acres."[2] At the turn of the century, William Osler, North America's leading internist, urged physicians to follow the precept that "education is a life-long process."[3] Practitioners wanted their peers and patients to view them as up-to-date, and as the pace of discovery accelerated, the challenge increased. In 1936 one medical writer warned, "Within five years after graduation, every textbook used in medical school is out of date." He urged doctors to read journals regularly and "attend all medical meetings possible."[4]

Postgraduate education and *continuing medical education* are terms for the various activities doctors undertake to maintain and increase their knowledge of medicine after completing formal residency or fellowship training. During the first half of the twentieth century, brief postgraduate courses served as the path to specialization for many doctors, including most practitioner cardiologists. Residency and fellowship pro-

TABLE 6-1
Major Types of Continuing Medical Education Activities (1955)

Reading: medical books, periodicals, pharmaceutical company literature

Informal personal contacts: colleagues, consultants, pharmacists, pharmaceutical representatives

Local hospital meetings: staff meetings, clinicopathological and radiological conferences, journal club

Medical society meetings: national, state, and local meetings of general or special medical societies

Formal postgraduate courses: sponsored by medical schools, teaching hospitals, and medical societies

SOURCE: Adapted from D. D. Vollan, *Postgraduate Medical Education in the United States* (Chicago: AMA, 1955).

grams ("graduate medical education") expanded as more physicians sought formal specialty training after several certifying boards began to establish standards for credentialing specialists around 1930.[5]

In 1940 Willard Rappleye chaired a commission on medical education that defined postgraduate education as "any type of systematic, supervised educational activity, formal or informal, that helps the physician to keep abreast of the developments in his own field of practice." He emphasized that postgraduate education was not intended to qualify a doctor "to enter a new field."[6] Paths to specialization were being demarcated, and various organizations (primarily the specialty boards) were trying to patrol them.

Demand for continuing medical education surged as American doctors returned to civilian life after World War II. San Francisco doctor Douglas Vollan supervised a study of the subject for the American Medical Association (AMA) in the 1950s (Table 6-1). His detailed, 184-page report provides valuable insight into the status of postgraduate medical education when the American College of Cardiology (ACC) entered the field in 1951.[7] Vollan based his conclusions on a survey of 481 individuals affiliated with 222 institutions (medical schools, hospitals, and societies) and 4,923 practicing physicians. Continuing medical education was portrayed as a means to address a perceived mismatch between the production and utilization of new knowledge. "Medical science has been developing at an increasingly rapid rate in recent years. The problem of bringing this new medical knowledge into the daily practice of medicine has become a matter of great concern."[8]

Each practitioner chose whether and how to participate in continuing medical education activities. In 1949 the dean of the University of Pennsylvania School of Medicine protested that only one-quarter of American physicians "really attempt to keep up." He thought this was due partly to a lack of educational programs, but he also blamed doctors who were "unwilling to spend time and money."[9] Although the expense of travel, tuition, room, and board was an issue, time away from practice was often the major impediment in an era when most doctors were solo, fee-for-service practitioners. However, travel options expanded in the 1950s and 1960s when airplanes replaced trains as the primary mode of long-distance transportation in the United States.

Doctors who made the effort to attend formal continuing medical education programs hoped their patients and colleagues would value the new knowledge, strategies, and techniques they brought back with them. These practitioners did not want "refresher" courses; they wanted to learn something new. Vollan found that 95 percent of the 2,085 courses offered by 160 organizations in 1952 were designed to "expand the physician's understanding of one narrow field or aspect of his own area of practice." Doctors thought programs put on by medical schools and specialty societies were usually better than those sponsored by general medical societies, hospitals, and the federal government.[10] Vollan's study also revealed that "part-time specialists," doctors who "give special attention to one aspect of medicine in which [they] generally [have] limited formal training," were "the largest consumer of [continuing medical education] programs limited to a special field of medicine."[11]

Most of America's practitioner cardiologists were part-time specialists when Vollan commenced his study in 1952, just as the ACC was entering the field of continuing medical education. Cardiology was expanding rapidly, and practitioners were struggling to keep up with new developments in diagnosis and treatment. Doctors at the 1950 American Heart Association (AHA) meeting heard academic cardiologist Edgar Allen predict, "If the conquest of [cardiovascular diseases] continues at the rate which characterized the fifteen years just past, within the lifetime of physicians now living there will be no cardiovascular disease which cannot be prevented or corrected."[12]

The annual meetings of the AMA and the American College of Physicians (ACP) in the mid-1950s included a few papers on cardiovascular subjects,[13] but the annual meetings of the AHA and the ACC

TABLE 6-2
Selected Medical Statistics—United States (1955–1956)

American Medical Association (AMA) membership	160,387[a]
AMA meeting attendance (1956)	27,321[a]
Internal medicine specialists	17,608[b]
Board certified internists (cumulative)	10,710[c]
American College of Physicians (ACP) members	9,200[d]
ACP annual meeting attendance (1956)	6,380[d]
ACP postgraduate program attendance (1956 total)	1,400[d]
Board certified cardiologists (cumulative)	563[c]
American College of Cardiology (ACC) members	1,444[e]
ACC annual meeting attendance (1956)[e]	
Physicians	384
Guests and spouses	70
Exhibitors	97
American Heart Association (AHA)	
Annual meeting attendance (1956)[f]	
Physicians and scientists	1,983
AHA and AHA affiliate staff	312
Hospitals (short-term nonfederal)	5,237[g]
Population (millions)	166[h]
Persons with hospital insurance (percent)	61[h]
U.S. medical school graduates	6,977[i]
National Heart Institute budget ($million)	18.8[j]

SOURCES: [a]American Medical Association Archives, Chicago. [b]R. Stevens, *American Medicine and the Public Interest* (New Haven: Yale Univ. Press, 1971), table 1, p. 162. Full-time specialists in internal medicine in all kinds of practice (in 1955); includes virtually all practitioner cardiologists, since cardiologists were counted as internists at this time. [c]H. R. Kimball [President, ABIM] to W. B. Fye, 26 October 1993. Includes a detailed listing of "Diplomates certified by the ABIM broken down by year." [d]E. C. Rosenow Jr., *History of the American College of Physicians: Executive Perspectives 1959–1977* (Philadelphia: ACP, 1984), p. 11. [e]ACC Archives. [f]"[AHA] Attendance Annual Meetings, 1953 through 1964," AHA file, Nelligan Papers, ACC Archives. [g]R. Stevens, *In Sickness and in Wealth: American Hospitals in the Twentieth Century* (New York: Basic Books, 1989), table 9.2, p. 230. [h]Ibid., table 10.1, p. 259. [i]W. G. Rothstein, *American Medical Schools and the Practice of Medicine, a History* (New York: Oxford Univ. Press, 1987), table 125.1, p. 284. [j]*National Heart, Lung, and Blood Institute Fact Book. Fiscal Year 1993* (Bethesda, Md.: NHLBI, 1994), p. 63.

were dedicated exclusively to cardiovascular medicine and surgery. In addition, because they attracted many heart specialists, the AHA and ACC meetings provided numerous opportunities for networking. Although both annual meetings included scientific and clinical presentations, the AHA emphasized research reports, whereas the ACC scheduled clinical lectures or scientific presentations more relevant to practitioners (Table 6-2).

Physiological, academic, and public health cardiologists were much more likely to attend the AHA sessions, but internists and practitioner cardiologists tended to go to the ACC meetings. AHA leaders such as Louis Katz and Howard Sprague who were hostile to the college had succeeded in discouraging most academics from participating in ACC programs. As a result, during the 1950s most speakers at AHA meetings were academics while those at ACC meetings were practitioners.[14] Whereas ACC meetings were devoted to the continuing medical education of physicians, AHA meetings also scheduled events for nonphysicians, reflecting the association's status as a voluntary health organization. Both practitioners and academics sensed the difference between the reorganized AHA and the new ACC.[15]

Strategies for educating practitioner cardiologists

Tinsley Harrison, immediate past president of the AHA, unintentionally acknowledged in 1950 that the association was not doing all that it could to help practitioners cope with the "rapid progress made in the cardiovascular field during the past decade." The public was "entitled to receive promptly the benefits of new discoveries" in cardiovascular medicine and surgery. Innovative teaching methods were required to facilitate the transfer of new knowledge and techniques from academics to practitioners—from the "ivory tower to the practical care of patients." Harrison thought this could best be accomplished "through some plan which brings medical research and medical education closer to the profession."[16]

The ACC founders created the college to help address this very problem. They envisioned their continuing medical education programs as a link between the academics who created knowledge and the practitioners who used it. In 1951 ACC president Bruno Kisch explained that the organization was formed to "try to give as many physicians as possible . . . instruction in cardiology" by uniting "for the first time in this country the clinician and the scientist in common work and exchange of opinion in our meetings for the best of the suffering cardiac patient."[17]

Franz Groedel, the founder of the ACC, had argued that "every technic recognized as valuable for cardiovascular diagnosis must be exercised by the cardiologist himself as soon as the technic is fully developed and can be applied without undue risk." He predicted that "every cardiologist" would perform cardiac catheterization and angiocardiography when they were refined and made safer.[18] Kisch returned to the diffusion theme during a 1952 ACC symposium on graphic recording techniques. The electrocardiograph had convinced a generation of heart specialists that technology had important implications for them and their patients. Kisch argued that a practitioner must adopt new "methods and instruments" so as to "not lose face and value in the eyes of his colleagues and his newspaper-reading patients." He explained that the college could help practitioners decide whether and when to incorporate new diagnostic tests and treatment strategies in their practices. "Every clinician wants to know whether or not it seems warranted to burden physician and patient with new apparatuses, with new expenses and with new factors in the calculation of diagnosis and prognosis."[19]

Practitioners appreciated the ACC's pragmatic approach to their educational needs. This fact was not lost on AHA leaders who had received complaints from doctors that many papers presented at the association's annual meeting were esoteric and irrelevant. Immediate AHA past president Howard Sprague concluded in 1951 that "it may well be necessary to divide our scientific program into a part which will appeal to practitioners and another for those carrying on more fundamental work."[20] The AHA responded to these concerns by creating the Section (later Council) on Clinical Cardiology (CCC) in 1952. Its official purpose was to "facilitate and encourage investigation, prevention, treatment and education in the field of clinical cardiology."[21] The following year, CCC chair Carleton Ernstene of the Cleveland Clinic "discussed the activities of the American College of Cardiology" with members of his executive committee and "stressed the importance of initiating, as soon as possible, an active program of professional education."[22]

Sprague's plan to hold simultaneous sessions was tried at the 1952 AHA meeting, but many papers not scheduled during the "basic science sessions" might well have been they were so esoteric.[23] Although the AHA meeting reverted to a single session in 1953 and 1954, CCC leaders kept pressing to separate clinical from scientific presentations. Under their plan (inaugurated in 1955), their council would sponsor clinically oriented sessions each day covering "as broadly as possible the entire cardiovascular field." Besides "purely clinical papers," these sessions would include "original papers or selected lectures and panels on investigative developments, if they apply to the clinical field."[24]

By now the AHA had created six councils reflecting the growing intellectual and functional diversity of cardiology: Basic Science, Circulation (formerly the Section for the Study of the Peripheral Circulation), High Blood Pressure Research, Rheumatic Fever and Congenital Heart Disease, Cardiovascular Surgery, and Clinical Cardiology.[25] These councils also wanted space on the program, so it was decided that the CCC would plan a session for practitioners that would run simultaneously with the research-oriented programs sponsored by other councils. The non-CCC sessions would consist of "more esoteric" talks targeted at "investigators and those clinicians who are interested in the details and technical aspects of current investigations." Traditionally, many AHA presentations summarized the results of basic and clinical research. But the CCC executive committee thought "the content of such papers, although exceedingly important, is often of very limited interest to the practicing physicians who want practical clinical education."[26]

During the 1950s, the ACC held two national scientific meetings each year: an "annual" spring meeting and an "interim" fall meeting. Both consisted of a single session with no concurrent presentations. College leaders selected two or three major topics for each meeting and asked speakers to present papers that emphasized recent developments of interest to clinicians. The focus was on new knowledge, diagnostic tests, and operative procedures. Nearly a third of each meeting was devoted to cardiovascular surgery. Many pioneers of this field presented papers or participated in panel discussions at college meetings during the decade.[27]

In 1955 ACC president Walter Priest explained that he liked the meetings because they didn't include "a 'rehash' of already published literature . . . [or] a parade of 15-minute papers on a vast array of subjects." He applauded the college's approach, which prevented "cerebral confusion and gluteal numbness."[28] Several innovations were introduced at college meetings during the 1950s: scientific exhibits distinct from industry exhibits (1953); simultaneous "fireside conferences" that allowed small groups of doctors to interact with one or more mentors (1955); scheduled visits to cardiac clinics, local hospitals, and catheterization laboratories (1956); and medical motion pictures during the luncheon recess (1958).[29]

Many Americans—doctors, heart patients, and healthy citizens— found themselves thinking about cardiovascular disease after President Dwight Eisenhower suffered a heart attack in 1955. When the ACC sponsored a one-day symposium on acute myocardial infarction at the Waldorf-Astoria Hotel two years later, the response was overwhelming. College secretary-treasurer Philip Reichert boasted that "the huge attendance" at this regional meeting (more than 2,500 physicians participated) "highlighted the importance and success of the educational program of the college and helped to increase its prestige."[30] When the ACC held its annual scientific sessions in Washington three months later, Eisenhower (who had survived both his heart attack and a reelection campaign) cabled, "As an association of physicians, you have successfully brought dedicated talent and training to the problem of heart disease. The achievements in this area of medicine are a credit to you and an inspiration to all who seek to strengthen the health of the nation."[31]

The financial success of the New York symposium, underwritten by Lederle Laboratories (a pharmaceutical firm), contrasted sharply with earlier college meetings. Because the ACC did not raise funds from the public, it was dependent on dues and income from exhibits at its meetings and advertisements in its journal. Money was a constant problem for the ACC during its earliest years, as it had been for the AHA before it became a voluntary health organization in 1948. When Reichert told the trustees in 1960 that the annual meeting realized a "tremendous profit" of $9 thousand, they applauded.[32] He knew that "the business of education, like any other business, runs on money."[33]

The ACC and the AHA controlled two income-producing educational vehicles (meetings and journals). Both venues offered pharmaceutical companies, equipment manufacturers, and publishers an opportunity to display and advertise their products. Reichert thought pharmaceutical advertising was a useful educational tool. Following World War II, he worked part-time for the J. Walter Thompson advertising agency and the Hoffmann-La Roche drug company to develop pharmaceutical advertisements.[34] Reichert encouraged firms to participate in both ACC venues by linking them: journal advertisers were given priority when exhibit space was assigned.[35]

Companies were willing to pay competitive rates to get advertising or exhibit space to reach doctors who could prescribe their products and encourage their hospital administrators to purchase drugs and equipment. For doctors, the ACC and AHA exhibits were merchandise marts where they could compare the latest medical equipment, learn about (and receive samples of) new drugs, and review current text-

books. Heart specialists, ACC and AHA leaders, and industry representatives were pleased as the exhibits grew steadily over the years.[36]
Reichert told the trustees in 1960 that the pharmaceutical companies
"have come to our support and are very anxious to get into the
convention."[37]

However, a few voices expressed concern about the money that
pharmaceutical companies spent on promotion. Charles May, a pediatrician at Columbia University, warned in 1961 that the "traditional
independence of physicians and the welfare of the public are being
threatened by the new vogue among drug manufacturers to promote
their products by assuming an aggressive role in the 'education' of
doctors." He questioned the wisdom of the profession's becoming
"greatly dependent upon pharmaceutical manufacturers for support of
scientific journals and medical societies." Claiming that they spent $750
million on promotion (including $125 million on journal ads and direct
mail) in 1959, May urged "ethical drug firms" to "reconsider the
appropriateness of attempting to influence physicians by subtle infiltra-
tion into the educational process."[38]

Just as federal funds fueled research and academic medicine in the
United States, grants from industry stimulated the continuing medical
education field. During the second half of the twentieth century, many
medical organizations (the AHA and ACC included) became dependent
on financial support from drug companies and other industries to
maintain their educational programs and develop new ones. Although
guidelines had been developed to assure the profession and the public
that this funding was acquired and used in an ethical manner, complaints were voiced periodically.[39]

One of the original "objects" of the ACC, outlined in its constitution, was "to make available free postgraduate training in cardiology
and angiology."[40] This goal became impractical as the trustees sought to
expand the number and scope of their continuing medical education
offerings and attract academic cardiologists as speakers while keeping
their dues in line with other professional organizations. The college
began to charge tuition fees for its continuing medical education programs in 1961.[41] Costs escalated when the ACC began to cover the
expenses of some speakers during the late 1950s. John LaDue, a New
York practitioner cardiologist who chaired the ACC program committee, explained in 1959 that the college had begun to reimburse speakers
"in full-time academic work who couldn't afford otherwise to attend
the meeting and instruct us."[42]

Academic cardiologist Eugene Braunwald was chief of the cardiology branch at the National Heart Institute (NHI) when he presented a paper at the 1963 ACC annual meeting. "I recall . . . their paying my way to come from Bethesda to Los Angeles to present a fifteen minute abstract on congenital aortic stenosis." But the college was still trying to overcome the AHA's informal sanction against academics participating in its programs. Braunwald recalls that the college "was considered a very, very, very poor relative of the American Heart Association" at the time. "I mean, it was not really considered a mainstream group . . . in the first few years." In this context, the college used financial incentives to encourage academics to participate in its meetings. Braunwald explained, "It was a seller's market as far as the college was concerned. But how the situation has changed over the years, how it has changed."[43]

ACC past president George Meneely, an academic cardiologist at Vanderbilt, supported this practice. In 1959 he told the trustees, "No one ever goes anywhere and gives an address for nothing. They do it either for the personal prestige involved, or they do it for the likelihood of it enhancing their professional reputation, or they do it for the likelihood that some increase in patient referral may generate, or something of that sort." He continued, "For those of us who are in full-time academic work, I can tell you very candidly that it is perfectly possible to be honored into a starvation situation. Even if your expenses to a meeting are paid, you still lose money." Meneely protested, "I think it is grossly unfair for a solvent organization of clinicians to take advantage of people" by inviting them to speak "and then farm them off with the concept that this is such an honor that they ought to pay their own way."[44]

More income was necessary if the ACC's educational programs were to grow in quality and number. At one time, past president Robert Glover, a heart surgeon, wondered whether it was realistic to expect that college meetings "should pay for themselves entirely from what we get from the technical exhibits and things of that sort."[45] This seemed to be a reasonable goal; it meant that other worthwhile money-losing continuing medical education programs could be continued. Reichert told the trustees in 1962 that more companies participated in the college's annual meeting since it was "now rated as a 'hot' convention by the Medical Exhibitors Association." In contrast to the early years, "where we regularly lost money" despite "good attendance," the income from sixty exhibitors at the 1961 meeting yielded a $10 thousand profit.[46]

Noting an "upsurge of interest in postgraduate medical education," a British academic physician analyzed American continuing medical education efforts in 1963. He criticized the standard medical convention, which usually consisted of a "series of lectures by experts whose subjects are the narrow fields to which they devote their lives." With typical British candor, he protested, "The whole arrangement is more that of a prima-donna and her theatre audience than a teacher-learner relationship." Complaining that the "audience is purely passive," he acknowledged that American medical educators were becoming "increasingly aware of the importance of learning as opposed to teaching, and are striving for more participation by the audience . . . as opposed to 'sitting and listening.'"[47]

The college recognized these concerns and adapted the structure of its annual meeting accordingly. The popular evening fireside conferences begun in 1955 focused on the management of common cardiac problems and encouraged active interchange between "experts" and practitioners. Sixty fireside conferences (thirty held twice) were scheduled during the 1962 meeting. Demand for this small-group format led the program committee in 1963 to offer participants four simultaneous "luncheon panels" each day in addition to the fireside conferences. By this time the ACC annual meeting had expanded to six formal sessions over three days.[48]

The college first offered simultaneous scientific sessions in 1966. This decision reflected growing pressure to put more papers on the program, the participation of more scientists and academic cardiologists in the meetings, and increasing specialization within cardiology. Some attendees were more interested in research, whereas others wanted to hear clinical topics. Acknowledging the increasing involvement of researchers in the college and its meetings, two evening "basic science forums" were added to the program. Meanwhile, practitioners were becoming more specialized in their clinical interests and activities. It was no longer realistic to expect all attendees to listen to a half-day symposium on congenital heart disease or operative techniques, for example. Most doctors wanted to learn about new procedures they could perform and medicines they could prescribe.

The ACC in print: New cardiology journals

Although the ACC's main mission was education, college leaders knew that only a fraction of the nation's heart specialists and internists attended their annual meeting. They decided to use another standard educational vehicle—the medical journal—to reach a larger audience. There were actually two goals: to disseminate knowledge and to publicize the college. Periodicals have long been the main format for diffusing innovations. Writing a century ago, medical administrator and bibliographer John Shaw Billings explained that since 1800 journals had been the "principal means of recording and communicating the observations and ideas of those engaged in the practice of medicine."[49]

America's cardiology journals followed an established pattern. New specialty societies often create periodicals to print papers written by (or of interest to) their members. These official journals usually include other items relevant to the field (e.g., meeting announcements and book reviews). Between 1925 and 1950, the AHA's official journal, the *American Heart Journal* (AHJ), was the only periodical devoted to cardiology published in the United States. Association leaders set the stage for the appearance of additional cardiology journals in 1950 when they ended their sponsorship of the AHJ and inaugurated *Circulation* (which the AHA owned) because they no longer wanted to share the profits with the publisher, C. V. Mosby.[50]

ACC founder Franz Groedel knew about the AHA's plans. In 1949, shortly before the college was incorporated, he and other members of the New York Cardiological Society (NYCS) discussed the possibility of assuming editorial control of the AHJ when the heart association dropped it. Mosby was not interested in having the NYCS sponsor the AHJ and invited Canadian academic cardiologist Jonathan Meakins (one of Thomas Lewis's earliest North American pupils) to form a new editorial board and continue the AHJ as an independent journal.[51] Meakins and Paul White had been friends from the time they worked together in Lewis's laboratory before World War I. White, an AHA loyalist, expressed no concern about possible competition between the AHJ and *Circulation*. He thought that with "proper editorial guidance" the AHJ could "serve a useful purpose in helping to keep abreast of the increasing amount of cardiovascular work that is going on."[52] Meakins agreed and told AHJ readers that progress in cardiology "both in volume and in scope, has outstripped the capacity of one journal."[53]

When it appeared in 1950, *Circulation* reflected the AHA's new commitment to research. Its title acknowledged the influence of Irving Wright, Irvine Page, and other association leaders who were interested in the cardiovascular system, not just the heart. Still, most practitioners preferred clinically relevant articles to research reports. In 1951 a New

Hampshire practitioner cardiologist complained to AHA president Howard Sprague that *Circulation* was "rather insignificant in regard to carrying on my practice. There are very few articles in it which can be used to improve the treatment of my patients or to aid in the diagnosis." This Harvard Medical School graduate explained that he was "interested in diagnosis and treatment rather than in vague scientific experiments on dogs."[54]

Speaking for other disgruntled practitioners, he warned Sprague, "I know many men who are dropping the journal for the simple reason that it does not get down to earth and give them help in their daily practice."[55] Sprague was stung by the criticism. A few weeks later, he told Tulane cardiologist George Burch that some doctors were dropping the journal because they thought it was too "high-brow." Sprague thought the AHA should create a separate research journal and make *Circulation* more clinically relevant so practitioners would continue to subscribe.[56]

When they formed the ACC, Groedel and several other NYCS members renewed their commitment to publish a journal. The ACC founders agreed that "the publication of an official journal of the society and the widened scope of its activities may be considered mutually interdependent." This journal would be the "voice" of their new college.[57] The ACC constitution included a pledge "to edit and publish a journal . . . pertaining to cardiology and angiology."[58] *Transactions of the American College of Cardiology,* an annual volume that included most of the papers delivered at the college's national meetings, was published between 1951 and 1957. Its editor, Bruno Kisch (who succeeded Groedel as college president), had already founded two journals: *Cardiologica* (1937), when he was still in Europe, and *Experimental Medicine and Surgery* (1943), shortly after he arrived in America. Kisch sent one hundred copies of the *Transactions* "to prominent journals for review" in order to "bring added publicity to the college." Meanwhile, he wanted to mail the ACC's monthly newsletter, *American College of Cardiology Bulletin* (January 1951) to five thousand doctors to acquaint them with the college.[59]

Although the *Transactions* evidenced the ACC's educational mission, it was not a traditional journal. For this reason, the trustees again explored the possibility of acquiring the AHJ, but Mosby declined.[60] College president-elect Simon Dack, a cardiologist at New York's Mt. Sinai Hospital, succeeded Kisch as editor of *Transactions* in 1955. When he became president, Dack appointed a committee to help the ACC inaugurate a traditional journal to replace *Transactions*. College members learned in 1957 that they could look forward to receiving the *American Journal of Cardiology* (AJC) the following year.

Dack, who would edit the new journal, informed them that it would be "devoted to clinical cardiology" and "directed primarily to the practicing cardiologist and internist." Aware of criticisms that had been voiced about *Circulation,* he explained that clinical research papers would be considered, but "abstruse scientific material" would be rejected. Dack encouraged members to submit manuscripts, because he believed there was "sufficient scientific talent within the college to produce papers and clinical reports of high caliber."[61] He assured prospective authors that the editorial process would be unbiased and that decisions would be made on the basis of a manuscript's content and quality rather than its source.[62] A Connecticut doctor applauded the college's decision to publish a journal "dedicated to clinical cardiology. How badly we clinicians need it!"[63] Potential advertisers were told that AJC would have a monthly circulation guarantee of 5,500 and represent "a new approach to the needs of the cardiologist, internist and general physician by presenting clinical cardiology in an easy, readable form."[64]

Ignacio Chávez, Mexico's foremost cardiologist, wrote the lead article for the first issue of AJC, a historical survey of the development of cardiovascular diagnostic techniques. Other prominent authors contributed to the inaugural issue: Samuel Levine on angina pectoris; Myron Prinzmetal on myocardial infarction; Claude Beck on the surgical management of coronary artery disease; and Charles Bailey on the operative treatment of mitral stenosis. The journal was a success—there was room for three heart journals. By 1960 *Circulation* had 8,800 subscribers, the *American Journal of Cardiology* 6,000, and the *American Heart Journal* 5,882.[65]

In 1964 Reichert told the AJC publisher, "Beginning with nothing more than an idea, my best wishes, Simon Dack's devotion, and your own sweat, a property was built up that is tops in its field." The income (split with the publisher) which the journal's ads provided was welcome, since it allowed the college to expand its educational programs. Reichert joked that even the Internal Revenue Department (as it was then called) had "awakened to the fact that the advertising pays the bills."[66] The journal diffused more than cardiological knowledge; it spread the college's name. In 1965 Reichert claimed that the journal "has put our name in a prominent spot in places where the college, without the journal, would hardly be known."[67]

Another publishing project demonstrated the breadth of the ACC's educational agenda. President-elect Ashton Graybiel had proposed in 1953 that the college produce a comprehensive encyclopedia of cardiology.[68] Two years later, Aldo Luisada, an Italian immigrant who directed the cardiology division at the Chicago Medical School, was selected to edit the encyclopedia. Published between 1959 and 1962, the five-volume, twenty-three-pound work entitled *Cardiology: An Encyclopedia of the Cardiovascular System* included contributions by more than 250 authors.[69] Dack thought the encyclopedia was the "best and most definitive reference work on cardiovascular diseases in the English language."[70]

New educational programs narrow the gap between town and gown

A few medical schools had begun to sponsor short postgraduate cardiology programs in the 1920s. The ACP began to offer two-week courses on cardiology (and other topics) in conjunction with selected medical schools in 1938.[71] This type of program became increasingly popular after World War II. In 1955 Joseph Wolffe, an ACC founder from Philadelphia, proposed that the college sponsor "clinical workshops" where members could spend a few days with academic cardiologists and heart surgeons. Small groups of practitioners (usually fewer than five) would visit medical schools and teaching hospitals to watch academic cardiologists and surgeons at work in the ward, cardiac clinic, catheterization lab, operating room, and research laboratory.[72]

Wolffe told Paul White that the goal of the workshop program was to allow "physicians interested in cardiology to observe advanced clinical and/or research projects at work, and to rub elbows in a sort of 'preceptor' relationship with pioneers in the field." He explained that the concept was unlike "the usual type of postgraduate course consisting of lectures to large groups or attendance at crowded clinics." Wolffe thought the informality of the program was one of its strengths.[73] After consulting with AHA president Cowles Andrus and his Harvard colleague Edward Bland, White declined Wolffe's invitation to participate. Andrus worried that "individuals who attended such a 'workshop' would be encouraged to exploit that experience."[74] White told an academic cardiologist in Philadelphia that the college's "workshops and pilgrimages are nothing new. They have been in progress informally for many years. This looks like a bit of window dressing."[75]

Despite the cool response from AHA loyalists, the ACC workshop programs were successful. During the first year (1956–1957), seventy-three workshops were held at teaching institutions around the nation, including Duke University Hospital, Emory Hospital, Johns Hopkins Hospital, the Mayo Clinic, Peter Bent Brigham Hospital, and the University of Montreal. Such prominent figures as Richard Gorlin, Samuel Levine, Myron Prinzmetal, Hans Selye, and Helen Taussig were among the dozens of preceptors who participated.[76] College leaders were pleased with the educational value of the workshops and thought the program had the added benefit of familiarizing academic cardiologists with the college.

The logistics of organizing so many courses was more than Wolffe and the college's small staff could handle, however. Within five years, the workshop program had evolved from a large number of informal programs with a few participants to a limited series of structured programs with multiple speakers and many attendees. The first large, college-sponsored, medical center-based symposium was held at the Peter Bent Brigham Hospital in Boston in 1961. Heart surgeon Dwight Harken organized a three-day workshop attended by sixty-six college members. The ACC sponsored five other programs that year. When the Brigham symposium was repeated in 1962, participants heard fifteen didactic presentations, attended medical and surgical clinics, and watched two heart operations.[77] These large symposia became a major part of the college's continuing medical education program. In 1962, 862 physicians attended ten symposium-style workshops. Five years later, the college sponsored thirty-four courses attended by 5,413 physicians, not counting the annual meeting.[78]

Leaders of the AHA's Council of Clinical Cardiology felt the need to compete with the ACC's popular symposium program. The association had cosponsored postgraduate courses with some local affiliates for several years, and they now wanted to expand the effort. In 1963 the CCC began organizing "interim courses" in cities that were too small for the annual AHA meeting but had a "strong medical community."[79] The first "Three Days of Cardiology" course, held at Emory University in 1963, consisted of lectures and panel discussions by local faculty and prominent guest speakers. During the next three years, similar courses were held at more than a dozen academic medical centers.[80]

ACC leaders were not complacent. When Grey Dimond, an academic cardiologist trained by Paul White, became ACC president in

1961, he challenged the organization to develop new educational programs because it was "youthful and able to experiment; lines of administration are short and flexible."[81] Dimond did not draw the logical corollary: the AHA had become a complex and bureaucratic organization as a result of its transformation into a voluntary health organization. Discussing the AHA and the ACC recently, Eugene Braunwald used a naval metaphor to distinguish these "two very important organizations." Comparing the AHA to a "great big battleship" and the ACC to a destroyer, he explained, "A battleship is powerful, but it moves very slowly and is not agile. The destroyer is smaller, it doesn't have the same fire power, but it can sure get there faster, and it can get into lots of tight places and do things quickly and easily."[82] Braunwald, who first presented a paper at an ACC meeting in 1957, feels that the ACC "introduced continuing education into the field" of cardiology and the AHA "got on the band wagon and copied it."[83]

The geographical scope of the ACC's postgraduate programs expanded significantly in 1961 as a result of the combined efforts of Eliot Corday, Grey Dimond, and Philip Reichert. The concept of sending American physicians abroad to lecture was not new. Shortly after the World Health Organization (WHO) was formed in 1948, it began sponsoring overseas "teaching medical missions." During the next five years, WHO sponsored visits to seventeen foreign countries.[84]

Mariano Alimurung, ACC governor for the Philippines, provided the stimulus for developing the formal "International Circuit Course" program in 1961. He had been one of Paul White's cardiac residents at the Massachusetts General Hospital shortly after World War II. Dimond (a White trainee at the same time) recalls that Alimurung "saw himself as a bridge between the United States and his country and was an unceasing ambassador."[85] Alimurung knew the ACC had organized small workshop programs in Buenos Aires, Montreal, and Mexico City and hoped it would sponsor a large postgraduate course in the Philippines.[86] Reichert was enthusiastic about the idea and asked the college's postgraduate education committee (chaired by Corday) to consider it.[87]

Meanwhile, Corday independently urged the ACC to sponsor lectures in Europe. Two world wars and persistent economic problems had seriously disrupted medical education and research on the Continent. Meanwhile, America had become the world's leader in cardiology and cardiac surgery. During a trip abroad in the late 1950s, Corday "was impressed with how far behind the countries of Spain, Portugal,

France, Italy, Greece, and Austria were in their knowledge of the recent advances in the field of cardiology." Citing recent American innovations such as open-heart surgery, he urged the college to undertake "missionary work" to "disseminate" new knowledge about the diagnosis and treatment of cardiovascular disease. Corday thought "teams of four or five outstanding, nationally known physicians and surgeons" could present lectures and "demonstrate new surgical techniques in these European countries."[88]

When Reichert learned of Corday's proposal, he told him about Alimurung's concept for a symposium in the Philippines. Corday formed a "Foreign Workshop Committee" and began planning an international "circuit course" to the Far East. The term *circuit course* was derived from a program popularized by William Middleton, dean of the University of Wisconsin Medical School, several years earlier. He and other medical faculty members had traveled throughout the state giving lectures and visiting with rural practitioners. Dimond himself had adopted this teaching approach in rural Kansas in the 1950s.[89]

The president of the Philippine Medical Association was enthusiastic about the college's program.[90] The nation's health secretary claimed it would be the first program of its kind in the Far East.[91] Former ACC president George Calver, physician to Congress, helped Corday gain access to the State Department to request federal funding for the international circuit courses. Government officials were interested because the proposal was in the spirit of the Peace Corps program that President John Kennedy had established a few months earlier. When State Department officials suggested that one or two doctors would be enough, Corday was miffed. He explained that what he had in mind was "like sending a ball team." At least five faculty members were necessary for a successful one-week program; "it was not enough to send a pitcher and a catcher."[92]

Corday and Dimond (now the college's president) understood politics. Dimond communicated with Janet Travell, President Kennedy's private physician, in an attempt to "reach his ear directly." Meanwhile, Dimond's longtime friend Franklin Murphy (who had recently become chancellor of the University of California at Los Angeles) put him in touch with "the proper people in the State Department."[93] Paul White, known for his interest in international cardiology, told his former pupil that the plan was worthwhile because "anything that brings people together" fostered "better international relations."[94]

The first international circuit course visited the Philippines and Taiwan in October 1961. It lasted five days and was funded by grants from the State Department and the Eli Lilly pharmaceutical company. In addition to Corday and Dimond, this first ACC team included heart surgeon Walton Lillehei, Tulane cardiologist George Burch, and AJC editor Simon Dack. Other prominent academic cardiologists and heart surgeons went on subsequent missions. The international programs, described by a *New York Times* writer as "a medical Peace Corps," enhanced the image of the college at home and abroad.[95] Proud of the effort, Corday emphasized that it had been "hard work, working through congressmen, nagging the State Department and the local embassies."[96] Government officials were pleased with the program. In 1964 Secretary of State Dean Rusk (whose department helped to support the missions) noted that the participants served "without compensation and at considerable personal inconvenience."[97] Vice President Hubert Humphrey thought the college "can be very proud of the circuit course program."[98]

Within five years participants in seventeen circuit courses had visited forty-four countries. There were some problems, however. In 1966 Corday explained that when the circuit course program was organized, the State Department asked surgeons not to operate abroad, because few overseas hospitals were equipped for heart surgery and the visitors would not be available to supervise postoperative care. Despite this prohibition, one surgeon operated in several cities during one circuit course. When some patients died following his departure for the next stop, Corday complained, "All the glory and glamour that he brought to [the country] was buried with the patients."[99] With this notable exception, the international circuit courses were successful, both as an educational vehicle and as a means of introducing several American academics to the college.[100]

As overseas cardiologists learned about the ACC through its journal, annual meeting, and international activities, some of them began to join the organization.[101] The college developed an innovative approach to impress new overseas fellows: the United States ambassador to the newly elected fellow's country would present the ACC certificate to him or her. British cardiologist Dennis Krikler was impressed that he and his family were invited to the U.S. Embassy in London in 1971 to be photographed receiving his ACC fellowship certificate from ambassador Walter Annenberg. Although "Annenberg hadn't heard of the

American College of Cardiology . . . he had been asked to do it by somebody fairly high up . . . and I thought it was a tremendous way to get [the certificate]."[102] By 1967 the college's membership roll of 3,200 physicians included individuals from fifty nations.[103]

Attempts at rapprochement between the ACC and the AHA

More academic cardiologists began to participate in the ACC as its educational programs flourished during the 1960s. This helped ease the tensions between the AHA and the ACC. These organizations had achieved a working relationship by the mid-1960s, although it had taken more than a decade to accomplish this goal. Shortly after the ACC launched its membership drive in 1951, Franz Groedel told AHA medical director Charles Connor that he would be happy to "arrange an official conference with your representatives to achieve mutual cooperation between our two organizations."[104]

The first formal meeting between ACC and AHA officers took place in 1952, a few months after Groedel's death. Bruno Kisch, Robert Glover, Ashton Graybiel, Seymour Fiske, and Philip Reichert represented the ACC. Irving Wright, Howard Sprague, and Robert King represented the AHA. The issues raised at this meeting would continue to cause friction between the two organizations. Sprague criticized the college's practice of issuing membership certificates, claiming that "certification" was a function of the American Board of Internal Medicine (ABIM), with major AHA input. Wright proposed that the ACC join the AHA as its clinical cardiology section. Graybiel resisted the concept of amalgamation because he felt competition between the two organizations was healthy.[105]

Sprague considered infiltrating the college leadership, an approach the AHA had used when immigrant pathologists Otakar Pollak and Wilhelm Hueper had formed the American Society for the Study of Arteriosclerosis (ASSA) five years earlier. Pollak and Hueper had sought Louis Katz's advice as they planned their organization. Katz, active in arteriosclerosis research, worried that ASSA might undertake a fund-raising campaign and compete with the AHA. From the outset, AHA leaders participated in ASSA and helped set its agenda. Cowles Andrus, Louis Katz, William Kountz, and Irvine Page served on the boards of both organizations. These AHA loyalists were in a position to influence the policies of ASSA, whose board consisted of just nine members. ASSA merged with the AHA in 1959 to become the Council on Arteriosclerosis.[106]

Still, some early ACC presidents were willing to consider a merger between the college and the AHA. Heart surgeon Robert Glover, the college's third president, told AHA president-elect Robert King in 1952 that the ACC's board was willing to consider the idea.[107] That year, Arthur Master (a prominent New York cardiologist who had chaired the cardiology division at Mt. Sinai Hospital for two decades) discussed the ACC situation with AHA past president Howard Sprague. Later, Sprague told King that Master wondered "if he and some others should join it with the idea of controlling the college eventually into some sort of amalgamation with the American Heart Association."[108] After three joint meetings in 1952, negotiations between the two organizations stalled. Voting not to participate in "joint programs" or "combined ventures" with the college, the AHA leaders sent a clear signal to the ACC.[109]

During the 1950s and 1960s, ACC leaders recruited academics hoping to improve the college's educational programs and enhance its image. Some officers and trustees advocated offering incentives to attract prominent cardiologists who, in turn, might influence others to join. The issue came to a head in 1956 when ACC past president Ashton Graybiel acknowledged that he had promised Los Angeles cardiologist Myron Prinzmetal that he "would gradually be promoted up to president" if he joined. A prolific researcher and a member of the influential National Advisory Heart Council (NAHC), Prinzmetal was associate professor of clinical medicine at UCLA. Some trustees resented this approach and were especially annoyed that Prinzmetal was nominated for office even before his membership application had been received.[110]

Graybiel argued that Prinzmetal would bring in other cardiologists from southern California, an area with many heart specialists but few ACC members. College president Walter Priest agreed that they needed a "truly key man in that area." He warned the trustees that if they did not elect Prinzmetal vice president, "we definitely [will kill] any chance that we will ever have of accomplishing anything on the West Coast." Glover also urged the trustees to support Prinzmetal: "We still are fighting a little bit of a battle for this organization." Their arguments were compelling: a majority of the trustees agreed and elected Prinzmetal.[111]

These dynamics reflected the pragmatic approach ACC leaders adopted to ensure the growth of their organization. They thought it could achieve its full potential only by recruiting both academics and practitioners from across the country. Although the ACC was expanding and its educational programs were successful, many academics still honored the AHA leaders' admonition not to join. Some of them feared their AHA research grants would be jeopardized if they joined the college. One of Simon Dack's friends resigned from the ACC after being "threatened" by an AHA loyalist in the 1950s. Dack recalls him saying, "I have been told that unless I resign . . . my grant will be discontinued."[112] College leaders persisted because academicians were a critical part of their educational mission. Philip Reichert told the board of governors in 1957 "that basic science men, professors and university men, [should] be encouraged to enter the college and meet with the clinicians so that the college would be set 'at the crossroads between clinic and laboratory.'"[113]

One source of friction between the AHA and the ACC during the 1950s was the lingering stereotype of the college as a second-rate organization founded and controlled by a group of dissident immigrants. As new ACC leaders emerged during the decade, some of them confronted this issue in an attempt to improve relations with the AHA. When he became college president in 1954, Paul White's former trainee Ashton Graybiel announced to members that he advocated abolishing the policy granting lifetime board terms to college founders and former presidents. He thought this was necessary to encourage the "infusion of new men with fresh ideas into the policy-making group." They would replace trustees who "because of changing interests and increasing age, no longer contribute very much to the welfare of the college."[114] But the real issue was not what the founders did or did not contribute; it was how they were viewed by AHA leaders.

Graybiel's suggestion went nowhere until the founders were diluted by new trustees. By 1957 a group of reformers on the board adopted his proposal as part of a plan to improve the college's image. They used their influence and their votes to change the college bylaws to reduce the power and visibility of the founders. That year, the fellows supported the reformers' agenda and passed an amendment by a four-to-one margin that transformed the founders from lifetime trustees with voting privileges to honorary trustees without a vote after a decade of service or at age sixty-five.[115]

Arthur Bernstein, a Newark, New Jersey, cardiologist present for the vote at the annual business meeting, recalls, "After a few years . . . the German group was just pushed out, made emeritus or something on the board, but not with power. . . . The attitude was simply that these are not our people and this is the American College of Cardiology and the Americans must take over."[116] Bernstein did not know many of the founders personally, and he accepted the AHA stereotype of them as Germans. However, although nine of the college's fourteen founders were from Europe, Groedel was the only one born in Germany, and he had died in 1951. Bruno Kisch had been on the medical faculty at Cologne but was born in Prague. The other foreign-born founders were from Italy (four), Austria, Russia, and Poland.

It is not surprising that some ACC founders were irritated by the decision. Seymour Fiske, an American-born Protestant, protested that it was "a little bit unkind for the majority of the men to vote us out." Glover attempted to reassure Fiske that he and the others "haven't been thrown out of the organization or out of the board of trustees." Unimpressed, Fiske declared, "You are emasculating us."[117] Reichert, an American-born Jewish cardiologist and part-time advertising consultant from New York, retained his influential position as secretary-treasurer. Five years later, he interpreted the 1957 coup as an indication that "the old team should not continue to dominate the meetings, and that the strength of the college depended upon the new team having complete freedom of action."[118]

After the revolt, the ACC and the AHA renewed discussions to explore areas of possible cooperation. George Meneely, Osler Abbott, Ashton Graybiel, and Philip Reichert (all American-born officers) represented the college. Edgar Allen, Carlton Ernstene, Irvine Page, George Wakerlin, and Stewart Wolf spoke for the AHA in a series of meetings in 1958. The AHA delegates saw that their predecessors' fears that the college might launch a competing public fund-raising drive were unfounded. Four years earlier Graybiel had announced to college members that he was "strongly opposed" to such a campaign or to supporting research projects, because that was the role of the AHA.[119] Meanwhile, the AHA had become financially secure; its 1958 income was $22 million.[120] College leaders had already agreed to limit certificates to full or honorary fellows. Now seemed to be the time to demonstrate to America's heart specialists that the organizations were entering a new phase. Acknowledging their shared interest in postgraduate education, the representatives agreed to combine the annual AHA scientific session with the interim ACC meeting in 1959.[121]

As ACC and AHA representatives planned the joint meeting, college president Osler Abbott, a heart surgeon at Emory, told Alfred Blalock that the liaison committee meetings had resulted in a relationship "of mutual respect and trust."[122] Most observers thought the joint 1959 meeting in Philadelphia was a success. There was one combined ACC-AHA scientific daytime session, and several heart association loyalists participated in the college's evening fireside conferences. When some college members worried that the joint meeting meant that amalgamation with the AHA was imminent, Reichert reassured them, "Our purpose is definitely to remain an independent College."[123]

But there was activity behind the scenes, and there were several agendas. Just after the joint meeting, ACC president-elect Grey Dimond informed his mentor Paul White that a "quiet revolution" had taken place in the college. Dimond admitted that he had "associated with the group with considerable hesitation," but he had decided two years earlier "to gamble and try to make a useful organization of it by working from within." By now, a few academic cardiologists had joined the college. "Friends in my own age group have been coming into the organization this year, and with luck I can anticipate the day that the American College of Cardiology will become the identifying group for the men who actually practice the specialty of cardiology." Dimond closed by explaining that the college "has had a revolution and Sam Bellet, Bob Grant, John LaDue, and I are trying to change its reputation— perhaps at the risk of our own."[124] In another letter, Dimond told White that his goal was to "upgrade" the college "to the place where there can be no possibility of criticism from any related organizations."[125]

Applauding Dimond's efforts "to change its character," White confided to his former trainee that the college "was at the beginning, of course, a miserable organization but I can well see that perhaps like the American College of Physicians it is headed for better days."[126] White had expressed this view three years earlier to former AHA president William Stroud. Although he then characterized the college as "an inferior organization," White thought it was "becoming respectable with time." He told Sprague, "This happened, you may remember, with the American College of Physicians. At the beginning, it was a society of people who could not get into the Association of American Physicians, but it became quite respectable."[127]

There were similarities between the founding of the ACC and the ACP. In 1928 ACP president Frank Smithies acknowledged that when the organization was created by New York internist Heinrich Stern (a German immigrant) thirteen years earlier, "in some quarters . . . doubt was held regarding whether or not the college was properly launched." Smithies continued, "the harshest criticism came from those who were least familiar with the venture." During its first five years, the ACP drew most of its members from New York and other cities in the Northeast, but Smithies joked that a "careful search of the roster of the early members fails to disclose a single scoundrel or irregular practitioner." He continued, "I mention this, because, during its early days, the college [ACP] faced such accusations and some even stronger, the echo of which injustice may be recognized even today if one has his ear close to the ground." The parallel between the elitist attitudes of some AHA leaders toward the ACC and some Association of American Physicians members toward the ACP is evident.[128]

White appreciated the efforts of his former pupils Ashton Graybiel and Grey Dimond to cultivate the ACC. In 1960 White told the AHA's medical director that he was aware of the "constantly improving status of the college due to the membership of a good many of the leading medical and surgical cardiologists in this country."[129] During the previous year, the ACC had successfully recruited four prominent AHA members (Francis Chamberlain, Irvine Page, George Herrmann, and Helen Taussig) by offering them honorary fellowships. Taussig accepted because she thought the college was "really trying to set high standards now and it will help them if some others come in."[130]

Although they were pleased that these influential cardiologists joined, the ACC reformers wanted to induct America's most influential cardiologist—Paul White. Between 1951 and 1960, at least four college presidents (Groedel, Graybiel, Abbott, and Dimond) had urged him to accept an honorary fellowship in their organization. If White joined, it would send a signal to all AHA loyalists and academic cardiologists that the ACC had become respectable. He resisted their efforts, however, telling a friend, "I think I will accept fellowship only on condition that the American College of Cardiology joins up as a council of the American Heart Association."[131]

Even if they could not recruit White, their college had something to offer America's growing population of young and ambitious academic cardiologists. These full-time faculty members were employed in university-affiliated institutions where their success (measured in terms of academic rank, influence, and income) depended mainly on their research productivity. These academics needed outlets for their research findings to prove that they were prolific and to enhance their chances for advancement. The college offered them a widely circulated journal and a national meeting that was growing in popularity each year.

The ACC annual meeting gradually expanded to include more clinical *and* scientific papers. The college's ambitious program of symposia provided another vehicle for academics to network with peers in other teaching institutions and meet clinicians who might refer them patients with complex and interesting heart problems. Increasingly, academic cardiologists saw the college's mission and programs as serving their needs. Meanwhile, a new generation of practitioner cardiologists had been exposed to research during their training and taught to think about cardiac diagnosis and treatment from a physiological point of view. A 1965 poll of ACC members found that a majority wanted the college's continuing medical education programs to include more information on basic and clinical research.[132]

The ACC's recruiting successes and their implications

During the 1960s ACC leaders succeeded in doubling the size of their organization; there were 4,225 people (2,781 fellows, 908 associate fellows, and 536 members) enrolled in 1970.[133] This growth encouraged them to raise the requirements for fellowship. Referring to previous liberal fellowship criteria, ACC president Osler Abbott told the college governors in 1960 that he did not "see how we could assume a position of integrity until we clean house." One governor responded that the college should "temper justice with mercy," noting that in its early years the organization was "glad for every member that we got, because every member meant 'X' dollars in the treasury, and we were really trying to live up to a champagne taste on a beer pocketbook." He assured Abbott that "these old fellows will fade away eventually."[134] A few weeks later, Reichert told a Massachusetts physician who had been turned down for fellowship that the ACC was no longer encouraging internists to join. The organization now wanted to attract "full-time specialists in our discipline" in order to be "a college of recognized cardiologists."[135]

In 1961 Osler Abbott (now credentials committee chair) told members, "As the college has developed into a fellowship of truly or potentially qualified cardiologists, the requirements for admission have become increasingly stringent and specific, especially so in regard to younger men." The qualifications for college fellowship in 1961 were (1) board certification in the physician's primary discipline (internal medicine, pediatrics, thoracic surgery, or radiology) and (2) continued activity in cardiology so that the candidate was either certified or eligible to be certified in cardiovascular disease.[136]

One way to recruit qualified heart specialists was to interest cardiology fellows in the ACC during their training, an approach Grey Dimond championed in 1960. When the college started recruiting members nine years earlier, there were very few formal training programs and few trainees. As government funding caused academic medicine to blossom in the 1950s, the number of programs and trainees increased dramatically to seventy-two cardiology training programs by 1960 (Table A9). Dimond thought the college should send "dignified literature" to every cardiology fellow in the United States inviting them to join as affiliate members. In this way, they "would capture the intellect coming along in American cardiology."[137] Reichert agreed and wrote to every program director asking them to encourage their fellows to join. He explained that "men who are being trained in the surgical, radiological or pediatric aspects of cardiology would be equally welcome."[138]

As part of Dimond's effort to attract aspiring heart specialists and enhance the scientific portion of the annual meeting, he urged the trustees to offer a prize for the best research paper submitted by a trainee. "Let us not give all of our gifts to old men; let's try to stimulate some of the younger men to compete for a prize." Dimond thought the college's "most precious weapon as the years go by is the young men who will compete."[139] The discussion of Dimond's proposal had the air of an auction. One trustee declared, "$50 is enough." Another proposed $250. A third interjected, "plus a bronze medal!" Dimond protested, "I am from California. $1,000 is an afternoon's income." After this animated exchange, the group agreed on a $1,000 prize and a medal.[140] After the meeting, college president Louis Bishop Jr. and Philip Reichert decided to ask a pharmaceutical company to underwrite the prize. Hoping Dimond appreciated their rapid action, Reichert told him, "the college has always been quick to act on something that looked good, and this idea looks very good to us."[141] Twenty-six researchers submitted papers and ten finalists presented their work during the Young Investigators Award session inaugurated at the 1961 meeting.[142]

Now several ACC leaders renewed the effort to recruit Paul White. Academic cardiologist George Griffith became president-elect of the college in 1962, just four years after he joined the organization. He had studied under White in the 1930s and had served as head of the postgraduate division of the University of Southern California School of Medicine from 1946 to 1949.[143] Griffith was initially hostile to the ACC, but his interest in continuing medical education and the ACC's growing involvement in this area finally led him to accept an invitation to join. Harken characterized him as a "highly respected disciple" of Paul White and as "Mr. Cardiology on the West Coast."[144] David Carmichael, a cardiologist in San Diego at the time, thinks that Griffith's decision to join the college gave the organization "strong legitimacy in southern California."[145]

With Grey Dimond and college president John LaDue, Griffith tried to get White to accept an honorary fellowship in the college. He assured the Harvard cardiologist that the college was committed to "education and attainment" and claimed there was no longer any conflict between the AHA and the ACC "except those which may be made by personalities." Referring to the coup to demote the founders, he assured White that "the antagonistic personalities" in the ACC were no longer influential in the organization.[146]

Even if they could not convince him to accept a fellowship, Griffith, Dimond, and LaDue wanted White to deliver the convocation lecture in Los Angeles in 1963. Recognizing the AHA loyalists' attitude toward ACC founder Franz Groedel, they persuaded the trustees to change the name of the "Groedel Lecture" to the innocuous-sounding "Gold Medal Lecture."[147] White vacillated, but the ACC officers persisted. Griffith reminded him that several of his former pupils were now college leaders. Finally, White agreed and informed Dimond that he hoped his participation in the meeting would "be helpful in bringing cardiologists together all over the country."[148]

But giving a lecture was not the same as becoming a member—and White was not ready to go that far until one of his Harvard colleagues forced the issue. White had referred patients to heart surgeon Dwight Harken for a quarter century. Harken had joined the college in 1957, had become a vice president the following year, and was president-elect in 1963. Known for his assertiveness, Harken was determined to get White to join the college during his term as president. He told White that he had been offered the presidency of the ACC, "a very large, highly efficient, permanent, important, and, I believe, honorable organization." Repeating the reformers' rhetoric, Harken assured him, "The old criticisms and even names are gone. They are even unknown to most of the modern membership." In a bold move of the sort he was famous for, the Harvard surgeon gave White an ultimatum: "If things are so fundamental and serious that you will not be associated with the organization, then I should refuse to be president."[149]

White responded, "By all means, go ahead and accept the presidency, for I believe that I shall join up myself before very long."[150] White not only delivered the convocation lecture in 1963, he also joined the ACC as an honorary fellow. AHA loyalist Louis Katz also accepted an honorary fellowship that year. Oglesby Paul, a former AHA president who knew them both very well, thinks they joined "because they felt . . . their membership in it might help to further upgrade something which wasn't going to go away."[151] Simon Dack credits Harken with winning over "practically all the big shots" in the AHA and views White's and Katz's honorary fellowships as "the culminating event" of that effort.[152] But there was a hidden agenda. White and Dimond hoped that the improved relations between the two societies would lead to "a reopening of negotiations" regarding a possible amalgamation.[153] Although Dimond continued to encourage a merger between the AHA and the ACC as late as 1968, there was essentially no support for the concept among ACC members.[154]

During his term as president, Harken launched an ambitious campaign to bring leading heart specialists into the college. With the help of the trustees, he developed two "blue ribbon lists" of cardiologists and cardiac surgeons who would be invited to join as fellows and would not be required to participate in the formal convocation ceremony. Since one of the goals was to expand the ACC's geographical representation, Harken explained that "ordinary clinicians" whose credentials justified admission were sought in addition to "people of distinction." The trustees were selective: only 81 of 278 individuals suggested were invited to join (63 accepted).[155]

While some prominent AHA members were joining the college, others were concerned about its growing size and influence. The association's Council on Clinical Cardiology (CCC) had been formed in 1953 to compete with (and possibly absorb) the college. When it became obvious that amalgamation was unacceptable to ACC members, CCC leaders renewed their efforts to compete with the college for practitioner cardiologists. Some thought that an incentive, the designation "fellow," would encourage leading clinicians to join the CCC. In 1961 AHA president-elect Scott Butterworth thought the CCC should be reorganized to "provide for a more select core, composed of those who are certified in the cardiovascular subspecialty," analogous to the fellowship category in the college. Sensitive to earlier criticisms that the AHA was elitist, CCC chair Wright Adams was opposed to forming such a "super group," however. He thought the CCC "should be a rallying point for cardiologists, but at the same time it must keep in mind the interests of the general practitioners and not downgrade them."[156]

AHA executive director Rome Betts agreed. He worried that doctors who did not qualify for fellowship would resent the formation of an elite. The organization had already felt the wrath of many physician members when it created the Scientific Council fifteen years earlier. But times had changed. The CCC executive committee concluded that unless the AHA began "to move in this direction, physician membership may not carry the prestige that a large national organization should be able to confer on its professional members." What they really feared was that practitioner cardiologists would join the ACC rather than their CCC.[157] AHA medical director George Wakerlin shared the CCC leaders' belief that the addition of a fellowship category would "establish the council as a rallying point for practicing cardiologists and assure vigorous leadership in clinical cardiology as a primary function of AHA." When the plan was discussed at the 1962 CCC business meeting, "a number of leading clinicians expressed their enthusiastic support of the proposed reorganization."[158]

As these events unfolded, AHA president Oglesby Paul assured Paul White that the association was aware of the college's growing influence. He admitted that the AHA had "been deficient in attracting clinicians" as members because it was "not the usual type of professional organization in that we have such a large lay representation." Paul explained that they were considering a plan of "upgrading professional membership . . . so that it will be competitive with other groups, and offer essentially the type of fellowship given by the American College of Physicians." But the stimulus for offering fellowships in the

CCC was not the ACP, it was the ACC. Referring to the ACC, Paul claimed, "Perhaps this type of competition is healthy for us and maybe it will do the whole field good."[159]

The AHA board of directors approved the CCC executive committee's request to establish a fellowship category in their council. Fellows would get a certificate, but there would be no designation analogous to the F.A.C.C. credential that signified fellowship in the college; the AHA board did not approve of this concept. The CCC leaders were gaining confidence and influence; theirs was already the largest of the AHA's eight councils. The following year, CCC chair Lewis January boasted, "The council has assumed leadership in the field of cardiology, maintains professional standards of training in practice, and represents the cardiologists and their interests to other professional groups, to the public and to the government."[160]

By the mid-1960s the AHA was secure in its position as the sole national voluntary health organization for cardiovascular disease. But the ACC's steady growth proved that most clinical cardiologists now identified the college as their professional organization. Largely due to Dimond, Griffith, and Harken's ambitious recruiting efforts, it was attracting academic cardiologists and heart surgeons as well as formally trained practitioner cardiologists. The AHA leaders acknowledged that the college was a legitimate professional society that sponsored a broad range of innovative and clinically relevant continuing medical education programs. In 1964 the AHA and the ACC established a joint committee to encourage cooperation in the area of postgraduate education.[161] Two years later, officers of both organizations met at the Summit Hotel in New York and agreed to meet annually "to discuss better coordination and cooperation between the two associations."[162]

Most academic cardiologists now viewed the college as a credible organization that they and their trainees should join. Even though a $50 initiation fee was introduced in 1964, more than 400 applications for membership were processed the following year. In 1966 college president Eliot Corday told the trustees that this level of interest "indicates the high regard with which the cardiologists hold the college." He explained that "membership in the college is now so highly sought for that each rejection calls forth a host of complaints."[163]

The field of continuing medical education was also flourishing. In 1965 President Lyndon Johnson's Commission on Heart Disease, Cancer, and Stroke declared that "continuing education is a categorical imperative of contemporary medicine."[164] More doctors than ever before chose to participate in an increasing number of traditional and innovative educational programs.[165] Meanwhile, the technologies of information transfer continued to evolve. The carousel projector made lantern slides obsolete, and these static image techniques would be supplemented eventually by television and videotapes. Government funding for military and defense research in communications accelerated the pace of discovery and invention in audio and video technology during the 1950s and 1960s. In this context, the ACC considered new learning techniques to supplement their annual meeting, journal, and clinical symposia.

In 1953 the California Medical Association had inaugurated *Audio Digest,* a continuing medical education program consisting of edited tape recordings. George Griffith served on the *Audio Digest* board and had encouraged the AHA to use the approach to supplement their traditional educational programs. He became frustrated, however, because "they absolutely dragged their feet."[166] The AHA committee on professional education surveyed the status and objectives of the association's continuing medical education effort in 1961. Their 47-page report devoted just sixteen lines to audiovisual teaching aids, which they viewed as adjuncts to standard didactic presentations; "when used alone they may lack warmth and the human touch."[167]

By this time Griffith was active in the ACC. He encouraged the college to develop an audiotape program in the early 1960s and was pleased when the trustees supported academic cardiologist Bill Martz's concept of a such a program in 1968.[168] Martz knew that *Audio Digest* and a similar audiotape program in Great Britain were successful. He thought that recent technological advances (e.g., small, battery-powered cassette tape players costing less than $50) would encourage more doctors to subscribe to an audiotape series.[169] The ACC launched an audiotape journal ACCESS (American College of Cardiology Extended Study Services) in 1969. The tapes included excerpts from the annual scientific meeting and college-sponsored symposia as well as concise reviews of published articles. Introducing the first tape, an announcer told listeners that they should find the program useful whether they listened "while relaxing at home, at the office, or perhaps use them to retrieve time otherwise lost riding in your car, or eating lunch."[170]

ACCESS was a spectacular success, in part because it offered doctors much more flexibility than structured courses. They heard concise summaries of clinically oriented presentations without the expense and inconvenience of traveling to meetings. Within six months, there were more than two thousand subscribers, only one-third of them college members. An 86 percent first-year renewal rate and a profit of $30 thousand reinforced the impression that the new program was a winner.[171]

In 1972 the name was changed to ACCEL (American College of Cardiology Extended Learning) when it was learned that a corporation held the copyright to the acronym ACCESS. Grey Dimond edited the series for several years and shared Martz's commitment to deliver a quality product. Dimond once told the trustees that 323 "uhs" were edited out of a twelve-minute tape on high blood pressure because the speaker "'uh'ed' hypertension to death."[172] ACCEL had 4,600 paid subscribers by 1974, and Dimond claimed to have "pretty well harvested those who call themselves cardiologists" in marketing the tapes. He also reported that his committee was planning to develop a videotape continuing medical education series. The college issued its first videotape program in 1973. During the next three years, it sold 674 copies of a ten-videotape continuing medical education program.[173]

By the mid-1960s the ACC had established a variety of successful continuing medical education programs that appealed to practitioner cardiologists who wanted to learn about innovations to help them care for patients—and to compete for them by offering state-of-the-art services. The college's programs also served the needs of academic cardiologists who wanted to transmit new knowledge while enhancing their curriculum vitaes. Meanwhile, the population of both groups of cardiologists increased steadily thanks to generous funding of cardiology training programs by the National Institutes of Health (NIH). The government's enormous impact on academic medicine and research contributed to the growing demand for continuing medical education programs: there was more to learn, there were more academics to teach, and there were more practitioners to read and listen.

CHAPTER 7

Washington, Medicine, and the
American College of Cardiology

Throughout the 1950s scientists and academics reassured politicians (who in turn reassured their constituents) that Washington's massive investment in biomedical research would produce results: not only new insights into the mechanisms of disease, but improved health. But as government-sponsored research led directly and indirectly to discoveries and innovations, concern grew that new knowledge was diffusing too slowly from academic medical centers and research institutes to community hospitals and doctors' offices. By the 1960s many voices called for new federal programs and policies to facilitate the transfer from academics to practitioners of knowledge and advances that might benefit patients. Congress listened and passed laws in the mid-1960s designed to accelerate the practical application of new knowledge and to make health care more available to older and indigent Americans. In this context, the American College of Cardiology (ACC) moved to Washington and established links with the National Heart Institute (NHI) and other government agencies.

By 1965 the NHI had spent more than three-quarters of a billion dollars supporting its mission, and it could point with pride to many practical discoveries made by researchers it had helped fund. Meanwhile, the ACC had established itself as *the* national organization committed to the continuing medical education of practitioner cardiologists. When college leaders decided to move their headquarters from New York to suburban Washington in 1965, they signaled ACC members, American Heart Association (AHA) leaders, NHI scientists, and politicians that the organization's agenda was expanding beyond its traditional focus on education. Still, the college entered the area of government relations cautiously, and only after Lyndon Johnson signed several laws dealing with medical research, education, and practice.

In a general sense, the Constitution justifies the federal government's involvement in health care. Article I, Section 8 empowers Congress to "provide for the common defense and general welfare of the United States." Although the government has enacted health legislation for two centuries, the number of bills passed has increased steadily (and dramatically) in recent decades.[1] Some of these laws, like the 1948 National Heart Act, directly affected cardiology, as discussed in earlier chapters. Other events continued to draw attention to the problem of heart disease.

When President Dwight Eisenhower suffered a heart attack in Denver in 1955, the nation was transfixed. Unlike earlier presidents who had been secretive about their health, Eisenhower wanted the public to know the details of his illness. Reflecting standard practice, Paul White (called to Denver to care for the president) kept Ike confined to a hospital bed for three weeks. Moreover, the Boston cardiologist ordered the commander-in-chief not to return to Washington for a month and a half. During that time, the public received regular briefings on Eisenhower's recovery. They also read editorials and articles that debated whether he should return to office or run for reelection.[2]

Eisenhower was not the only prominent politician with heart disease in this era. Congressman John Fogarty, a Rhode Island Democrat and powerful ally of the heart lobby, had suffered an acute myocardial infarction two years earlier, and Senate majority leader Lyndon Johnson had one just a few months before the president. Congress, composed almost exclusively of middle-aged and older men, took notice. Eisenhower was sixty-four years old when he had his heart attack, but Fogarty was just thirty-six and Johnson only forty-six. Paul White recalled in 1971 that prominent members of Congress "became especially interested in our work when they themselves developed heart disease (as many of them did) and became our patients."[3]

Members of the heart lobby appeared regularly before congressional committees to plead for additional research funds. For citizen-activist Mary Lasker, finding cures for chronic illnesses like cancer and heart disease was a moral cause. She told a reporter she was opposed to heart attacks "the way I'm opposed to sin." Lasker's enthusiasm was infectious. This reporter characterized her as a "catalyst" and an "indispensable mobilizer of the public and congressional will."[4] Sensing the public's interest in medical research and responding to the rhetoric and promises of influential academic physicians and scientists, Congress appropriated more money each year for medical research in general and heart research in particular during the 1950s. The National Institutes of Health (NIH) appropriation more than tripled between 1955 and 1958 (from $60.8 million to $189.3 million), reflecting the influence of the research lobby and the impact on politicians and the public of dramatic innovations like the Salk polio vaccine and open-heart surgery.[5]

Medical research was a growth industry in the United States. In 1957 the government provided $109 million to support medical research at America's medical schools and universities (two-thirds of their research budgets).[6] The following year it was estimated that almost twenty thousand "professional research workers" staffed the nation's growing "medical research enterprise." Not surprisingly, a group of academic physicians and scientists told the Secretary of Health, Education, and Welfare that "the expansion of medical research and education required in the national interest will be costly and should not be restricted by lack of funds."[7]

John Fogarty told Congress in 1958 that "the returns for the investment" in cardiovascular research had been "unusually high" and had "resulted in lives saved and lengthened, in suffering and disability relieved, and in the economic benefits of decreased medical care and increased productivity." He cited advances in cardiovascular surgery and the introduction of antihypertensive drugs and anticoagulants as specific examples of the practical benefits of research.[8] And the list of innovations kept growing. Two years later Fogarty boasted about the introduction of transistorized cardiac pacemakers, artificial heart valves, and closed-chest cardiac massage. NHI grants had supported much of the research that led to those and other significant advances.[9]

Democratic Senator Lister Hill of Alabama created a Committee of Consultants on Medical Research in 1959 to determine "whether the funds provided by the government for research in dread diseases are sufficient and efficiently spent in the best interests of the research for which they were designed."[10] Chaired by Boisfeuillet Jones, vice president and administrator of health services at Emory University, the committee concluded that federal funds had been efficiently spent and declared that "the present level of support is far from adequate to permit the great advances essential for the future." Generous federal research funding was crucial, because "the doctor is dependent on the ammunition that medical research puts into his hands and which has enabled him to treat or prevent diseases such as tuberculosis, syphilis, pneumonia, poliomyelitis, rheumatoid arthritis, and many forms of congenital heart disease against which he was almost helpless at the beginning of the century." These conclusions are not surprising, because Jones's twelve-member committee consisted mainly of academics, including Baylor cardiovascular surgeon Michael DeBakey of the heart lobby and Harvard pathologist Sidney Farber of the cancer lobby. Several members of the committee "were old friends in the cause of medical research," according to historian Stephen Strickland.[11]

Some members of the research lobby assumed it would be even easier to get larger NIH appropriations after the nation elected both a Democratic president and a Democratic Congress in 1960. They worked openly and behind the scenes to maintain the momentum of the prior decade, which had seen the NIH's annual appropriation increase tenfold to $343 million. But despite some notable and widely publicized advances, they had to acknowledge that relatively little progress had been made against the two chronic diseases responsible for more disability and death than any others: heart disease and cancer. But this admission could also be used to justify *more* money for *more* research.

In March 1961 President John Kennedy invited a group of clinical investigators and basic scientists from major academic medical centers and research institutes, the directors of the National Cancer and Heart Institutes, and the medical directors of the American Cancer Society and the AHA to participate in a conference to plan a "national attack on the two major causes of death in our country." Michael DeBakey was among the twenty-five doctors and scientists who attended the President's White House Conference on Heart Disease and Cancer the following month. Reflecting its influence in the area of cardiovascular research, the AHA was well represented. Four former AHA presidents (Cowles Andrus, Irvine Page, Paul White, and Irving Wright) attended.[12]

The draft summary the conference participants sent to the president included rhetoric the heart and cancer lobbies had used regularly to justify increased government expenditures for research. But now, sensing the administration's interest, they argued for much more than the standard annual increase in the NIH appropriation. A "vast expansion of medical research" and "thousands of additional research scientists" were required if there was to be "a successful offensive against these dread killers." Driving their message home, the academics and scientists claimed that heart disease was "no more inevitable than the infectious diseases which medical research has almost wiped from the face of this country."[13]

The 1961 conference participants wanted their government to go beyond supporting the traditional NIH intramural research and extramural grant programs. They urged Washington to place "great emphasis" on the development of "strong programs for research and training in urban medical centers throughout the country." This agenda reflects, in part, the makeup of the panel. Academics outnumbered the NIH representatives from Bethesda by ten to one. Emphasizing that research alone was inadequate to combat heart disease and cancer, the participants insisted that the "manpower problem" was central to "progress in the health field." Although more researchers were needed, better-trained (and continuously retrained) clinicians were also critical if the battle was to be won. "In order to bring optimal medical care to cancer and cardiac patients in this country, much more must be done towards providing for the *continuing education of the practicing physician.*"[14] NIH director James Shannon, whose institute had provided research grants to 293 institutions in 1960, acknowledged that there was a significant problem "communicat[ing] hard research facts pertaining to the clinical problems the physician meets on a day-to-day basis."[15]

Although these issues resonated in Bethesda, on Capitol Hill, and in the nation's academic medical centers, there was no action, because of what Stephen Strickland refers to as a "tug-of-war" between NIH officials on one hand and the chronic disease lobbies and their powerful congressional allies on the other.[16] Kennedy's successor Lyndon Johnson established the Commission on Heart Disease, Cancer and Stroke in 1964 to recommend "steps to reduce the incidence of these diseases through new knowledge and more complete utilization of the medical knowledge we already have." With characteristic bluntness, Johnson challenged the commission members assembled at the White House: "Unless we do better, two-thirds of all Americans now living will suffer or die from cancer, heart disease or stroke. I expect you to do something about it." This was not simple political rhetoric. Johnson, a heart attack survivor, knew that the problem was real. Coronary artery disease alone was responsible for the death of more than one-half million Americans annually (one-third of all deaths).[17]

Michael DeBakey chaired the president's commission, which included former AHA president Irving Wright and Johnson's cardiologist Willis Hurst of Emory University. At this time, DeBakey was a trustee and former vice president of the ACC, and he kept college leaders informed of the commission's deliberations. Although commission members appreciated the NHI programs, they sought new approaches to combat the chronic diseases that killed and disabled millions of Americans each year. During World War II, DeBakey had been impressed with the specialized centers for care that the military developed in the European Theater where personnel, facilities, equipment, and patients with specific injuries were concentrated. He recalled recently that the center concept "stuck with" him and that Vannevar Bush's report on science in postwar America had a "tremendous impact" on his attitude about research. During the 1950s DeBakey became, in his words, an "activist" in the heart lobby and a vocal advocate for "research centers."[18]

Although Wright's subcommittee on heart disease acknowledged that research had "yielded a high return on the public investment," it saw a "pressing need" for applying the advances in practice "so the American people can receive the full benefit of what medical research has accomplished." To address a perceived shortage of specialized personnel and facilities, the subcommittee recommended establishing at least twenty-five regional heart centers "in selected universities and medical research institutions throughout the country."[19] Wright, an academic physician and clinical investigator, decried existing policy guidelines that forced the NHI to support only "research oriented" training and urged that "greater emphasis" be placed on training superior clinicians. His subcommittee claimed that there was a "critical shortage of medical manpower" and predicted it would get worse.[20] They demanded new funding to train heart specialists who would be "ultimately responsible for carrying the fruits of research to the majority of the American people."[21]

The DeBakey commission report stimulated controversy and concern as various interested observers tried to determine how its recommendations, if implemented, might affect them and their institutions. Dwight Harken, the ACC's immediate past president, told college trustees that although he liked most aspects of the report, he saw it as "a blueprint of, and a road map to, government direction of medicine partially controlled through academic medical channels."[22]

In Washington, legislation and appropriations are necessary to breathe life into committee reports and operationalize their recommendations. DeBakey's ally in Congress was Lister Hill, a longtime influential supporter of the heart lobby. Hill introduced the "Heart Disease, Cancer, and Stroke Amendments of 1965" (S596) into the Senate in order to implement many of the DeBakey commission's ambitious proposals.[23] Irving Wright told Hill's subcommittee that twenty-five regional "heart disease centers" would cost $166.2 million, and 160 "heart stations" (which would include coronary care units) in cities and towns throughout the nation would cost $117.5 million over five years.[24] Wright stressed that this regional medical center approach would complement rather than undermine the NIH's traditional mission of supporting research and training programs in academic medical centers.

Some private practitioners worried that the proposed new federal program might jeopardize their traditional role in caring for heart and cancer patients. Republican Representative William Springer of Illinois challenged DeBakey regarding the makeup of his twenty-eight-member commission, charging that all but one of its fourteen physician members were academics. When DeBakey responded that he practiced in an academic setting, Springer was unimpressed. The senator speculated that the commission's recommendations would have been very different if one-half of its members had been "doctors who do nothing but practice medicine." He claimed that there was not a single practitioner in his district who supported the plan.[25] DeBakey insisted that the proposals were designed to improve the heart care available in many of the nation's hospitals, not just a few elite academic medical centers. Springer's concerns were symptomatic of a larger issue; many doctors were alarmed about the federal government's expanding role in medicine. Fogarty assured the congressional committee that private physicians had nothing to fear from the proposed legislation, since it would not interfere with the "patterns, or the methods of financing, of patient care."[26]

DeBakey asked the ACC trustees to "help him get this bill through," but the college leaders decided not to issue a formal statement. Although they supported certain aspects of the legislation, the trustees expressed concern that it would lead to excessive government interference in medical practice.[27] A modified bill, carefully worded to placate critics, passed in 1965 (PL 89-239). Its stated purpose was to encourage research in (and the diffusion of new knowledge about) heart disease, cancer, and stroke.[28] Former AHA president Irvine Page later claimed that the legislation signaled "the biomedical community that money was available for the asking." He continued, "The medical schools were quick to act upon that signal. Soon a cadre of professional mendicants sprang into being, many with permanent 'chairs' in Washington."[29]

After Congress passed the bill, the NHI initially planned to establish approximately ten "centers of excellence" for cardiovascular research and training.[30] But several institutions and politicians expressed concern about the limited impact such a program would have. Gradually, the original concept of a few federally supported centers of excellence was being replaced by a decentralized model that would be inclusive rather than exclusive—egalitarian instead of elitist. It would provide funds to locally designed programs called Regional Medical Programs that would seek to "assure the maximum utilization of existing resources including facilities and manpower." The goal was to "provide the opportunity to physicians and hospitals throughout the United States to deliver the latest advances in diagnosis and treatment" to patients with cardiovascular disease or cancer.[31]

The Regional Medical Programs bore little resemblance to De-Bakey's original concept, which would have directed the new federal subsidies to a few academic centers. Instead, many institutions and communities were free to use federal funds in ways they thought would enhance the care of their patients and the health of their citizens. The result was a patchwork quilt of programs that ranged from health surveys to transtelephonic courses and plans for new coronary care units. In 1968 Republican Congressman Melvin Laird of Wisconsin (a strong supporter of the NIH) told more than fifty representatives of Regional Medical Programs that their presentations at a national conference demonstrated "that this program is finally getting started. It has got a long way to go, but at least you are defining the problem."[32] Despite Laird's cautiously optimistic appraisal, tensions persisted. Later that year, academic cardiologist Tinsley Harrison warned that the Regional Medical Program strategy might fail "either because of the mutual lack of confidence between the profession and the federal government or as a consequence of 'town and gown' bickering."[33]

By 1973 the political support necessary to continue funding the Regional Medical Programs was eroding. Speaking of federally funded programs generally (and the Regional Medical Programs specifically), Stephen Strickland concludes that "they cannot fully succeed without consistency of purpose and steadiness in implementation and funding." These critical ingredients were lacking in the Regional Medical Programs. Although more than $500 million was spent on a multitude of separate projects, there was no unifying theme or agenda. What was to have been a coordinated effort to diffuse knowledge and enhance patient care turned into a series of disconnected demonstration projects. Funding ran out in 1975 as Washington's priorities continued to change and it became apparent that no consensus regarding the program's value had developed. The main legacy of the Regional Medical Programs, according to Strickland, was that they enhanced communication and cooperation among health care providers and educators.[34] DeBakey's vision of a few well-funded centers for cardiovascular research, education, and patient care would never come to fruition.

Medicare: A social program that revolutionized American medicine

Although the impact on American cardiology of the Heart Disease, Cancer, and Stroke Amendments of 1965 (PL 89-239), which established the Regional Medical Programs, was limited, that would not be the case with another bill that Lyndon Johnson also signed into law in 1965. The Social Security Amendments of 1965 Act (PL 89-97) established Medicare, a program that entitled all citizens sixty-five years of age and older to government-funded hospital insurance benefits, and Medicaid, a program that paid for care delivered to indigent Americans. These social programs had a major effect on medical practice in the United States.[35]

The passage of Medicare was a high-water mark for the national health insurance movement in the United States that originated before World War I.[36] Often acrimonious, the political debate about the government's role in insuring Americans against illness has continued for three generations. The concept was discussed actively during the Roosevelt administration, and Harry Truman worked hard (but failed) to secure passage of national health insurance legislation after winning the 1948 election. Truman once stated that his biggest disappointment as president was his inability to overcome the organized opposition to national health insurance, led by the American Medical Association

(AMA).[37] President Lyndon Johnson respected Truman's effort and chose to sign Medicare into law in Independence, Missouri, with the former chief executive at his side.

America's unique social and political context during the early 1960s set the stage for the passage of Medicare. Democrats, some of whom had lobbied for national health insurance for years, now controlled Congress and the White House. In his first State of the Union Address, President Kennedy proposed that older Americans should be provided with health insurance through the nation's Social Security program. A month after Kennedy's inauguration, Senator Clinton Anderson and Representative Cecil King introduced a health care bill into Congress that would provide health insurance for older Americans through a program called "Medicare." The ensuing political debate (a process Woodrow Wilson once termed the "dance of legislation") resulted ultimately in passage of the 1965 law.[38]

Medicare Part A paid for hospital-based diagnostic and treatment services provided to older Americans who were guaranteed "free choice" to "obtain health services from any institution, agency, or person qualified to participate."[39] Medicare Part B covered many physicians' services through a voluntary "supplementary medical insurance" program eventually administered by nongovernment third-party payers (Table 7-1).[40] This aspect of the plan had important implications for heart specialists, because it provided payment for office-based services and outpatient diagnostic tests—an area of cardiology that would expand rapidly during the 1970s as a result of technological innovations and liberal reimbursement policies.

Although the dramatic expansion of private health insurance during the middle third of the twentieth century and the advent of Medicare and Medicaid affected all medical practitioners, the impact varied among specialties. These differences related mainly to the frequency of specific diseases in various segments of the population, the number and types of specialists who cared for patients afflicted with them, and the availability (or invention) of relevant diagnostic and therapeutic approaches. Medicare (and other third-party payer reimbursement schemes) especially benefited procedurally oriented specialties like cardiology and cardiac surgery. Two things contributed to Medicare's disproportionate impact on heart care. Cardiac disease was common (especially among the elderly), and cardiology was becoming increasingly procedure- and technology-oriented.

TABLE 7-1
Outline of Medicare Legislation (1966)

MEDICARE PART A: HOSPITAL INSURANCE

Beneficiaries:	All Social Security eligibles over 65
Benefits:	Sixty days of hospital coverage per benefit period; post-hospital skilled nursing home services
Financing:	Payroll tax on current workers and their employers
Administration:	Federal (Social Security Administration), through fiscal intermediaries

MEDICARE PART B: SUPPLEMENTAL MEDICAL INSURANCE

Beneficiaries:	Persons eligible for Medicare who pay monthly premiums
Benefits:	Physician services (excluding physical checkups)
Financing:	Premiums, general revenues, patient costsharing
Administration:	Federal (Social Security Administration), through fiscal intermediaries

MEDICAID: FEDERAL-STATE GRANT PROGRAM FOR POOR FAMILIES AND
THE MEDICALLY INDIGENT

SOURCE: T. R. Marmor, "Reflections on Medicare," *J. Med. Philo.* 13 (1988): 5–29, table 1, p. 11. Reprinted by permission of Kluwer Academic Publishers.

By insuring the elderly against acute illness, Congress created a system that favored cardiology, which, by the mid-1960s, was focused on diagnosing and treating acute flare-ups of chronic disorders such as coronary artery disease. Influenced by a coalition of scientists, academic physicians, and concerned citizens, politicians had chosen to direct research funds toward chronic diseases such as cancer, heart disease, and arthritis after World War II. When their investment in research began to pay off, they chose to guarantee that the nation's older citizens would benefit. Even though laws were passed during the 1960s that provided support for maternal and child care and nutrition, far more money was spent on the elderly in the Medicare program. Had the government chosen to invest the money spent on Medicare ($4.7 billion in 1967) on maternal health or child care instead, cardiology would have grown more slowly.[41]

Heart specialists active both before and after the inception of Medicare provide a valuable perspective on its impact on cardiology. Responding to the question "How do you think the introduction of Medicare affected cardiology?" former ACC president Charles Fisch said, "It made cardiologists rich, as simple as that."[42] Physiological cardiologist Lewis Dexter thinks Medicare's effect on American medical practice was "tremendous." One unfortunate result, in Dexter's opinion, was that it contributed to the transformation of medicine from "a profession into a business."[43] It is important to recognize that the progressive expansion of private health insurance as a fringe benefit of employment after 1940 also fueled the growth of cardiology. The financial impact of public and private health insurance plans grew steadily after the advent of Medicare. Between 1965 and 1980 there was a tenfold increase ($9.6 billion to $105.7 billion) in the amount private insurers and Medicare paid for health claims (Table A10).[44] A significant portion of these funds would go to heart specialists for diagnostic tests they performed and care they delivered. By 1992 cardiologists received 8 percent ($2.84 billion) of total Medicare expenditures.[45]

Initially, cardiologists, like other physicians, did not expect Medicare to increase their incomes significantly. When Medicare was being debated three decades ago, most physicians were opposed to the government program. Congressman Wilbur Mills, an Arkansas Democrat, played a major role in crafting Medicare Part B, which reimbursed physicians for their services on a fee-for-service basis that came to be known as "usual, customary, and reasonable" or UCR. This portion of the Medicare program was part of a political compromise that addressed concerns raised by many practitioners, the AMA, and Republican members of Congress. Recalling how doctors and the AMA were initially opposed to Medicare, Mills remarked several years later, "Now I think they realize its a gold mine."[46] Health policy analyst Odin Anderson emphasizes that Congress, "in order not to antagonize physicians unduly . . . . enshrined the principle of usual, reasonable, and customary as a basis for determining fees" when it passed Medicare. "Hospitals were also held in some awe by Congress," according to Anderson, who notes that "providers were given in effect, an open-ended budget."[47]

The case of cardiothoracic surgery provides an extreme example of the impact that the advent of health insurance, combined with technological and procedural innovations, had on some specialists' incomes. Prior to the expansion of private health insurance and the introduction of Medicare and Medicaid, doctors and hospitals provided a significant amount of charity care, especially during the Great Depression.[48] In 1936 Ethan Butler, a Mayo Clinic–trained surgeon and past president of the American Association for Thoracic Surgery who practiced in New York State, discussed the financial implications of specializing in thoracic surgery—heart surgery's precursor field: "There is an economic aspect in the practice of thoracic surgery that cannot be ignored. It is fair at this time to warn the young man who hopes to make thoracic surgery his one and only field of professional endeavor that 75 to 90 percent of all thoracic surgery must be done without hope or expectation of financial remuneration. Those, therefore, who engage in this work to the exclusion of all else must either be subsidized or independently wealthy."[49]

Butler's admonition reflected economic conditions during the depression and the fact that many of the patients thoracic surgeons then cared for had tuberculosis. Not only did tuberculosis occur more frequently in poor people, it caused working people to lose their jobs and depleted their resources.[50] But it is also important to note that fewer than 5 percent of Americans had any form of health insurance when Butler issued his warning. His specialty and health care financing would change dramatically during the next four decades. A series of surgical innovations and the advent of liberal reimbursement policies for heart operations radically transformed the financial outlook for cardiothoracic surgeons. One writer estimated that the average annual gross income of heart surgeons in 1981 exceeded $500 thousand. In 1990 Medicare would pay these surgical specialists nearly $1 billion.[51]

Medicare and private health insurance reimbursement policies helped transform cardiology from a technology-oriented into a technology-dominated specialty. The field was poised for growth in the 1960s as new equipment and techniques were invented, often with the help of NIH funds, indications for their use were liberalized, and access to them was enhanced by expanding health insurance coverage. Meanwhile, the focus in cardiology and cardiovascular surgery research and practice had shifted from congenital and rheumatic heart disease (uncommon conditions) to coronary artery disease and its complications (problems that affected millions of older Americans) (Table 7.2).

Although most physicians welcomed the increased reimbursement they received for their services as a result of expanding health insurance coverage and the UCR payment paradigm, a few expressed concern. Academic cardiologist George Burch, chief of medicine at Tulane from 1947 to 1975, was annoyed that Medicare's fee schedule encouraged procedures and codified charging practices he detested. In a 1977

TABLE 7-2
National Heart Institute Research Grants by Disease Area (1966)

DISEASE AREA	TOTAL GRANTS	TOTAL FUNDS ($MILLION)
Atherosclerosis	387	16.3
Heart failure and shock	530	14.8
Hypertension	332	12.8
Myocardial infarction	166	8.2
Cardiopulmonary disease	178	7.3
Congenital heart disease	106	7.2
Rheumatic heart disease	75	3.0
Cerebrovascular disease	55	1.8
Other cardiovascular	210	8.4

SOURCE: J. A. Shannon, *The Advancement of Knowledge for the Nation's Health: A Report to the President* (Washington, D.C.: GPO, 1967), p. 91.

editorial, he complained that the government paid only $20 for a history and physical examination by a "master physician," when it paid $65 for interpreting an echocardiogram, $85 for monitoring a cardiac stress test, and up to $450 for performing a cardiac catheterization. A "super cardiologist" got just $20 for spending an hour with a patient, while "any surgical procedure of one hour duration provides an income of several hundred dollars."[52]

Burch complained that "people (all taxpayers included) are being hurt financially by this system of financing the care of heart disease" and charged that "the cost of cardiac care needs careful scrutiny." The diffusion of technology also frustrated this academic, known for his conservatism as well as his candor. He argued that "expensive, hazardous, and even fatal or permanently crippling diagnostic and therapeutic procedures have not only entered the practice of cardiology in special centers but are employed extensively throughout the nation, even in small, rather poorly equipped areas."[53] But Burch's assessment overlooked the public's demand for the tools and techniques of "modern" cardiology. Congress saw things differently and provided funding to help develop, diffuse, and pay for new technology and procedures useful in the diagnosis and treatment of heart patients.

Government research grants and health insurance programs also catalyzed the nascent biomedical technology industry. Earl Bakken, founder of Medtronic, Inc., a pioneering medical electronics firm incorporated in 1958, explains that before Medicare his company sometimes found it difficult to get reimbursed for their pacemakers, which were usually implanted in elderly patients with limited resources. There were "fund raisers, dances, or picnics or whatever to raise money so that the person could buy their pacemaker." The advent of Medicare "boosted sales a great deal," according to Bakken. Policy analysts agree that the structure of America's health care reimbursement system in recent decades has fostered the development and diffusion of medical technology.[54]

The federal government would not treat all chronic diseases equally. Patients with kidney failure (end-stage renal disease or ESRD) benefited from a special program introduced in 1973 (as part of PL 92–603) to cover the cost of purifying the blood by dialysis using the artificial kidney machine—in all afflicted people, not just the elderly. But the number of patients with kidney failure was small compared to the number of people with heart disease. In 1977 thirty-five thousand patients received government-subsidized care for chronic renal failure, but one hundred times as many Americans had coronary artery disease. Shocked by the unexpectedly high cost of the ESRD program, Congress resisted calls to extend this health care model to other chronic diseases.

The federally sponsored dialysis program had an important impact on one medical specialty, however. Clinician-historian Steven Peitzman writes, "The implications of dialysis for nephrology as a subspecialty have been staggering." It created new clinical opportunities for nephrologists (specialists in kidney diseases). Dialysis, according to Peitzman, was "not viewed as part of the required skills of the general internist." Once kidney specialists had a powerful therapeutic tool (dialysis) and received liberal reimbursement for their specialized services, nephrology flourished.[55]

The ACC moves to Washington

During the 1950s and early 1960s, practitioner cardiologists did not have a voice in the debate about Washington's role in medical research funding and health care financing. The AHA represented the interests of scientists and academics, while the ACC focused exclusively on continuing medical education. The AMA theoretically spoke for all American physicians, but only half of them belonged to the organization. Most AMA members were office-based practitioners, and many academics and specialists in group practices chose not to join.

ACC leaders exhibited no interest in political or socioeconomic issues during the organization's first decade. Busy recruiting members and establishing educational programs, they saw no compelling reason to enter these areas. College founder and longtime executive director Philip Reichert proudly told college members in 1958 that their organization did not have a legislative committee. "We are working strictly along the basis of what we are supposed to be doing, which is the dissemination of information in cardiology."[56] Although college president George Meneely agreed that the college did not need such a committee, he warned members not to be complacent. He thought they had "a positive responsibility with regard to legislation" related to medicine and research. This academic cardiologist challenged ACC members to "take personal steps to influence this legislation" by talking to their elected representatives.[57] Future college leaders concluded this approach, which encouraged individual action but insulated their organization from government affairs, was inadequate.

The 1960s would be a period of transition for the ACC. By the end of the decade, the organization would have a new executive director, a new headquarters, and a government relations committee. These interrelated developments set the stage for the college to expand its agenda beyond continuing medical education. Between 1949 and 1953, the officers ran the organization out of their New York apartments. When Philip Reichert hired the ACC's first full-time employee in 1953 (administrative secretary Maude Crafts), he leased a "very dark" two-room apartment up a "long flight of winding stairs" at 140 West 57th Street. In 1955 the college moved into a two-room office in the Empire State Building. When more space was needed two years later, Reichert leased a corner suite on the building's twenty-seventh floor.[58]

All but one of the ACC founders lived in New York City, but that was irrelevant after the 1957 coup (discussed in Chapter 6) limited their influence within the organization. Four years later, Grey Dimond and his circle of reformers saw an opportunity to put even more distance between *their* college and the founders, whom some AHA loyalists still portrayed as dissident immigrants. Dimond was college president in 1961 when the trustees first discussed moving the college headquarters out of New York. At the time, Dimond and Los Angeles cardiologist Eliot Corday were working with State Department officials to get funding for the ACC's international circuit courses. George Calver, a recent college past president who was physician to Congress, helped them meet government officials who might facilitate their request for federal funds. Dimond created a State Department Contact Committee in 1961 to acknowledge Calver's activities on behalf of the college. Chair and sole member of the "committee," Calver was understandably enthusiastic about moving the ACC headquarters to Washington, since he was born, lived, worked, and was well connected there.

Dimond strongly supported moving the college headquarters to Washington. Rents were cheaper there, and the college might be able to afford space for a library and museum as well as its offices. Even New York native Philip Reichert acknowledged that a Washington location "would give us an excellent and a central setup . . . in the place where the college had originally been incorporated."[59] He served, with Calver and Washington cardiologist Irving Brotman, on a special building committee created in 1962 to explore alternatives for relocating the college.

As the ACC leaders discussed the options, they considered practical issues such as rent, cost of living, availability of qualified staff, and access to transportation. They debated the merits of staying in New York, moving to Washington, or choosing a more central location such as Chicago (where the AMA, the American College of Surgeons, and several other professional organizations had their headquarters). Although most trustees favored Washington, the relocation discussions were complicated by "personalities, ambitions, hidden agendas, and hidden hostilities," according to Dimond.[60] George Griffith, Dwight Harken, and Dimond were anxious to enhance the image of the college in the eyes of academic cardiologists, especially the influential AHA leaders. Dimond characterized their efforts to further reduce the visibility of the New York founders by moving the college to Washington as a "bloodless coup."[61]

Meanwhile, Philip Reichert was sixty-five, and there was concern that soon he would be unable to cope with the growing demands of his job as the college's executive director because he was hearing-impaired and had a progressive eye disorder that had made it nearly impossible for him to read.[62] When he became president-elect in 1963, George Griffith hired a management consultant firm, George Fry & Associates, to evaluate the ACC and advise its leaders about their operations, office staff, and agenda. Griffith also wanted them to suggest methods of improving the "national image of the college."[63]

The consultants sent Griffith a 52-page report in May 1963. After interviewing eight college leaders and attending the annual meeting in Los Angeles, they had concluded that the ACC needed to develop a "more precise plan of organization, better structured procedures, and expanded central office services." The consultants were impressed, however, that in just fourteen years the college had "grown from a small, local society to an internationally respected institution . . . [that] appears to be only a few years away from universal recognition as the symbol and motivator of excellence in cardiology." Although they identified "two schools of thought" with respect to relocating the headquarters, the consultants heard repeatedly that "the combination of the college's history, the heavy concentration of membership in the New York area, and the New York office location tends to orient the college excessively to New York interest."[64]

Finding a successor for Reichert was the college's "most urgent problem." The Fry consultants suggested hiring "a relatively young" administrator with experience dealing with professionals and public relations skills.[65] Grey Dimond knew just the person for the job. Between 1955 and 1960 he had worked closely with a young man in the University of Kansas Medical School's continuing medical education department. William Nelligan was not a physician; he was a thirty-nine-year-old administrator with a journalism degree from the University of Kansas and experience in advertising and continuing medical education programming.[66] Dimond had hoped to hire Nelligan to replace Reichert two years earlier when he was president of the college, but the first opportunity arose after the Fry report outlined a strategic plan for the college. Griffith, Corday, Harken, and other college leaders were impressed with Nelligan when they interviewed him during the ACC's 1965 annual meeting in Boston. Although the move to Washington seemed certain by this time, Dimond wanted to be sure nothing went wrong and urged Nelligan to link his acceptance to a firm commitment from the college to relocate there.[67]

A native of a small Kansas town, Nelligan did not want to move his family to New York. Dimond informed trustee George Burch that Nelligan would accept the job only if the college moved to Washington. "I am very much in favor of this and hope you will use your trustee vote to back it."[68] Corday told Nelligan that he, Dimond, Griffith, and

Harken were trying to overcome the influence of "certain people in New York" who were "opposed to moving the college."[69] Nelligan applauded "the tremendous amount of personal time and effort" that Corday was dedicating to the effort. "I hope that we can look back some five years from now and say that the Washington location was the best, not only for the Nelligans, but also for the future growth and maturing of the college."[70] Nelligan got the job and would play a major role in building the college during the twenty-seven years he served as its executive director. His influence reflected his management skills and his long tenure in an organization where part-time presidents serve just one year.[71]

The reformers had won: a solid majority of the trustees backed the move to Washington. When Dwight Harken created an Office Relocation Committee in 1965, the ACC agenda still focused exclusively on continuing medical education. Members were told that "the college realizes that it needs to develop and maintain closer relations with other organizations primarily interested in higher education—organizations in most instances, with headquarters in Washington."[72] Other associations had moved (or were considering moving) to the nation's capital. In a widely circulated strategic plan, a consultant urged the Association of American Medical Colleges in 1965 to "establish regular representation in Washington" because this would "enhance relationships with the United States government and with many educational and scientific organizations now located in the capital."[73]

But just where in Washington should the ACC move? A downtown location would place the college near the State Department, which was supporting the international circuit courses. The logical alternative was to select a site near the NIH campus in Bethesda, a Maryland suburb about ten miles from downtown Washington. Calver strongly supported a downtown location, mainly because he resented the NIH, claiming they had once "snatched" some of his personnel. Calling Bethesda a "honky-tonk sort of town," he tried unsuccessfully to form a coalition to "oppose the absorption of the college" by the NIH.[74] Another factor complicated the debate. Irving Brotman, a vocal member of the relocation committee, wanted the college to buy a property he owned on 22nd Street near "Embassy Row." Motivated in part by economic self-interest, Brotman characterized Bethesda as a "small, main street town with cheap restaurants, hot dog stands, automobile dealers, cheap moving picture theaters, motels and chain grocery stores."[75]

Condemning Brotman's lack of objectivity, the trustees voted to move to Bethesda in June 1965. Within six weeks, Corday's lawyer had negotiated an early release from the Empire State Building lease; Reichert, Crafts, and Nelligan had packed up the college's records; and movers had transported them to Bethesda. The trustees had decided to rent space in a stone mansion on the grounds of the Federation of American Societies for Experimental Biology (FASEB) near the NIH campus.[76] Delighted with the chain of events, Dimond informed his mentor Paul White, now an honorary ACC fellow, that he had been "successful (with the help of others) in moving the national headquarters of the College of Cardiology to Bethesda and in putting a good friend of my Kansas days in as executive director."[77]

The move to the Washington suburb was both symbolic and substantive. It demonstrated that the college's future was tied to academic endeavors epitomized by the NIH and the National Library of Medicine, which had moved to Bethesda three years earlier. College visitors were struck by the contextual change. From New York's busiest commercial building, the headquarters had moved to FASEB's eleven-acre campus. A year after the move, Corday remarked, "When we compare the academic atmosphere of our new offices with that of the Empire State Building, where we were sandwiched in between girdle manufacturers and hosiery mills, it's quite a change."[78]

While the ACC's new Bethesda location set the stage for collaboration between the college and the NIH, it also meant that the organization was close to most federal agencies, the Surgeon General's office, and Capitol Hill. Former ACC president Samuel Fox recalled recently that the move gave college leaders "opportunities to engage in things with the federal government, because we were right up the avenue, so to speak, from the headquarters of many of the relevant agencies." There was another benefit: "the membership looked on the college increasingly as a very cosmopolitan group and not just . . . a rather provincial group serving the interest of people in practice in New York City."[79]

Dimond, Griffith, Harken, and Corday had emerged as dynamic and ambitious college leaders. Their common interest was postgraduate education, but each of these strong personalities had a distinct vision of what the college should be. By now, the ACC's educational programs were well established and participation in them was increasing. Shortly before the move to Bethesda, Nelligan told Corday that he was "certain that there are ways in which we can help NIH and they can help us." He continued, "At the least, we should make them *aware* of our aims and objectives and that the college is the spokesman in cardiology for medical education."[80] Nelligan's assessment also reflected the facts that academic cardiologists and their trainees were joining the college in record numbers and the organization's relations with the AHA were improving.

Corday, who became ACC president in 1965, was eager to extend the college's agenda beyond continuing medical education programming. The air in and around Washington was heavy with talk about the federal government's increasing role in medical education, research, and patient care. As politicians on Capitol Hill debated several bills with important implications for practitioners, Corday created a committee "to advise Congress, the NIH, and the Surgeon General on cardiovascular matters." The AHA had been testifying before Congress for a quarter of a century, but Corday and some college trustees thought the association had a conflict of interest. He argued that this was "a natural function" of the college, since the organization could advise the government "without having a vested interest because of the fund-raising aspect."[81] Tulane cardiologist George Burch agreed: "There will be no financial axes to grind since the college is not concerned with large quantities of government money except the support that we receive from the State Department for the overseas courses."[82]

Dimond, whose sole focus was education, saw things quite differently, but his influence in the ACC declined when he completed his final term as a trustee in 1965. Opposed to Corday's idea of a legislative committee, Dimond recalled recently that he had "fought the college going into that arena . . . for a number of years." Unlike Corday and Burch, he thought the AHA was the proper organization to represent cardiology on Capitol Hill. Still hopeful that the AHA and the ACC might eventually merge, Dimond worried that Paul White and other heart association leaders would resent any attempt by the college to inject itself into government affairs. There was another issue. From Dimond's perspective, Corday (a Los Angeles cardiologist whose practice included several celebrities) did not conform to the new academic image of the college he and George Griffith were trying to create to impress White and his circle.[83] But other college influentials thought Corday was an effective leader, and they shared his interest in government relations. Momentum was on the side of a new generation of college leaders who supported a broader agenda for their organization.

The ACC as a consultant to the federal government

The ACC's first interactions with the federal government reflected the organization's educational mission. Shortly after moving to Bethesda, the ACC established a link with the NHI that capitalized on the college's experience in continuing medical education programming. This collaboration was encouraged by Congress's growing impatience with delays in the diffusion of new knowledge as discussed earlier in this chapter. The Senate Subcommittee on Communications told Lister Hill's Senate Subcommittee on Health in 1965 that "knowledge unused is knowledge wasted." The government "has been given a clear mandate and substantial resources to support the generation of health knowledge through biomedical research. The results of this policy have been the great scientific advances that characterize our time." Subcommittee members thought it was "strange" that the "government has not been given a similar mandate and similar resources to support the transmission of medical knowledge to its point of application . . . the meeting place of physician and patient." Because knowledge was a significant factor in determining the "success of their encounter," educating practitioners about innovations was crucial. The subcommittee challenged the government to "develop a partnership" whereby federal and nonfederal agencies and organizations would "work together to transmit the urgent messages upon which health depends."[84]

Corday seized the opportunity to establish a formal relationship between the college and the government. ACC members were informed that "a congressional inquiry into NIH research funding brought forth a recommendation that 'Ivory Tower' research must be applied more promptly to clinical practice." Corday thought the college could "play a vital role in overcoming the time lag" by coordinating occasional meetings on cardiology topics between government officials and nongovernment experts.[85]

Fifteen people met at the college's new headquarters on the FASEB campus in November 1965 for the first "Bethesda Conference," which was devoted to physical fitness standards for aircraft pilots. Selected college members met with high-ranking officials representing military aviation, the Federal Aviation Agency, the Public Health Service, and

United Airlines during the two-day meeting. Corday, who helped organize the conference, explained recently why government and industry were interested in the topic: "Pilots were dropping dead on the stick. They'd find nitroglycerin in their pockets. So we realized they had to have a better workup."[86]

The second Bethesda conference, held the following month, had far greater implications for cardiologists and heart patients. It dealt with techniques for training nurses to work in coronary care units. Hughes Day, the Kansas cardiologist who had created the nation's first coronary care unit three years earlier, chaired the conference. Twenty-five people participated, including James Jude (who had helped invent closed-chest cardiopulmonary resuscitation), Thomas Killip and Bernard Lown (academic cardiologists who headed coronary care units), four NHI representatives, and five nurses. The college strongly supported "the expanding role of the nurse" in the coronary care unit and wanted to help formulate protocols to train them.[87]

A comprehensive summary of the Bethesda conference on training coronary care unit nurses was published in the *American Journal of Cardiology,* and 12,000 reprints were circulated to doctors, members of Congress, and others in "interested government agencies." Corday told the trustees that the publication not only "rendered a service to medicine," it also "helped the image of the college." Impressed by the ACC report, Mary Lasker arranged for Corday to visit Senator Lister Hill to discuss the college's recommendations for training nurses to recognize life-threatening cardiac arrhythmias and initiate cardiopulmonary resuscitation.[88] Hill applauded the college's efforts and added a provision for training coronary care unit nurses to the "Allied Health Professions Personnel Training Act of 1966" (S3102). For almost two decades, Hill had listened to the heart lobby stress the importance of reducing cardiac disease mortality. He told Corday that he was very impressed with the Bethesda Conference conclusion that adequately equipped and properly staffed coronary care units could save up to 45,000 lives a year.[89]

The ACC was off to a good start in its new Bethesda location. A year after the move, Nelligan told the trustees that the college was now "in a position to offer advice and counsel to the various agencies of the federal government, such as the National Heart Institute and the legislative groups on the hill." He explained that the college's state governor structure had already been used effectively to influence senators and representatives with respect to animal care legislation, a major concern of researchers and academics.[90]

In the eight years since Reichert had acknowledged the college's indifference to legislative matters in 1958, it had become obvious that the federal government was increasing its involvement in health care delivery. In addition to supporting research at the NIH and academic medical centers, Congress had signaled that the government might attempt to coordinate certain aspects of heart care (through Regional Medical Programs) and would surely become a major purchaser of medical care (through Medicare and Medicaid). With Medicare on the horizon, the ACC began receiving requests from members regarding fee schedules—a phenomenon that was not unique to the college or cardiology. Medical sociologist Eliot Freidson emphasizes that the advent of Medicare led many professional associations representing physicians to turn their attention to reimbursement because of its "critical economic importance" for their members.[91]

In 1966 an ACC member from Philadelphia asked the trustees to review reimbursement policies for heart tests. "As you know," he wrote, "professional colleges of the radiologists and the pathologists have greatly aided their respective members in negotiating contracts under the Medicare Program." Although this practitioner acknowledged that the college's mission was postgraduate education, he thought the organization "could be of real service" to its members if it formulated guidelines "for an equitable Medicare fee schedule for electrocardiograms and other cardiac diagnostic procedures performed in a hospital."[92]

This was a thorny issue. It was impossible to deny that economic self-interest motivated some members who urged the college to enter the political arena on behalf of heart specialists. Past president George Griffith still did not want the college to get involved in pocketbook issues. He told Nelligan, "We must stay out of the field of socioeconomics. It leads to the death of enterprise and excellence in education."[93] Following Griffith's lead, Nelligan informed the Philadelphia cardiologist that the trustees had decided recently that the college would not get involved in socioeconomic issues that other organizations such as the American Society of Internal Medicine (ASIM) were addressing.[94] The ASIM had been created in 1956 as an advocate society for internists. It focused on reimbursement issues and published materials designed to educate the public about the role of internal medicine specialists and how internists differed from general practitioners. Although some leaders of the American College of Physicians (ACP) thought their organization should fill this role, they were outnumbered by those who wanted to maintain the focus on continuing medical education and remain aloof from socioeconomic issues.[95]

As government involvement in medicine escalated and new leaders emerged within the ACC, the organization moved cautiously into the unfamiliar and unpredictable world of medical politics. College leaders chose to enter the fray as advocates of research funding rather than take on the more controversial subject of physician reimbursement. When Mary Lasker asked the college to add its voice to the heart lobby, Corday responded. By 1966 the college was speaking to Congress on behalf of academic cardiologists whose research and training programs were dependent on government grants. Academics, many of whom now belonged to the college, felt especially vulnerable when the House and Senate reduced the NHI appropriation by almost 15 percent between 1963 and 1965.[96]

Senator Lister Hill, one of the heart lobby's most effective allies on Capitol Hill, welcomed the college as a new partner in his campaign to promote basic and clinical investigation as a means to improve the health of Americans. When Corday, Nelligan, and college president William Likoff appeared before Hill's Subcommittee on Appropriations in 1967, the senator expressed concern that voluntary health organizations (like the AHA) "don't talk too much about what the government is putting up" because they raised funds from public campaigns.[97]

Hill had a point. AHA public relations director Fred Arkus warned participants in a 1967 "public relations workshop" that the association was facing "major new challenges" that would determine its "growth and even survival during the next twenty years." Citing the "emergence of government as a leader in the cardiovascular field" and the fact that the AHA could not "proceed on the *traditional* basis that we are . . . territorial commander in the CV field," Arkus declared, "We cannot afford to bask in the sunshine of past accomplishment."[98] The AHA was justifiably proud of its record of research funding and public education, but it depended on donations from the same people whose tax dollars supported the government's research agenda. In 1967 the AHA committed approximately $17 million to fund cardiovascular research, but the NHI budgeted ten times that amount.[99]

Lister Hill wanted the ACC to tell the American people just how much the government had done—and was doing—to support research and promote their health. The college representatives agreed to help spread the message. Nelligan, whose first job was selling advertising for the *Kansas City Star and Times,* told the senator, "We can be salesmen for this." Hill responded, "That is what I am trying to enlist you as right now: salesmen." Likoff assured Hill, "You have just enlisted the American College of Cardiology." Nelligan explained that the college had a governor in each state: "I think through these Governors, we can carry this message to the people."[100]

Likoff, chief of cardiology at Hahnemann Medical College, expressed concern that the House had approved only a 2 percent increase in the NHI budget, "the lowest increment offered to any of the institutes." He argued that the major problem with respect to heart disease "is not the failure to apply facts; it is the lack of facts to apply." Adopting standard heart lobby rhetoric, the Philadelphia academic cardiologist assured the senators that the ACC "supports sensible appropriations for effective endeavors that will eventually elevate the health of the public. Basic research is the foundation of this effort. Clinical investigation explores the practicality of theoretic concept." Alluding to the Regional Medical Programs, Likoff claimed that "community programs extend the results of clinical investigations to the field of public health."[101]

Academic cardiologists could see that the ACC was a vocal new ally in their effort to expand their research and training programs. They responded by joining the college in increasing numbers; it already provided them with opportunities for teaching and publicizing their research results. Reflecting on this era, Nelligan recalled recently, "the leadership of the organization at that point was tending much more to academic cardiovascular medicine. . . . those individuals relied very, very heavily on the National Institutes of Health and particularly, at that time, the National Heart Institute for funding of their projects, fellows, training grants, and so forth."[102] Houston surgeon Michael DeBakey, an influential member of the heart lobby, had become a college trustee in 1963. Three years later, he and Corday were appearing together before Congress to urge increased funding for the NHI. DeBakey feels the college had become, by the late 1960s, the strongest voice in the field of cardiac disease, "much more so than the American Heart Association."[103]

DeBakey rejected the view (articulated most forcefully by Dimond and Griffith) that the college should devote itself solely to educational efforts. He argued that the college's new role in lobbying Congress to support research was a natural extension of its original mission. In 1967 he told the ACC trustees that it was "research funding which provides the basis for this postgraduate education. . . . This is where knowledge comes from, research, and you've got to have funding for research." And the ultimate goal—better patient care—depended on research *and* education. Corday strongly supported DeBakey's position. He told the trustees, "I don't think we appreciate really what Mike is doing for medicine in our time. When Mike appears before a congressional committee they listen."[104]

Nevertheless, Corday worried about the future of the heart lobby and wondered what would happen "when these people are out of the picture; who is going to make the appeal?"[105] His concerns were well founded. Fogarty had died a few months earlier of a heart attack at the age of fifty-three, and Lister Hill was seventy-three. DeBakey was also worried: "You would think that in all the House of Representatives there would be one good spokesman for health, but there isn't. Mr. Fogarty died, and now we have no more spokesman for health."[106] The issue of who spoke for cardiology and heart research mattered to these men. Reflecting on this era, Nelligan thought the most compelling reason for the college to get involved in governmental affairs was because its leaders "wanted to be recognized as the principal voice for cardiovascular medicine. We weren't going to rely on the American College of Physicians or the AMA or somebody else to speak for cardiology."[107]

Although the college adopted the philosophy and traditional rhetoric of the heart lobby (previously dominated at an organizational level by the AHA), there was another dimension to the ACC's involvement. Unlike the heart association, the college was a professional society that represented America's practitioner cardiologists—always the organization's main constituency. The government's increasing involvement in medicine was a compelling reason for the college to become active in medical politics. In 1967 Likoff warned ACC members that if their college was "unwilling or unable to . . . [be] a forceful instrument of action, the responsibility most certainly will fall to remote agencies." He knew that many members worried that "government control, political direction, and influence by subsidy" would significantly change the practice of medicine.[108] Other professional organizations—even some leaders of the traditionally conservative ACP—shared these concerns. Two years later, ACP president Marvin Pollard warned that "the territory of medicine has been invaded by government" and urged "a more aware medical profession to establish . . . its own programs in order to resist successfully the territorial invasion that can have so disastrous an effect on our profession."[109]

As the government began to direct its attention away from research to physician workforce issues in the late 1960s, academics and practitioners became increasingly concerned. Full-time faculty members worried about losing grant support, and clinicians sensed that additional government involvement in medical practice was inevitable. In 1969 Dimond conceded that it was impossible to "rebuild the powerful team that once protected the National Institutes of Health. The era of Lister Hill, Fogarty, Mary Lasker, Jim Shannon, and others is over." He predicted that "any new grouping of such power will be around the delivery of health services and the production of health personnel."[110] Dimond was right, and the transition was already causing consternation among academicians, most of whose jobs had been created as a result of federal research funding. But the competition for government appropriations was becoming increasingly intense. The escalating war in Vietnam and the spiraling cost of Medicare led Congress to reassess its commitment to research and its involvement in health care delivery.

Louis Katz's son Arnold, a promising young cardiac physiologist, told Dimond, "The NIH has been the major source of financial support for the medical revolution that has taken place since World War II." He predicted that if that support were "withdrawn to the extent mandated by proposed NIH budget cuts, the future of American scientific medicine is in serious danger." Katz warned, "We all know how easy it is to destroy a first class medical scientific community, World War I destroyed Vienna as a scientific community, and World War II virtually wiped out Europe as a leader in world medicine. Can we let the Vietnam war do that here?" This scientist hoped the ACC would "take a strong stand for continued high level support for the NIH."[111]

Practitioner cardiologists also wanted their college to take a stand— on their behalf. During the early 1970s the ACC moved cautiously beyond its ritualistic support of grants for the NHI and the National Library of Medicine. In 1970 the college's Liaison Committee with Congress, the Surgeon General (Public Health Service), and the NIH was renamed the Committee on Governmental Relations, and Dayton,

Ohio, cardiologist Sylvan Weinberg succeeded Corday as its chair. Weinberg, a forty-seven-year-old practitioner, challenged the trustees, "We haven't taken any official positions except on matters that are sort of God and Country." Acknowledging that the practice environment was changing rapidly, the trustees again debated whether the ACC should become active in or remain aloof from socioeconomic issues. Weinberg reminded them that the ACP had "in a sense backed away from some of the problems that it thought it was above and found another organization [ASIM] growing up to take a role that perhaps they now wish that they had gotten into."[112]

Weinberg and a new generation of ACC leaders did not want to abdicate the areas of medical politics and socioeconomics to another group, because they affected all college members. Meanwhile, government involvement in health care continued to escalate, and it did not seem to matter which political party controlled the White House. Between 1965 and 1972 academic and practitioner cardiologists were affected directly or indirectly by several new laws, including Medicare (1965), the Heart Disease, Cancer, and Stroke Amendments (1965), the Health Manpower Act (1968), the Radiation Control for Health and Safety Act (1968), the Comprehensive Health Manpower Training Act (1971), and the National Heart, Blood Vessel, Lung, and Blood Act (1972).[113]

Citing this flurry of medical lawmaking, Weinberg told the ACC trustees in 1972 that it was "extremely important" that they hire a legislative assistant. Reassuring skeptics that the person would not be a lobbyist, he argued that it was crucial for the college to be aware of—and react to—legislation that related to the cardiovascular field. Why? Because the college must "represent the interests of the membership."[114] A legislative assistant would have the added benefit of enhancing the college's visibility in Washington "so the committees of Congress, agencies of the federal government, [and the] executive branch" would think of the ACC as the principal resource for information and advice regarding cardiology.[115] The medical climate had changed, and cardiologists now expected their professional society to track, interpret, and respond to new developments. Recognizing this, the trustees approved hiring a part-time legislative assistant to help the Government Relations Committee analyze "the many health related bills in Congress, and [serve] as liaison with the various agencies and committees of the federal government."[116]

The ACC hired Ray Cotton, a Washington lawyer familiar with the workings of the federal government, in 1973. During the next year, the college expanded its involvement in the area of government relations, "in scope and tempo, in keeping with a similar increase in government activities and legislation that affect cardiology from the point of view of teaching, research, and practice."[117] Cotton was a listening post; he gathered and interpreted information on pending legislation and federal regulations that might affect the college's five thousand members. Increasingly, information flowed both ways. Within a decade, the college would become the main resource for government agencies seeking data about cardiology. AHA leaders had traditionally been influential participants in the heart lobby, but their role was diluted as ACC officers (most of them academics by the 1970s) assumed a dominant role in representing the specialty in the government arena. At the same time, the original heart lobby evolved into a larger, more inclusive group that came to view the ACC leaders as allies.

An internal AHA decision also catalyzed the college's entry into the area of government relations in the 1970s. In 1972 the association decided to move its headquarters from New York to Dallas. The AHA needed more space and was concerned about the practical issues of availability and cost. In 1972 the association's income was $50 million, and it had a solid record of supporting productive researchers. After considering several cities for their new national headquarters, the AHA leaders chose Dallas, in part because they were promised free land for their building. Although the new AHA national center was attractive and functional, its Dallas location had implications for the association's future role in government relations.[118]

Michael DeBakey, a longtime influential member of the heart lobby, thought the AHA's decision to move to Dallas was a mistake. "With all due respect, they missed the boat."[119] Although the AHA's influence in Washington was diluted by distance, the association maintained its prominent role in the heart lobby. The AHA leaders, like those at the college, recognized government's increasing influence in medicine. Association president Gerald Austen stated in 1978, "In the past several years, public policy has become a major concern not only of the [AHA] president but also of the affiliates, the Scientific Councils, and other subdivisions within the association." Heart association leaders continued to appear regularly on Capitol Hill in support of funding for biomedical research and training grants.[120]

Heart House: The embodiment of an educational ideal

Despite the ACC's entry into the area of government relations, the organization's primary agenda was still education. President-elect William Sodeman put it simply in 1970: "We are in the business of continuing education."[121] Some ACC leaders framed their organization's involvement in medical politics as a natural extension of its educational mission (as DeBakey had in 1965). They thought the college had a responsibility to educate legislators and government officials about heart disease and cardiology practice. As the college extended its agenda and increased its continuing medical education offerings, more staff and space were required.

Grey Dimond sensed that there was an opportunity to recapture some of the organization's momentum. He urged the college to incorporate a sophisticated educational facility, a "learning center," in its proposed new headquarters building and suggested the name *Heart House* for the complex.[122] This would make it possible for the college to sponsor educational programs in its own facility, which would be equipped with state-of-the-art audiovisual equipment to facilitate learning. Heart House would transform the organization: the "college without walls is now to have walls."[123]

In 1968 the trustees authorized borrowing money to purchase a 9.8-acre parcel of land one block north of the NIH campus in Bethesda for $525 thousand.[124] College leaders still had to develop a strategy to raise several million dollars for the land, building, and furnishings. Their informal agreement with the AHA precluded a public fund-raising campaign, and it seemed unlikely that the members would donate enough money to construct and equip the elaborate facility. Dwight Harken, Simon Dack, and George Griffith, co-chairs of the fund-raising committee, asked ACC governors in 1970 to try to attract tax-deductible contributions from members, interested citizens, industry groups, and private foundations.[125]

The Heart House project was controversial, and tensions became apparent shortly after the fund-raising appeal was launched in April 1970. The college's governor for Ohio warned that doctors were "not very ardent or enthusiastic fundraisers." He was reluctant to try to raise money for Heart House "without having some very definite goals and objectives in mind."[126] Kentucky's ACC governor informed the fund-raising committee that his constituents were asking how contributions to Heart House would "serve Kentucky, our local community, and me as an individual?"[127] Some governors argued that the ACC should choose a more central location or build more than one learning center if the intent was to enhance the college's educational agenda.

But college leaders were committed to a single location in Bethesda. They wanted their innovative educational-administrative facility to be close to the NIH, the National Library of Medicine, and the federal government. Dimond, Griffith, and Bill Martz (an Indianapolis cardiologist who chaired the Heart House Committee) thought the proposed facility could also serve as a laboratory for experimenting with new technologies to aid the learning process. The government was especially interested in innovative educational methods and programs to facilitate the transmission of new knowledge from researchers to practitioners.[128] Moreover, cardiology was a specialty that challenged the senses. Simple examination of the heart included observation, palpation, and auscultation with a stethoscope. Special equipment was envisioned that would allow learning center participants to take advantage of new technologies to improve their diagnostic skills and learn about advances in cardiology.

But the educational facility Dimond and Martz envisioned would be expensive, and many college leaders worried the members would not support such an ambitious proposal. Although Corday thought that, "to argue against Heart House as a college headquarters is like arguing against motherhood," he warned that "the membership will balk if the primary need is for an educational facility in Bethesda with a price tag of $6 million."[129] Reflecting this pragmatic assessment of the problem, the college also sought donations from philanthropic foundations and industry, emphasizing the "unique opportunity to develop the finest continuing medical education learning center to be found anywhere."[130]

Between 1971 and the dedication of Heart House six years later, several brochures were produced to educate college members and potential donors about the philosophical and practical aspects of the project. Sensitive about the issue of "What's in it for me?" one of the earliest booklets explained that the "services" of Heart House would not be limited to "those physicians who are fortunate enough to spend time studying in Bethesda." Members were assured that Heart House would contribute to the education of physicians everywhere through the development and distribution of a variety of educational materials, including "tapes, slide sets, manuals, films, and self-assessment examinations."[131] Sensing the ambivalence about the centralized learning center concept, Nelligan explained, "We're asking the membership to build the headquarters and foundations and others to build the Learning Center."[132]

Although Heart House would be unique in American cardiology, it drew part of its inspiration (in both structure and philosophy) from the headquarters of the American Society of Clinical Pathologists, which college leaders had visited as they planned their own facility. Bill Martz had also been impressed with a high-tech continuing medical education facility he had seen in Denmark.[133] In 1974 Deputy Assistant Secretary for Health Theodore Cooper told Harken that the government thought the Heart House project was important because the "so-called crisis in health care" was due in part to the lag between the discovery of new knowledge and "its application to therapeutic and preventive medicine." Cooper thought Heart House could help bridge this gap by serving as a focus for dialogue "not only amongst scientists and physicians, but also amongst policy-makers and physicians."[134]

Two weeks after Heart House was dedicated in October 1977, the college held the first of an ongoing series of "learning center programs." The inaugural program, "The Bedside Art and Science of Cardiac Diagnosis," was taught by former AHA president Proctor Harvey and Antonio de Leon Jr. of Georgetown University Medical School. Although cardiac diagnosis now focused on an array of sophisticated invasive procedures and noninvasive tests, this first course highlighted the 150-year-old technique of auscultation. But Harvey had access to an array of advanced technologies to help him teach cardiac physical diagnosis in the building's auditorium. Other early Learning Center programs focused on innovations in the diagnosis and management of various types of heart disease.

The college, now comfortably situated in an attractive and functional building in the Washington suburbs, was transformed during the 1960s from a New York–based society composed almost exclusively of practitioner cardiologists into a larger and more sophisticated organization that also addressed the needs of academics. ACC-sponsored educational programs were flourishing, and the college's voice was heard around the world and on Capitol Hill. If success was measured in terms of members, the college was thriving. It doubled in size during the decade, from 1,987 members in 1960 to 4,305 in 1970. This increase signaled that college membership was becoming a standard step in the career path of heart specialists. It also reflected the vitality of cardiology, one of medicine's most rapidly growing fields.

~~~~~~~~~~~~

CHAPTER 8

Fueling the Growth of Cardiology: Patients, Procedures, and Profits

The rapid growth of the American College of Cardiology (ACC) during the 1970s was a reflection of the vitality of the specialty it represented. Between 1965 (when the ACC moved to Bethesda) and 1979, college membership tripled, to 9,360, and the number of board certified cardiologists increased sixfold, to 5,228. These statistics reflected a surge in the number of cardiology trainees and the fact that most of them now sought formal recognition that they were heart specialists. Market forces encouraged the diffusion of cardiologists and their technologies. Many factors—social, political, economic, medical, scientific, and technological—fueled the specialty.

Public health cardiologists continued to emphasize the prevalence of cardiovascular disease and produced statistics to show that it had increased between 1940 and 1960. But people wanted results rather than reports and rhetoric. Washington responded by renewing its commitment to conquering heart disease (and cancer). New diagnostic tests, such as coronary angiography, and therapeutic procedures, such as coronary artery bypass graft surgery, gave heart specialists powerful tools to care for cardiac patients. Meanwhile, the demand for heart care increased as more people were insured against the cost of acute illness. Medicare in effect encouraged hospitals to purchase technology and to recruit specialists to use it. Many interested observers—practitioners, hospitals, and industry—sensed that cardiology had entered a golden age. Heart disease was prevalent, new technologies were abundant, and cardiac procedures were liberally reimbursed.[1]

Cardiologists became increasingly wedded to technology during the second half of the twentieth century. It was potent and profitable. As in many other fields, cardiology benefited from advances in electronics as a consequence of weapons and space research. Examples include the totally implantable permanent pacemaker, nuclear cardiology techniques, and cardiac ultrasound. The migration of these heart care innovations from academic medical centers to community hospitals created many opportunities for cardiologists. During the 1970s and 1980s graduating cardiology fellows entered an expanding job market. Their specialty constantly evolved as new technologies and techniques (or enhancements of older ones) were introduced. This meant that new cardiologists possessed skills that hospitals and older practitioners wanted to offer their patients.

By the late 1960s some observers began to voice concern that all this technology and all these specialists—not just in cardiology, but in medicine generally—were too costly. The consensus that creating and diffusing sophisticated tests, procedures, and specialists should be a national priority was eroding. Academics, representatives of organized medicine, politicians, health policy analysts, and other interested parties struggled to find a politically acceptable and affordable balance between pragmatism and idealism as they negotiated the future of health care delivery in the United States. The ACC, positioned strategically in Washington, participated in the debate, especially as it pertained to technology and physician workforce.

Cardiology's thriving technologies

The coronary care unit concept was a new heart care paradigm that united high-risk heart patients, technology, and specialized staff— nurses and doctors—in a specific hospital environment. This innovation had implications for both doctors and patients. It was no longer possible simply to put a person with a heart attack in a quiet room, prescribe sedatives and blood thinners, and leave him or her unattended. Once they were admitted to a coronary care unit, heart attack patients found themselves connected to a monitor in a bright, noisy room with minimal privacy. Should the heart slow or accelerate drastically, an audible alarm triggered a race against time as nurses scrambled to the bedside to initiate cardiopulmonary resuscitation and defibrillate the patient if cardiac arrest had actually occurred.

The coronary care unit innovation spread quickly because it saved lives in a very visible and dramatic way. Proponents of the coronary care unit model did not want to wait for scientific studies to prove its

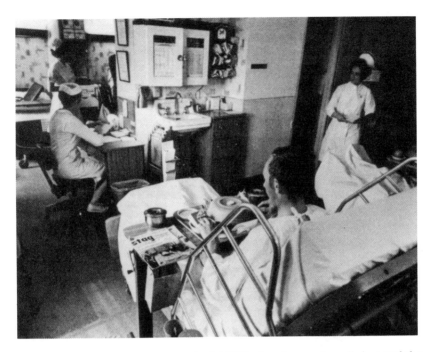

Four-bed coronary care unit in Maryland (1972). Curtains can be pulled around the patient for privacy.
SOURCE: C. W. Clipson and J. J. Wehrer, *Planning for Cardiac Care* (Ann Arbor, Mich.: Health Administration Press, 1973), p. 16.

efficacy. Urging the creation of more coronary care units in 1966, the chair of Baylor's department of medicine stated, "When human life is at stake, numbers are irrelevant."[2] ACC president Eliot Corday, a vocal advocate of coronary care units, claimed that one hundred thousand patients a year with hearts "too good to die" could be saved if they were cared for in them.[3] Early experience had shown that admission to a coronary care unit instead of a regular room conferred a significant survival advantage. Corday predicted that within a few years "all coronary patients will be admitted, as a matter of routine, to such units for surveillance and care." He urged cardiologists to convince their hospitals to develop coronary care units.[4]

Sixty percent of America's hospitals had fewer than one hundred beds, and most of these small facilities had no staff cardiologists (Table 8-1). Still, community hospitals could not ignore the advent of the "crash cart," the cardiac arrest team, and the coronary care unit,

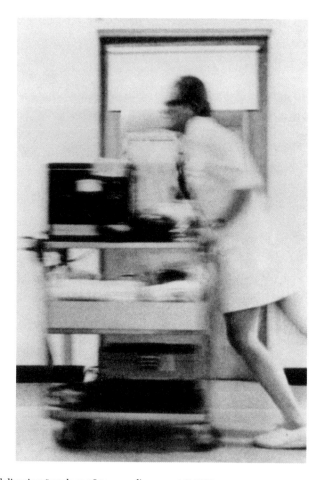

Nurse delivering "crash cart" to a cardiac arrest (1972).
SOURCE: C. W. Clipson and J. J. Wehrer, *Planning for Cardiac Care* (Ann Arbor, Mich.: Health Administration Press, 1973), p. 71.

because they admitted most of the nation's heart attack victims. Internists and general practitioners who cared for these patients knew that the stakes were suddenly higher. Corday warned that once a medical staff created a coronary care unit "it is holding a tiger by the tail." Establishing a cardiac arrest team and a coronary care unit meant that one or more doctors had to be prepared to drop everything to direct cardiopulmonary resuscitation whenever a cardiac arrest occurred. Once a "single resuscitation is started, the medical staff is rigidly tied down."[5]

The rapid diffusion of coronary care units into community hospitals expanded the cardiology job market during the 1960s and 1970s. Doctors generally supported hiring a specialist to create and run a coronary care unit if there was no one on the hospital staff to assume the responsibility. Practitioners did not want their office hours or hospital rounds interrupted by catastrophes. And beyond simple cardiopulmonary resuscitation, managing a cardiac arrest was a job for a cardiologist. General practitioners and most internists had not been trained to treat the spectrum of life-threatening arrhythmias or cardiogenic shock that might complicate a heart attack. In most larger hospitals, cardiologists took charge of the coronary care unit with its monitors, audible alarms, and high-risk patients.

The ACC held a Bethesda Conference on coronary care units in 1965. Two years later, the college cosponsored the National Conference on Coronary Care Units with the American Hearth Association (AHA) and the U.S. Public Health Service. There, data were presented that proved coronary care units saved lives. The participants concluded that ideally every unit should be staffed by a cardiologist.[6] Thomas Killip, chief of cardiology at New York Hospital and an early coronary care unit researcher, agreed. The following year he wrote that the "CCU was designed to provide the services of two specialists . . . the physician-cardiologist and the trained cardiac nurse" to patients with heart at-

TABLE 8-1
U.S. General Hospitals by Size (1965)

SIZE (BEDS)	NUMBER	PERCENT
Fewer than 25	562	9.8
26–50	1,445	25.2
51–100	1,480	25.8
101–200	1,107	19.3
201–300	539	9.4
300+	608	10.6
TOTAL	5,741	

SOURCES: R. Stevens, *In Sickness and in Wealth: American Hospitals in the Twentieth Century* (New York: Basic Books, 1989), table 9.2, p. 230. Copyright © 1989 by Basic Books, Inc. Reprinted by permission of Basic Books, a division of HarperCollins Publishers, Inc.
NOTES: The number and bed capacity of U.S. hospitals have changed very little since 1965. In 1991 there were 5,342 hospitals. See *Source Book of Health Insurance Data, 1993* (Washington, D.C.: Health Insurance Association of America, 1994), table 5.2, p. 104.

TABLE 8-2
Estimated Number of Coronary Care Units in the United States (1960–1972)

YEAR:	1960	1965	1967	1972
CCUs:	0	50	350	2,300

SOURCE: "Training technics for the coronary care unit," *Am. J. Cardiol.* 17 (1966): 736–747, and *Proceedings of the National Conference on Coronary Care Units* (Washington, D.C.: GPO, 1968). The 1972 number is an estimate. See L. E. Meltzer and J. R. Kitchell, "The development and current status of coronary care," in *Textbook of Coronary Care,* ed. L. E. Meltzer (Philadelphia: Charles Press Publishers, 1972), 3-25, p. 18.

tacks.[7] Other voices also called for cardiologists to direct coronary care units. "Every unit should be directed by a qualified cardiologist," insisted two public health physicians, because this "appeared to produce the best results as measured by patient selection, by disease outcome, by efficiency and by cost."[8]

If every hospital with more than one hundred beds created a coronary care unit and staffed it with a cardiologist, there would be 2,254 director positions (Table 8-1). But who would fill them? By 1965 the American Board of Internal Medicine (ABIM) had certified only 803 cardiologists and the ACC had just 2,818 members. Many community hospitals felt compelled to create a coronary care unit even if they did not have a cardiologist to staff it. Within a decade, more than two thousand were in operation (Table 8-2).

Patterns of care for heart attack patients had begun to change even before the advent of the coronary care unit. Between 1939 and 1969 there was a significant increase in the number of chemistry tests, x-rays, and electrocardiograms performed on heart attack patients in one community hospital, even though the length of stay did not change (Table 8-3). During the next twenty years, there would be a dramatic decrease in the length of hospitalization for heart attack patients; it is now about a week.[9]

Continuous electrocardiographic monitoring of heart attack patients in coronary care units also helped to clarify how they died. A heart attack results from sudden complete obstruction of a diseased coronary artery (coronary thrombosis), which prevents blood and oxygen from reaching the muscle supplied by the vessel. This event causes a variable amount of the heart muscle to die and may trigger abnormal and potentially lethal heart rhythms. Whereas cardiac arrhythmias were shown to cause almost one-half of in-hospital heart attack deaths, an equal number of patients died from shock and congestive heart failure due to muscle damage and resulting pump failure. Despite aggressive coronary care unit management of the cardiac arrhythmias that complicated heart attacks, the death rate during the 1970s remained around 20 percent.[10]

These findings led to new treatment strategies and stimulated research into ways to limit the size of heart attacks.[11] Physiology came to the bedside in 1970 with the invention of a balloon-tipped, flow-directed cardiac catheter that could be floated from a vein into the heart and used continuously to monitor intra-cardiac pressures. The "Swan-Ganz" catheter gave clinicians a powerful new tool to help them manage the sickest heart attack patients.[12] It also contributed to a trend that saw cardiologists gradually displace internists and general practitioners from the bedside of heart attack patients.

Although the advent of the coronary care unit transformed the care of heart attack patients and stimulated the job market for cardiologists, the nearly simultaneous expansion of indications for cardiac

TABLE 8-3
Hospital Care of Patients with Heart Attacks (1939–1969)

PATIENTS WITH MILD HEART ATTACKS

	YEAR			
	1939	*1949*	*1959*	*1969*
Days in hospital (survivors)	33.9	29.5	26.9	27.2
Chemistry tests	0.6	2.1	5.7	19.6
X-ray procedures	0.7	0.3	1.0	2.5
Electrocardiograms	2.0	3.5	4.5	6.2

PATIENTS WITH MODERATE HEART ATTACKS

	YEAR			
	1939	*1949*	*1959*	*1969*
Days in hospital (survivors)	32.3	25.8	22.7	28.4
Chemistry tests	0.6	2.2	5.2	18.4
X-ray procedures	0.3	1.8	0.5	3.3
Electrocardiograms	1.2	3.2	3.6	6.6

SOURCE: S. P. Martin, M. C. Donaldson, C. D. London, O. L. Peterson, and T. Colton, "Inputs into coronary care during 30 years: A cost effectiveness study," *Ann. Intern. Med.* 81 (1974): 289–293, tables 4 and 5. Adapted with permission.
NOTE: The data are the mean number of tests done during the hospitalization. See original article for a detailed discussion of the definitions and data.

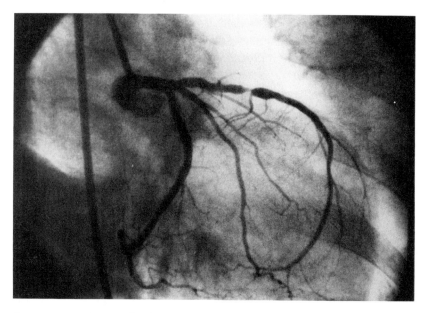

A coronary angiogram showing a severe narrowing in the left anterior descending coronary artery.

SOURCE: Marshfield Heart Care, Marshfield, Wis.

catheterization and angiography ("invasive" diagnostic techniques) had an even greater impact on the specialty. In 1961 about thirty thousand cardiac catheterizations were performed in the nation's 513 catheterization laboratories. At the time, 90 percent of America's hospitals (virtually all of those with fewer than 300 beds) did not have a catheterization laboratory.[13] The following year, Cleveland Clinic cardiologist Mason Sones published a description of his invention of selective coronary angiography. This procedure made it possible to demonstrate in living patients whether or not they had significant coronary artery narrowings. If they did, the test could identify the location, number, and severity of the blockages.[14] Recognizing the clinical relevance of coronary angiography, the ACC devoted a fireside conference to the technique at its 1962 annual meeting.[15] Three years later, one cardiologist remarked that "the clinical application of coronary arteriography is spreading rapidly."[16]

Coronary angiography changed the practice—and the profession—of cardiology, as the electrocardiograph had half a century earlier. The acceptance and use of a medical test relates to many things, but chief among them is its perceived value as an aid to diagnosis and treatment. A major stimulus for the diffusion of coronary angiography was the widespread adoption of a new surgical technique to treat angina pectoris, chest pain usually caused by narrowings in one or more of the heart's arterial blood vessels (coronary arteries). These blockages limit the amount of oxygenated blood reaching the heart muscle supplied by the affected artery. Medical treatment with nitroglycerin and other anti-anginal drugs is designed to relieve symptoms by (1) augmenting the heart's oxygen supply by increasing coronary blood flow and/or (2) decreasing the heart's oxygen demand by reducing its workload. Although it is often helpful, medical therapy rarely relieves symptoms completely.

Angina has psychological and physical consequences; most patients have to avoid strenuous activities and, unless treated, many are disabled by the condition. British physician William Heberden's original 1772 description of angina has not been surpassed. Stressing the "sense of strangling and anxiety" that accompanied angina, he explained that those "afflicted with it are seized while they are walking, (more especially if it be up hill, and soon after eating) with a painful and most disagreeable sensation in the breast, which seems as if it would extinguish life, if it were to increase or continue; but the moment they stand still, all this uneasiness vanishes."[17]

Mason Sones's Cleveland Clinic surgical colleague René Favaloro first described saphenous vein coronary artery bypass graft surgery (CABG) as a treatment for angina in 1968.[18] The goal of CABG is to provide blood to the portion of heart muscle supplied by an obstructed coronary artery. This is accomplished by connecting a piece of a leg vein between the aorta and the diseased coronary artery beyond the point where it is narrowed or blocked. The procedure was met with skepticism, because several earlier attempts to improve the heart's blood supply surgically had been ineffective. Five years before Favaloro's CABG publication, Cleveland Clinic surgeon Donald Effler acknowledged that surgical treatment for coronary artery disease was "in virtual disrepute in most medical centers today."[19]

Shortly after Favaloro reported his CABG procedure, Henry Zimmerman, a cardiologist at another Cleveland hospital, wrote a scathing attack on the surgical treatment of angina. Admitting that medical management "leaves a lot to be desired," Zimmerman claimed that

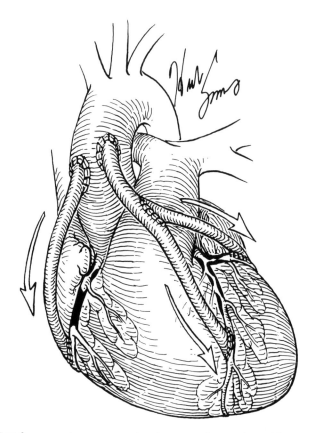

A "triple" saphenous vein coronary artery bypass graft operation with veins connected between the aorta and the diseased arteries beyond the point where they are narrowed or blocked.

Source: M. DeBakey and A. Gotto, *The Living Heart* (New York: David McCay, 1977), figure 75, p. 140.

"surgical management of coronary artery disease is in a state of almost total chaos." He protested that there was no consensus regarding the many operations developed for treating angina.[20]

Zimmerman's essay exaggerates only slightly the climate Favaloro faced when he introduced CABG in 1968. His chief Donald Effler complained to Zimmerman, "The fact remains that interest and enthusiasm for revascularization surgery is accelerating steadily as more and more qualified people participate in this surgical endeavor. Your diatribe may appeal to others who think as you do, but in no way will it change the direction of revascularization surgery."[21] There was cautious optimism but no consensus on the new CABG technique—there had been too many false starts. Matters were complicated by the fact that Favaloro had published an optimistic summary of the Cleveland Clinic's extensive experience with the controversial Vineberg internal mammary artery implant operation just one year earlier.[22] Despite these concerns, CABG quickly gained supporters because patients and doctors thought it worked.

In 1971 the National Heart and Lung Institute (NHLI) Advisory Council decided to evaluate CABG. Former ACC president Eliot Corday was a member of the committee, which was chaired by heart surgeon John Kirklin. They urged the NHI to sponsor a multicenter study of the risk, early results, and late outcome of CABG. Their committee acknowledged the "highly controversial and emotional nature of this subject," but they thought "by taking *no* position, some other perhaps less-knowledgeable branch of the government *will* soon."[23] Advisory council members hoped to contain the new operation—already gaining in popularity—until its safety and efficacy were known. Their deliberations resulted in the development of a multicenter randomized clinical trial, the Coronary Artery Surgery Trial (CASS), designed to compare CABG and medical treatment in patients with angina.[24]

Congress watched with interest. Warren Magnuson voiced his concerns about CABG in the Senate chamber in 1972. He told his colleagues that almost twenty thousand bypass operations were being performed annually, although the effectiveness, indications, and contraindications of the four-year-old procedure were unknown. The Washington Democrat argued that evidence must be gathered to support the claims made for the operation, because it had major implications for "manpower, operating rooms, catheterization labs, and so on." He understood the critical linkage that existed between medical and surgical heart specialists and the tools they needed to test and operate on patients suffering from such a common disease. It was estimated that almost three million Americans had angina.[25]

Even without hard scientific proof, many heart specialists (and their patients) were impressed by the benefits of the new bypass operation. People with significant angina welcomed anything—even major surgery—to cure their symptoms. Although nitroglycerin often relieved an anginal attack, there were no medicines that predictably prevented the spells.[26] Family doctors and internists referred their patients seeking relief from this distressing symptom to cardiologists,

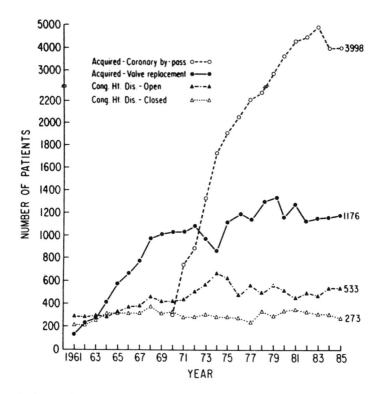

Cardiovascular surgery caseloads in New York (1961–1985).

SOURCE: J. R. Malm, "New York—a bellwether for thoracic surgery," *J. Thorac. Cardiovasc. Surg.* 92 (1986): 169–180, figure 11, p. 177.

who performed angiography to see if CABG was feasible. Doctors also hoped CABG would protect their patients from the most dreaded complication of coronary disease—heart attack with its risk of sudden death.

In 1972 New York cardiologist Charles Friedberg proclaimed CABG as the "current rage." Although he was optimistic about the operation, he thought it was "premature" for every heart surgeon to be performing it, and even less appropriate "for every hospital with available funds" to establish an open-heart surgery program.[27] Meanwhile, Johns Hopkins cardiologist Richard Ross pointed out that "economic factors" made it "difficult to be objective" about the merits of CABG. He explained that there "are cardiac surgical teams and hospitals in this country which have been doing only an occasional [open-heart] case—

one to two per week—who now, for the first time, see an opportunity to utilize the equipment and personnel and fully to profit economically from them."[28]

Coronary artery bypass surgery exploded during the 1970s as clinical evidence supporting it accumulated. In 1977 academic cardiologist Eugene Braunwald expressed concern about the "industry" that grew up around the operation; it was estimated that seventy thousand procedures would be performed in the United States that year at a total cost of nearly $1 billion. He thought the NHLI-sponsored CASS trial was a "particularly wise investment" because "the outcome will affect such a large number of patients and such a substantial fraction of medical resources." Soon, CASS and other large cooperative studies proved that the operation was safe and effective, especially for patients with severe coronary artery disease. Debate continued with respect to the relative benefits of medical versus surgical therapy for patients with angina who had less severe coronary artery disease as defined by a coronary angiogram.[29]

Who controls the catheter?

The advent of the coronary care unit, coronary angiography, and CABG helped transform cardiology into a field focused on coronary artery disease and cardiologists into "invasive" specialists whose unique tool was the cardiac catheter. But the path leading to a career as an invasive cardiologist was longer and better patrolled than the one aspiring heart specialists followed between the world wars. Then, an internist could become a cardiologist merely by acquiring an electrocardiograph and claiming proficiency in its use. Although AHA leaders received complaints about this phenomenon during the 1930s and 1940s, they were powerless to respond. America's small, disorganized community of heart specialists could not regulate the spread of the electrocardiograph, even had there been a consensus that they should try. Manufacturers were free to sell their electrocardiographs to any doctor who wanted to buy one; by the middle of the century, several inexpensive models were available.

The equipment and skills necessary to perform coronary angiography exceeded what was required to record and interpret an electrocardiogram, however. While many practitioner cardiologists and some internists bought an electrocardiograph during the middle third of the

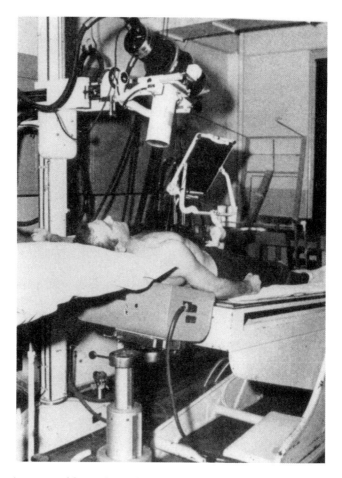

X-ray equipment used for cardiac catheterization and angiocardiography.

SOURCE: R. B. Dickerson, "Performance of angiocardiography and cardiac catheterization as a combined procedure," *Am. Heart J.* 47 (1954): 252–269, figure 2, p. 255.

century, catheterization and x-ray equipment was much larger, more complex, and extremely expensive. The technology for invasive cardiology would be purchased and managed by institutions, not individuals. Hospitals owned the equipment and eventually restricted its use to cardiologists whose fellowship directors certified that they were formally trained and qualified to use the cardiac catheter. Although all doctors own a stethoscope and many general internists interpret electrocardiograms, only 1.5 percent of American physicians currently perform cardiac catheterization.[30]

Coronary angiography would be controlled, and cardiologists would be the specialists who performed it. During the 1970s and 1980s America's large and growing community of cardiologists took possession of the cardiac catheter from the small group of invasive radiologists whose mentors had helped to invent angiography in the 1930s.[31] Whereas angiography in general and coronary angiography in particular were developed (and initially performed) mainly by radiologists, cardiac catheterization was developed by physiologists and performed by physiological cardiologists. Because cardiac catheterization and angiocardiography developed from separate traditions, two types of specialists initially performed them.[32]

The cardiologists who began doing angiocardiograms in the 1950s portrayed the move as a natural extension of cardiac catheterization that enhanced efficiency. In that era most catheterizations were performed in children born with abnormal hearts. Daniel Lukas, a

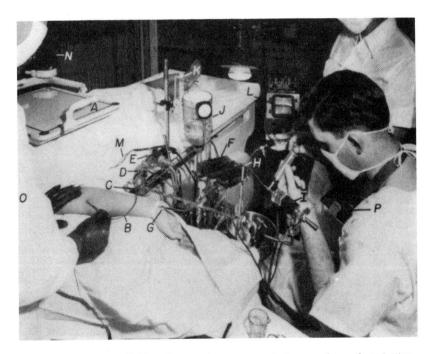

Apparatus for injecting fluids and measuring pressures during a cardiac catheterization.

SOURCE: E. H. Wood and H. J. C. Swan, "Catheterization of the heart and large vessels," in *Cardiology* (New York: McGraw-Hill, 1959) vol. 2, chapter 12, pp. 4-292 to 4-322, figure 4-164, p. 4-300. Reproduced with permission of McGraw-Hill, Inc.

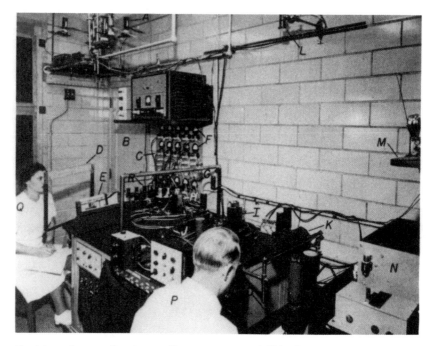

Equipment for recording intracardiac pressures, arterial blood pressure, and the electrocardiogram.

SOURCE: E. H. Wood and H. J. C. Swan, "Catheterization of the heart and large vessels," in *Cardiology* (New York: McGraw-Hill, 1959) vol. 2, chapter 12, pp. 4-292 to 4-322, figure 4-161, p. 4-296. Reproduced with permission of McGraw-Hill, Inc.

physiological cardiologist at New York Hospital, advocated combining angiocardiography with cardiac catheterization because injecting contrast into the heart's chambers could provide the cardiologist with a visual map of the blood's path through and out of the heart. "A catheter introduced into such a heart may in its wanderings resemble a rat in a psychologist's maze."[33] This combined approach would be the model adopted in most centers.

The relationship between the various types of specialists who participated in the evaluation of symptomatic cardiac patients evolved in parallel with the technology that helped to define their roles. Speaking of the diagnosis of congenital heart disease, radiologists Israel Steinberg and Charles Dotter warned in 1951, "The radiologist should not consider the stethoscope an 'antiquated instrument,' the pediatrician should not regard angiography as a traumatic procedure to be avoided at all costs, and the cardiac catheterizer should recognize his own diagnostic inadequacy in certain situations."[34] In adult cardiology, these tensions would be resolved as three specialists merged into one—the invasive cardiologist—a clinician who examined the patient and performed both cardiac catheterization and angiography.

Cardiology gained control of coronary angiography for several reasons: (1) cardiologists were *clinicians* who directed the workup of patients referred to them for chest pain; (2) coronary angiography was a procedure capable of causing cardiac arrest and death; (3) cardiologists were better trained to treat cardiac emergencies; (4) cardiology fellowship programs were poised to produce cardiologist-angiographers to meet the demand; (5) most radiology residency programs did not seek to train angiographers; (6) invasive cardiologists greatly outnumbered invasive radiologists; and (7) cardiologists outnumbered radiologists on national committees that established guidelines for the procedure.[35]

A few radiologists saw the new technique as an opportunity to advance their discipline. One cardiovascular radiology fellow urged in 1965 that all new angiographic techniques should be "the responsibility of the radiologist." He thought these advances offered "an unparalleled opportunity of increasing the stature of the radiologist as a clinician."[36] But most radiologists did not aspire to be clinicians. They defined themselves as imaging specialists who provided a valuable service, but they chose not to provide direct patient care. Although cardiologists viewed themselves as distinct from internists, they were clinicians who provided traditional patient care. They performed routine histories and physical examinations, proposed diagnoses, offered prognoses, and provided treatments.

Historian Harry Marks describes the phenomenon in a general sense: "Claims to know patients and diseases, not machines, generally underwrite physicians' rule over technologies. . . . Technical competence *per se* plays a minor role in establishing medical jurisdiction over a technology." He points out that the first radiologists were once able to use this fact to their advantage. When physicist Wilhelm Röntgen discovered x-rays in 1895, physicians claimed that their special knowledge of disease gave them the right to take over the medical applications of the powerful rays from the scientists and photographers who initially worked in the field.[37] Gradually, these practitioner radiologists were replaced by full-time radiologists who did not participate in traditional patient care but focused their activities on imaging techniques. One result of this decision was that radiologists lost control of the patients they examined.

Radiologists were skilled in imaging, but they were not trained to care for heart patients, especially patients undergoing a procedure that could cause life-threatening cardiac arrhythmias. Johns Hopkins cardiology chief Richard Ross warned in 1963 that coronary angiography "is not without hazard, and the investigator must be aware of the risks and be prepared to deal with emergency situations that may develop."[38] As experience with the procedure grew, it became apparent that the risks were acceptable but real: approximately three patients in a thousand died as a result of the procedure.[39] Nonfatal complications were more common. Radiologist angiographer Sven Paulin warned in 1970 that "cardiac reactions, such as ventricular fibrillation or rather long lasting electrocardiographic changes are often recorded."[40]

Bypass surgery was a powerful stimulus for the diffusion of coronary angiography, which provided crucial information for deciding whether angina patients should be treated with medicines or surgery. If an operation was feasible, angiography gave the surgeon a road map for the procedure.[41] By the early 1970s René Favaloro had published his technique of coronary bypass surgery, and as a consequence demand for invasive cardiologists increased dramatically. Coronary angiography and CABG transformed the management of patients with angina. Writing just before CABG was introduced, a British doctor claimed that coronary angiography "seems at present to offer little that cannot be more easily obtained by much simpler methods, such as good history-taking and electrocardiography." Once CABG was developed and accepted as a rational approach, coronary angiography had a distinct purpose.[42]

Five years later (and just three years after Favaloro described CABG), cardiovascular radiologist Harold Baltaxe claimed that coronary angiography had "become a routine procedure, even in the community hospital." He predicted the number of coronary angiograms would soon "skyrocket to the point where there will be an acute shortage of physicians capable of performing the procedure."[43] But America's cardiology training programs seized the opportunity and began producing large numbers of invasive cardiologists.

Radiologist Melvin Judkins, a pioneer of coronary angiography, was upset that cardiologists had taken over the procedure. In 1974 he complained that for a decade, "the nation has been training virtually every new cardiologist in the techniques of cardiac physiology and angiography, most with a somewhat limited experience in coronary arteriography." He was especially annoyed that each cardiologist "enters the field with the inalienable right to perform such unforgiving techniques." Addressing the rapid increase in the number of institutions performing cardiac catheterization, Judkins thought laboratories should be developed only if there was a "real need, rather than as a 'me too' prestige service."[44]

A 1977 study of eight community hospitals in the Seattle area revealed that of the nineteen persons who performed coronary angiography, seventeen were cardiologists and only two were radiologists.[45] America's rapidly expanding community of invasive cardiologists was gaining control of the catheter. But who was controlling the catheterizers? During the 1977 ACC annual session, three pioneers of coronary angiography (cardiologists Mason Sones and William Sheldon, and radiologist Melvin Judkins) created the Society for Cardiac Angiography (SCA). They had invited approximately twenty invasive cardiologists and cardiovascular radiologists to their organizational meeting. This new society illustrates that specialists define themselves in various ways; the doctors who created the SCA saw themselves as specialists who used a specific tool (the catheter) and a single technology (the x-ray) to evaluate one organ (the heart). This progressive fragmentation of cardiology into subdisciplines based on technology would accelerate during the 1970s (Table A5).

The SCA founders set an ambitious agenda: (1) establish criteria for training individuals in catheterization and angiographic techniques; (2) develop and maintain a database to track morbidity and mortality related to these procedures; (3) support research; (4) develop techniques for self-assessment and peer review; and (5) define requirements for diagnostic cardiac catheterization and angiographic facilities. Although membership in the new society was "strictly limited to individuals who had become experts in the broad field of cardiac catheterization and angiography," both cardiologists and radiologists were invited to apply. They could not be casual specialists; candidates had to have had at least five years of catheterization experience and to have performed at least one thousand diagnostic procedures.[46]

Three years later the SCA published standards that, de facto, transferred control of the cardiac catheter to invasive cardiologists in the

United States. They required that "a radiologist/cardiac angiographer who was operating independently must be trained to make a diagnosis and institute the proper therapy in a crisis situation." Radiologists who wanted to perform coronary angiograms had to be prepared to diagnose and treat all types of cardiac arrhythmias and "be familiar with all the modalities of cardiopulmonary resuscitation." Moreover, they had to do the work of a clinician, obtaining an adequate history and performing a "complete physical examination."[47] Radiologists were not interested in becoming cardiologists. They had chosen their specialty; radiology was a dynamic and lucrative field in its own right. The powerful new technique of computerized transverse axial tomography (the CAT scan) was introduced into America in 1973, noncardiac angiography was growing, and general diagnostic ultrasound was developing rapidly.[48]

The SCA committee that developed these guidelines included five cardiologists and four radiologists. Their conclusion was that a clinician rather than an imaging specialist should perform coronary angiography. And once cardiologists controlled the catheter for injecting contrast into the coronary arteries, they assumed responsibility for injecting into the heart's cavities (formerly the role of the radiologist-angiographer). The contest was over: cardiologists would perform both cardiac catheterization and cardiac angiography. A recent study of 187 hospitals in the United States found no radiologists performing coronary angiography.[49] They maintained responsibility for the x-ray equipment necessary to perform coronary angiography and often provided formal interpretation of the images the test produced, however.

Meanwhile, cardiologists competed with radiologists for control of another powerful diagnostic imaging technique, cardiac ultrasound (echocardiography). Diagnostic ultrasound evolved from military research which led to the invention of Sonar and Radar. An ultrasound machine transmits high-frequency sound waves (greater than 2 million cycles per second) that are reflected by solid objects. Some reflected sound waves return to their source, and the machine then transforms them into a visual image of the structures they hit. Although radiologists played a significant role in developing and diffusing general diagnostic ultrasound, some clinical specialists were active initially in organ-specific uses of the technology (e.g., cardiologists, neurosurgeons, and obstetricians).[50]

The technique was first used to image the heart in 1954 by physicist Helmuth Hertz and cardiologist Inge Edler of the University of Lund, Sweden. There was little interest in echocardiography for a decade, according to Edler: "The cardiologists were satisfied with the new invasive techniques: heart catheterization and angiography."[51] By the early 1960s several European groups were developing echocardiography as a clinical tool to detect mitral valve stenosis and pericardial effusion (fluid around the heart). The first publication on echocardiography in America appeared in 1962, when Edler contributed a paper on "ultrasonic cardiology" to the multivolume encyclopedia of cardiology published by the ACC. In it, he included ultrasound images of the aortic, mitral, and tricuspid valves as well as examples of mitral stenosis, pericardial effusion, and an intracardiac tumor. The technology migrated to the United States through the University of Pennsylvania, where biomedical engineers John Reid and Herman Schwann collaborated with cardiologist Claude Joyner to repeat and extend Hertz and Edler's work.[52]

Harvey Feigenbaum, a cardiologist at Indiana University, was America's most zealous promoter of echocardiography during the 1960s and 1970s. He was impressed with the ability of ultrasound to detect pericardial effusion, a potentially life-threatening condition. Standard approaches for diagnosing this problem were awkward or invasive (requiring catheterization).[53] The portable echocardiograph machine made it possible to detect a pericardial effusion promptly, noninvasively, and without risk. Feigenbaum popularized this in a widely read 1965 article in the *Journal of the American Medical Association,* which encouraged many hospitals to buy echocardiograph machines and cardiologists to learn to use them.[54]

The ACC helped to promote echocardiography. Feigenbaum and Joyner participated in a luncheon panel on the test at the college's 1966 annual meeting.[55] Feigenbaum emphasized the clinical and research value of echocardiography, trained many fellows in the technique, sponsored and participated in frequent continuing medical education courses on echocardiography, and published a popular book on the subject. In 1975 Feigenbaum organized the American Society of Echocardiography "to promote, maintain and pursue excellence in the ultrasonic examination of the heart."[56] He recalls, "We had to have some sort of quality control." The "potential for abuses was great" because the test was harmless and, unlike cardiac catheterization and angiography, could be performed in doctors' offices. There were no restrictions on who could purchase an ultrasound machine, and they cost less than $10 thousand. Feigenbaum feared inadequately trained doctors would buy one, "and there were plenty of companies around who would be willing to sell it" and "just go about their merry way."[57]

Echocardiography diffused quickly once it became apparent that it was useful for evaluating patients with common clinical problems such as heart murmurs and congestive heart failure. Although some practitioner cardiologists learned to interpret echocardiograms by attending continuing medical education programs, the technique was disseminated mainly by new cardiology graduates who had received formal training in it.[58] An active biomedical industry grew up around ultrasound imaging during the 1970s. Taking advantage of advances in electronics and computer technology, industry scientists and engineers collaborated with academics to invent "two-dimensional" echocardiography, which provided much better visualization of the heart than the original single-plane technique. ACC president Borys Surawicz predicted that this innovation would "fare better than the nearly defunct three-dimensional movies in our theaters."[59]

Surawicz was right. During the next decade, the diagnostic power of echocardiography was enhanced further with the introduction of color flow imaging (which could show whether the heart valves leaked) and quantitative techniques that could show whether the valves were obstructed. These innovations, based on the Doppler principle, affected patient care. Two-dimensional and Doppler echocardiography obviated the need for catheterization and angiocardiography in many cases of congenital heart disease and acquired valvular heart disease. These advanced echo techniques made it possible to assess whether or not valvular abnormalities were present, and if so, how severe they were. The heart's pumping function could also be acurately assessed using echocardiography.

Today, cardiologists control echocardiography, a goal that the ACC helped achieve through its continuing medical education programs and policy statements. College leaders understood the concept of turf. In 1973 ACC president Jeremy Swan warned, "to identify all imaging including echo techniques as being exclusive radiological territory would be disastrous to the field of medicine and patient care in general and to the sub-specialty of cardiology in particular."[60] Two years later, the college's Long Range Planning Committee approved a motion "strongly supporting the concept that echocardiography is the province of cardiologists."[61]

A few radiologists were concerned. The author of a 1978 essay entitled "Let us not lose echocardiography" urged academic radiologists to include echocardiography training in their residency programs.[62] It was too late; as with angiography, cardiologists controlled the patients. They could learn about echocardiography, buy a machine, and interpret the tests without any involvement by radiologists. By 1987 fewer than 5 percent of academic radiology programs had any responsibility for interpreting echocardiograms.[63]

Meanwhile, another noninvasive cardiac diagnostic technique gained momentum. The search for noninvasive alternatives to catheterization was motivated by a desire for less expensive and safer outpatient procedures useful to both clinicians and researchers. Nuclear cardiology (a variety of techniques that use radioisotopes injected into the bloodstream to test the heart's pumping function and its blood supply) gave doctors another tool for studying common clinical problems such as congestive heart failure and coronary artery disease.[64] Cardiologists wanted to have free access to this evolving diagnostic field, but they faced an obstacle that did not exist with ultrasound. The federal government had taken a strong regulatory stand on the use of radioisotopes because of increasing concern about the risks of radiation exposure.[65]

ACC past president Sam Fox told the college trustees in 1975 that it was crucial that cardiologists be able to learn and use nuclear cardiology techniques "without inhibition by others who feel this is in their guild area."[66] Seven years later, the college also challenged the government's Nuclear Regulatory Commission plan to extend the training period for physicians who wanted to use radioisotopes for diagnostic procedures from three to six months. With the AHA, the ACC issued a statement that this change would "discourage persons well trained in cardiology from participating in nuclear cardiology and, therefore, deprive the public of the expertise cardiologists offer in nuclear cardiology studies."[67] Although they would not dominate nuclear cardiology, cardiologists were not precluded from performing and interpreting the tests if they met the Nuclear Regulatory Commission training standards. Most heart specialists chose not to get involved, however. By the 1980s they were busy enough with angiography, echocardiography, and other diagnostic procedures. Nuclear cardiology became the shared domain of nuclear medicine specialists, cardiologists, and radiologists.

Technological innovations were not limited to diagnosis. Permanent electronic cardiac pacemakers were invented in Sweden and the United States in the late 1950s. University of Buffalo surgeon William Chardack reported the successful implantation of battery-powered pacemakers built by engineer Wilson Greatbatch in 1960.[68] This report heralded a new era in the treatment of patients with symptomatic heart block. Their symptoms ranged from dizziness and lightheadedness to fainting and seizures. Many symptomatic patients died. In 1951, before pacemakers were invented, Paul White advised injecting epinephrine intramuscularly "at intervals of every few hours as needed." But this approach, used for decades, was impractical for chronic therapy.[69] Many Americans learned about pacemakers in a 1961 article in the *Saturday Evening Post*. They read that "an amazing new pocket-size ticker sparks hesitant heartbeats and provides added years of near-normal life for many cardiac patients."[70]

The earliest permanent pacemakers were not developed in the laboratories of universities, research institutes, or large private firms. Greatbatch assembled his in a workshop in a barn behind his farmhouse. Earl Bakken founded Medtronic, today America's largest pacemaker manufacturing firm, in a garage where he repaired electronic equipment for the University of Minnesota. Bakken recalled recently that there was initially "a lot of skepticism" about pacemakers. The original models were not implanted under the skin. These external pacemakers consisted of wires attached to the heart connected through a skin incision to a large battery kept at the patient's side. Although Bakken's fledgling firm sold hundreds of external pacemakers between 1958 and 1961, business skyrocketed when a fully implantable system was invented. Within fifteen years, more than 150,000 pacemakers were implanted in the United States.[71]

This powerful therapeutic technology attracted cardiologists and heart surgeons. Pacemaker implantation is a surgical procedure. Some cardiologists performed or participated in the operation, but surgeons did many of them. The operator makes an incision under local anesthesia and inserts the pacemaker generator (the first ones were three inches in diameter and almost an inch thick) into a "pocket" fashioned under the skin. This battery is then connected to a flexible electrode that carries electrical impulses to the heart. The incision is closed and the pacemaker stimulates the heart to beat at a preset rate.[72] Although pacemaker implantation was a minor surgical procedure, many cardiologists chose not to perform it. Surgeons Seymour Furman, Dryden Morse, and Victor Parsonnet and academic cardiologist Warren Harthorne hoped to organize the field by founding the North American Society of Pacing and Electrophysiology (NASPE) in 1979.[73] Concerned that too many doctors were implanting pacemakers, Parsonnet thought NASPE and the ACC's pacemaker committee (which he chaired) should focus on quality of care.[74]

Staff and capital equipment costs limited the multiplication of catheterization laboratories and open-heart surgery programs, and government regulations restricted the spread of nuclear cardiology. These retarding influences were not operative in the case of pacemakers, which moved into community hospitals quickly because they cured a previously untreatable problem and were relatively simple to install and maintain. Parsonnet attributed the rapid diffusion to the "generous financial incentives for both the practitioner and the hospital" provided by private insurance and Medicare.[75] Manufacturers also benefited. Because most patients needing pacemakers were older, "innovators in this field had a federally subsidized market for their products," according to one policy analyst.[76]

How much technology and how many cardiologists do we need?

During the second half of the twentieth century, the new diagnostic technologies and therapeutic procedures for heart patients spread rapidly from academic medical centers and large multispecialty group practices such as the Mayo Clinic and the Cleveland Clinic to community hospitals across the country.[77] Market forces encouraged the migration. Cardiac disease was common in middle-aged and older people; more than a million Americans had heart attacks each year. Citizens were better informed about health care as the news media continued to emphasize medical "breakthroughs."[78] The accelerating suburbanization of America also encouraged the spread of sophisticated heart care. Between 1949, when the ACC was founded in New York, and 1970, when Heart House was being planned in Bethesda, the "urbanized" area of Washington, D.C., increased from 181 to 523 square miles. By 1980 two-thirds of America's dwelling units were single-family homes surrounded by a yard—and they were occupied by people who wanted health care nearby when they got sick.[79]

The increasing availability of health insurance as a benefit of employment also fueled the public's demand for specialized heart care. After 1965 all American citizens over the age of sixty-five (with few exceptions) and approximately three-quarters of other Americans had hospital insurance. For many patients with an acute illness that required hospitalization, cost was no longer a barrier to specialty care. If they had (or got) heart disease, insured patients wanted access to "modern" cardiac care close to home, and this meant technology and heart specialists. By the mid-1970s the nation's cardiology and cardiothoracic surgery training programs were producing a record number of practitioners to meet the demand. These doctors transferred innovations like coronary angiography, echocardiography, and open-heart surgery from academic centers to community hospitals across town and around the country.

Writing a decade before the invention of CABG, four surgeons from Asbury Park, New Jersey, declared in 1959 that "open-heart surgery is entirely within the realm of a great many small city and community hospitals." They justified their position by claiming that fifty thousand infants were born annually with some form of congenital heart disease and twenty-five thousand Americans had acquired valvular heart disease that could be treated surgically. This ambitious foursome demanded action. "Given the trained surgeon and an interested and dedicated group of workers in a community hospital," they wrote, "there may be excuses but there are no real reasons why this newest surgical innovation cannot be added to the protocol. Postponement . . . for supposedly better times, circumstances, conditions, or machines, may cost the hospital an opportunity to take a giant scientific step forward." Action benefited everyone, including patients who had a right to "this recent and effective treatment."[80]

Many surgeons and hospitals around the country shared this view and had acted on it. Although there were only 86 medical schools in 1961, there were already 513 catheterization laboratories, 777 closed-heart surgery programs, and 327 open-heart surgery programs.[81] Hospitals encouraged the diffusion of talent and technology. Administrators and board members wanted to enhance their hospitals' image and earnings by adding services and specialists to attract more patients. Manufacturers of diagnostic and therapeutic equipment were happy to cooperate; diffusion meant bigger markets and more profit. Initially, almost everyone believed this series of events served the public interest.

Many people framed the diffusion of specialty care and technology in terms of fairness. If sophisticated heart care was available only at academic medical centers, few Americans would have access to it.[82] In 1969 the Inter-Society Commission for Heart Disease Resources sought to "provide the opportunity to physicians and hospitals throughout the United States to deliver the latest advances in diagnosis and treatment" to cardiac patients. This recommendation reflected the ideology of the Regional Medical Programs Service, which funded the commission, and the heart lobby (represented by Irving Wright, who chaired the commission). Although the commission's ambitions and proposals seemed logical to many academics, they worried some health care planners.[83]

Just as government funding catalyzed academic medicine in the 1950s and 1960s, Medicare and other insurance plans now fueled the private sector (Table A10). Liberal "cost-plus" reimbursement policies made it easier for community hospitals to acquire expensive diagnostic equipment (such as catheterization laboratories), institute new programs (such as open-heart surgery), and attract specialists (such as cardiologists and cardiac surgeons). The real dollar value of shipments of x-ray and medical electronic equipment increased tenfold in the United States between 1963 and 1983, to more than $2 billion annually.[84] Some cardiologists and surgeons urged restraint with respect to establishing catheterization laboratories and open-heart programs. Their stated reasons included the underutilization of many existing facilities and the presumption that quality related directly to volume. The threat of competition was an unstated concern. Other heart specialists argued for diffusion, even if they were not seeking to establish a program out of self-interest or for the benefit of their trainees.

In 1970 Cleveland Clinic surgeon Donald Effler argued that the epidemiology of coronary artery disease demanded that both medical and surgical therapy should be "available at the local level." He explained, "The understandable tendency to divert coronary patients to a few established centers will, in the long run, be neither practical nor desirable." As a first step, Effler advocated introducing coronary angiography "to the community hospital," rejecting the "oft heard lament" that it was "highly dangerous and expensive."[85] Effler made these statements supporting the aggressive expansion of modern heart care just two years after his colleague Favaloro had reported the introduction of CABG. In that brief time, new surgical procedures (such as internal mammary-coronary artery anastomosis and multiple vein grafts) had been developed that promised to expand the pool of angina patients who might benefit from CABG.[86]

In 1973 the Inter-Society Commission for Heart Disease Resources raised concerns about the nation's cardiac surgery programs in its report on "optimal resources for coronary artery surgery." It charged that some heart surgery programs created during the past two decades "failed to function satisfactorily because of poor planning, inadequate staff and material resources or insufficient case loads." Moreover, "others remained in existence but with resources and case loads so marginal as to raise serious questions about their effectiveness, safety and economic soundness." The recent introduction of CABG heightened concern. "There is evidence that we may again see a proliferation of poorly conceived, poorly planned units with costly duplication of facilities and sub-optimal care."[87]

The commission proposed that heart surgery be restricted to hospitals performing at least four open-heart operations a week, and that community hospitals be prohibited from building a cardiac catheterization laboratory unless the projected volume exceeded ten procedures a week. The first proposal was problematic for surgeons and hospital administrators. In 1969 only 7 percent of the 518 hospitals performing open or closed cardiac operations achieved the recommended annual case load of two hundred procedures.[88] Another study revealed that the five hospitals in Seattle equipped for open-heart surgery performed a total of just 318 procedures in 1968, less than one-third of the recommended minimum. Although these hospitals had adequate capacity, they did not have the patients.[89] The proponents of diffusion argued that CABG would eliminate the underutilization, however.

Hundreds of hospitals had established their heart surgery programs before the enactment of the Heart Disease, Cancer, and Stroke Amendments of 1965 (PL 89-239) and the National Health Planning and Resources Development Act of 1974 (PL 93-641), laws designed, in part, to curb the spread of expensive new technology.[90] The government was now willing to take on the difficult issue of escalating health care cost. A report prepared by President Nixon's Council on Wage and Price Stability seven years after the advent of Medicare concluded that "the increased capability of physicians to treat illness, using more sophisticated and expensive techniques, increased the demand for better insurance protection. This in turn, probably assisted in the development and provision of still more sophisticated and costly care." They had identified the problem, and they knew that the government had contributed to it.[91]

As tensions mounted, some observers charged that Medicare reimbursement policies contributed to unnecessary construction and overutilization. Academic internist and former American College of Physicians (ACP) president Robert Petersdorf complained in 1976, "Visiting small communities in rural Washington, I often see a patient lounge ripped out to make room for a catheterization suite."[92] Two years later, ACP president Jeremiah Barondess, an academic internist at New York Hospital, charged that money was the "driving force in the diffusion and use of technologic capacity." He expressed concern that physicians and hospitals had "financial incentives to make heavy use of technology."[93]

Hospitals were major participants in the process. Community hospitals, like academic medical centers, wanted to increase their income. They were the institutions that built most of the catheterization laboratories and offered surgeons the facilities, equipment, and staff necessary to develop open-heart surgery programs. Reflecting on the 1970s, Petersdorf and Public Health Service cardiologist Thomas Preston charged that "ill-conceived chauvinism" had led America's medium and large hospitals to construct "facilities for coronary angiography and surgery."[94]

But their harsh assessment ignored a critical part of the equation—patient demand. Many practitioners and community hospital administrators would have considered the charge a manifestation of academic arrogance. Community hospitals were competing with teaching hospitals, and some were winning. They were transforming themselves into larger, more comprehensive institutions in order to compete in the marketplace. "Name inflation" was part of this process, according to health policy analyst and historian Daniel Fox. During the 1970s many community hospitals denoted themselves "medical centers," hoping to win prestige and patients by being "identified with education, research, and advancing technology."[95]

One hospital administrator complained in 1972 that "everybody wants to become a medical center. . . . Every hospital has taken the attitude that they are in pursuit of excellence and damn the cost, go ahead. . . . we've got to do everything for everybody."[96] That year Senator Abraham Ribicoff, former Secretary of the Department of Health, Education and Welfare under John Kennedy, predicted that the 1960s and 1970s would be remembered as "the years when the sky was the limit in medical costs." The Connecticut Democrat proclaimed that the "American health care industry attained a moment in the sun" when "it became a bigger business in the United States than national defense." A $27 billion industry in 1960 had grown to a $79 billion enterprise in 1972.[97] That year, about 38 cents of each health care dollar went to hospitals and 25 cents went to physicians.[98]

Doctors were a more important part of the health care equation than their direct cost share suggested. They supervised the patient's diagnostic workup and therapy and influenced where those activities took place. Hospitals hoping to develop a state-of-the-art heart care program needed more than catheterization laboratories, operating rooms, and a new name. Above all, they needed trained specialists to attract and admit the patients and perform the complex diagnostic and therapeutic procedures these people needed. Academic medicine re-sponded to the increasing demand for practitioners by turning out record numbers of cardiologists in the 1970s. Just as there had been no rules governing the spread of cardiac catheterization laboratories prior to the 1970s when certificate of need legislation, designed to restrict the purchase of major equipment, was enacted, there was no system to regulate the number of cardiologists produced.[99]

Along with this explosion of technology and hospital-based care, the number of physicians increased dramatically in the United States beginning in the early 1970s as a result of new government policies. By 1960 most opinion leaders agreed that America needed more doctors. The federal government first committed significant resources to aug-ment the physician workforce in 1963 with enactment of the Health Professions Educational Assistance Act (PL 88-129). By now, there were many complex forces affecting America's health care system. In a report prepared for the Association of American Medical Colleges (AAMC) in 1965, Lowell Coggeshall, an academic internist who was vice president of the University of Chicago, identified twelve major health care trends in the United States (Table A7). These "inextricably intertwined" trends were: (1) accelerating scientific advances; (2) an expanding (and aging) population; (3) increasing individual health expectations; (4) enhanced ability to pay for care; (5) unrelenting specialization; (6) diffusion of and growing dependence on technology; (7) progressive institutionalization of care (office and hospital rather than home); (8) increasing teamwork in health care delivery; (9) growing demand for physicians; (10) rising employment of other health personnel; (11) expanding government involvement in health care; and (12) rising costs.[100]

Although the Coggeshall report stressed the continuing trend toward specialization and its implications for health care delivery, it did not include a specific recommendation on physician workforce. In 1966 the AMA published a report on graduate medical education that did. Chaired by Case Western Reserve University president John Millis, Ph.D., the Citizens Commission on Graduate Medical Education challenged the "arrogance in specialized medicine" and urged a reaffirmation of the important role of the "primary physician." The Millis report supported training more physicians "competent and willing to offer comprehensive and continuing care" to counterbalance the "fragmentation" of care that had resulted from progressive specialization.[101]

Although the government was not yet prepared to regulate the process of specialization, it was convinced that the country needed more doctors. Congress gave medical schools more than $5 billion in direct funding between 1965 and 1971.[102] This led (as planned) to a dramatic increase in the number of both medical schools and students (Table A8). It also helped to swell the ranks of specialists. By this time, the academics who taught America's medical students and residents were not part-time practitioners or primary care physicians; they were full-time clinical scientists and specialists. Richard Ross, who witnessed this massive federal investment in medical education, recalls that the new medical schools recruited their faculties from research-oriented academic medical centers. Those individuals "went out and developed programs designed to replicate themselves. So we had this virus, if you will, of high-tech specialty medicine replicating itself in medical schools that really were built to . . . train practitioners."[103]

Cardiology was already growing when the government-financed infusion of more medical students supercharged the system. Between 1949 and 1960 the number of cardiology fellowship programs and trainees increased tenfold, and the trend continued during the next decade (Table A9). Just as NIH research grants had helped many academic medical centers build and equip catheterization laboratories during the 1950s, Medicare made it possible for more nonteaching hospitals to install them after 1965. This fueled the demand for invasive cardiologists across the country. Cardiology technology and trainees went hand-in-hand. Liberal government funding had created an academic infrastructure capable of rapid expansion, and cardiology training programs were poised to meet the growing demand for practitioner cardiologists to diffuse new diagnostic tools such as coronary angiography and echocardiography.

Calls for more heart specialists had echoed through Washington for two decades when Lyndon Johnson's 1965 Commission on Heart Disease, Cancer and Stroke decried the "critical shortage" of formally trained practitioner cardiologists.[104] Leaders at the NHI shared the commission's belief that the nation needed more clinical cardiologists. The following year, acting director William Zukel told Congress that cardiology was one of half a dozen specialties with "alarming manpower shortages." He explained that the institute had developed plans to provide specialized training for hundreds of clinical cardiologists over the next five years. Their training would emphasize "the latest methods of diagnosis, treatment, and patient care."[105]

Although the heart lobby had lost some of its strongest voices by 1969 (Fogarty had died of a myocardial infarction and Lister Hill had retired), Washington Senator Warren Magnuson emerged as a strong supporter of the cause. That year, this influential Democrat strongly urged his colleagues to increase the NHI's budget because "heart disease is clearly a major national problem." Magnuson was "particularly disturbed" that appropriations to support training clinical fellows were scheduled to be cut. He protested that although 55 percent of hospitalized patients had cardiovascular disease, "only hospitals in large cities have an adequate corps of well-trained cardiologists."[106] But this was changing as more fellows entered practice. Between 1961 and 1976 the number of cardiology training programs grew from 72 to 253, and the number of fellows increased tenfold from 142 to 1,409 (Table A9).

Several things contributed to this explosive increase. During this fifteen-year interval, the number of medical school graduates rose by 72 percent (Table A8). Meanwhile, the number of international (foreign) medical graduates entering cardiology training and practice in the United States also increased dramatically (Table 8-4). The tensions that Franz Groedel and other immigrant physicians faced when they came to America during the 1930s and 1940s had eased as a perceived doctor

TABLE 8-4

International (Foreign) Medical Graduates as a Percentage of Newly Licensed U.S. Physicians (1950–1975)

YEAR:	1950	1960	1970	1975
PERCENTAGE:	5.1	17.7	27.3	35.4

SOURCE: W. G. Rothstein, *American Medical Schools and the Practice of Medicine, a History* (New York: Oxford Univ. Press, 1987), p. 216.

glut turned into a doctor shortage after World War II. In this context, progressive changes in immigration and medical licensing laws made it easier for foreign-born physicians to come to America for postgraduate training and to stay afterwards.[107] The number of international medical graduate cardiologists increased by 228 percent between 1970 and 1985 in the United States (Table 8-5).

By the 1960s most graduates of United States medical schools were becoming specialists, and many were attracted to fields they perceived to be dynamic, interesting, and lucrative. Cardiology won on all three counts. Senator Ribicoff protested in 1972 that internists, family physicians, and pediatricians had come to be viewed as "medicine's second class citizens" as a result of unrelenting specialization.[108] But specialists were perceived to be "in the vanguard of scientific medical practice," according to a member of the National Academy of Sciences.[109] At the time, cardiology was seen as a prestigious specialty with many job opportunities. Sociologist Stephen Shortell asked a sample of Chicago physicians, patients, and business school students in 1974 to rank

TABLE 8-5

Birth Origin and Medical School Graduation of Self-Designated Cardiologists in the United States (1970–1985)

	1970	1975	1980	1985
Foreign-born, foreign medical school	909	1,280	2,072	2,985
U.S.-born and U.S. medical school	4,920	5,550	7,575	9,733
U.S.-born, foreign medical school	92	103	176	297
Total self-designated cardiologists	5,921	6,933	9,823	13,015
Foreign-born as a percentage of total	15	18	21	23

SOURCE: P. R. Kletke, W. D. Marder, and S. L. Thran, *Socioeconomic Characteristics of Cardiology Practice* (Chicago: AMA, 1988), table 3.3, p. 57.

forty-one medical specialties and paramedical fields "according to what *you personally* believe the prestige of that occupation to be." Cardiology fared well: physicians ranked it second (tied with neurosurgery; thoracic surgery was first), patients ranked it third (neurosurgery was first and thoracic surgery was second), and business students ranked it second (neurosurgery was first).[110]

At first, this proliferation of specialists seemed to be in the best interest of patients and the nation. Technology without specialists trained to use it properly was not only wasteful, it was potentially dangerous. Louder voices were beginning to challenge the traditional *laissez faire* approach to specialty training and technology diffusion. Senator Edward Kennedy urged the adoption of national health insurance and other reforms in his 1972 book, *In Critical Condition: The Crisis in America's Health Care.* Whereas Kennedy believed that doctors should have the "right to choose their style of practice, their specialty, and the location of their practice," he argued that citizens should have the "opportunity to influence the cost, quality, and organization of health care." The debate was relevant to cardiologists and other specialists. The Massachusetts Democrat proposed that the government should be able to offer "incentives" to encourage doctors to "practice in a manner, in a specialty, and in a place where the people's need is the greatest."[111]

Two years later, in a speech at Yale Medical School, Kennedy warned, "As the major investor, the American people have more than a passive interest in what you do and how you go about doing it." Because academic medicine was heavily subsidized by taxpayers, citizens "have the right to expect that their dollars will be wisely spent and used in the effort to address the major elements of the health care crisis." Kennedy argued that this extended to "the organization, delivery and financing of medical care, as well as in the search for new knowledge."[112]

Republicans were also concerned about health care costs. President Richard Nixon proposed important changes in the way government funded medical education and training in 1973. Under his plan, clinical research and training grants and faculty "career development awards" would be eliminated, and research grants would be cut except for cancer and heart disease. These proposals had profound implications for medical schools and teaching hospitals. Two academics predicted that "the immediate impact will be on the training of cardiologists, hematologists, gastroenterologists, and other subspecialists. Faculty positions will be lost."[113]

By this time, academic cardiologists viewed the ACC as an organization that understood their concerns and was willing to articulate their agenda. Cardiology programs had grown dramatically in size and number during the quarter-century since passage of the National Heart Act. Clinical demands had increased markedly with the introduction of coronary angiography, echocardiography, CABG, and other innovations. Richard Ross chaired the Johns Hopkins cardiology division between 1960 and 1975. He sees clinical demands as the driving force behind the striking expansion of cardiology training programs during that era: "Programs have grown because the service load has grown."[114]

Many academic cardiologists, whose rank and salary usually depended on their research productivity, had come to rely on trainees (who functioned independently) to do much of the routine clinical work. The proposed cuts in fellowship support threatened academic cardiology by depleting the supply of trainees. ACC's longtime executive director William Nelligan recalls many discussions about this dilemma among academic cardiologists: "They'd just throw up their hands and say, 'We can't operate without all the fellows. They're there to take care of people.'"[115]

When the Nixon administration proposed phasing out fellowship support beginning in July 1973, former ACC president Eliot Corday informed the trustees that government officials had told him the move reflected the belief that after completing federally subsidized specialty training, "cardiologists . . . go out into practice and earn $50,000 a year right off if they run cardiac catheterization labs." The government was becoming increasingly reluctant to "pump money into training programs" because most fellows entered practice rather than research careers.[116] No one could dispute the fact that most specialists entered practice after completing training usually partly or wholly subsidized by the government. According to Richard Ross, cardiology program directors often labeled their trainees as research fellows because that was "the way to get people funded."[117] They did research, but most of them, like nearly all medical school matriculants, wanted to become doctors rather than researchers or teachers.

The irony in the proposed cuts in clinical training grants was that just a few years earlier Congress had wanted to produce more practitioner cardiologists. Two influential members of the heart lobby, Irving Wright and Michael DeBakey, had claimed there was a "critical shortage" of cardiologists in 1965. As government funding cuts loomed on the horizon, tensions rose with respect to the allocation of what money might remain. Some academics—especially those not involved in demanding clinical specialties like cardiology, with its high volume of acutely ill patients—agreed with the politicians who wanted to eliminate clinical (and restrict research) training grants. Harvard Medical School dean Robert Ebert, an internist, argued in 1973 that the government should not support programs that were nothing more than a vehicle "for the training of future practitioners in the sub-specialties."[118]

In this context Senator Ribicoff made a proposal that helped set the stage for several medical workforce studies during the 1970s. The Connecticut Democrat urged the government to undertake "a series of studies and negotiations with the various specialty boards, from family practice right on up to neurosurgery, to try and determine what the future of medical manpower ought to look like."[119] There were no rules regarding the numbers and types of specialists trained in America's teaching hospitals. August Swanson of the AAMC charged in 1973 that politicians "in their frantic efforts to increase physician manpower, have focused with fevered intensity on expanding medical school enrollments [and] creating more medical schools." But no one tried to manage specialization. Rather than reflecting the nation's needs, Swanson claimed that the numbers of residency and fellowship slots were "determined by the aggressiveness of hospitals and service chiefs seeking to fill their manpower needs."[120]

When the ACC began to focus on the workforce issue in the early 1970s, there was no complete list of cardiology training programs, so the context, content, quality, duration of training, and number of positions were unknown. The college got an NIH grant to survey the nation's cardiology training programs, evaluate the professional activities of cardiologists, project future cardiology workforce requirements, and assess the educational needs of heart specialists. They defined "cardiologists" broadly and chose to include all physicians who indicated in the AMA directory that they had a primary or secondary interest in cardiovascular disease (Table 8-6).[121]

The ACC survey revealed that practitioner cardiologists were equally divided between those who devoted more than half of their time to cardiology and those who spent more than half of their time functioning as general internists. The surveyors found that only half of the self-designated heart specialists were certified in internal medicine and only 10 percent were certified in cardiology. These statistics reveal

TABLE 8-6
A Snapshot of U.S. Cardiology (1972–1973)

Self-designated cardiologists	10,691
Training programs (active)	280
Fellows graduated (1973)	793
Fellows enrolled (1973)	1,278
Cardiology faculty members (full-time)	1,513
Full-time faculty/training program	4.6
ACC members	5,468
ABIM certified cardiologists (cum. total)	1,718
Cardiologists per 100,000 population	5.6
Total physicians per 100,000 population	168
Cardiologists as a percentage of U.S. physicians	3%
Average age of cardiologists	48

SOURCE: N. O. Fowler, H. N. Hultgren, and H. D. McIntosh, "Training programs in cardiovascular disease," *Am. J. Cardiol.* 34 (1974): 429–438, and F. H. Adams, S. Abrahamson, and R. C. Mendenhall, "Development of the study," *Am. J. Cardiol.* 34 (1974): 394–396. The 280 number is derived from the published list of filled programs in 1972. ACC membership from ACC archives. Board certification data from ABIM. See also W. H. Pritchard and W. H. Abelmann, "Current status of manpower in cardiology," *Am. J. Cardiol.* 34 (1974): 408–416.

that the overwhelming majority of cardiologists saw no value in board certification. Although some of the men who created the ABIM in the 1930s assumed their examinations might be used eventually to restrict hospital privileges, that was still not the case four decades later.

The lingering practice of self-designation complicated attempts to define the cardiology workforce and plan for the future. In projecting future workforce needs, the ACC considered several variables: (1) the demand for services, (2) the spectrum of services provided, (3) the rate at which noncardiologists and paramedical personnel might assume responsibilities, and (4) the rate of change in the number of active cardiologists. Based on the survey results and their perception of trends in American medicine and cardiology, the college estimated that the nation would need approximately 4,600 additional cardiologists within three years—several hundred more than would be produced at the current rate.[122]

Academic internist Arnold Relman of the University of Pennsylvania characterized the ACC workforce survey as "an enormous step forward" and "a model of the kind of study that needs to be made by every medical subspecialty." Although Relman praised the survey, he worried about its conclusions. "Alarmed by the effects that . . . over-specialization may have on the future of internal medicine," Relman thought that "most unbiased observers" agreed that there were already too many specialists and too few primary care physicians. He favored setting limits on subspecialty training slots. But part of the equation was what each physician actually did, not just what he or she was called. With respect to cardiac disease, Relman thought "any well trained general internist or family practitioner ought to be able to provide good ambulatory care for patients with the common diseases affecting the cardiovascular system."[123]

In 1974 ACC president Henry McIntosh urged the college to support the government's goal of training more primary care physicians, in part because he thought most cardiologists did not want to provide primary care.[124] The following year Ray Cotton, the ACC's consultant for government relations, urged college leaders to "offer continually" their "views and expertise" to policy makers. He reminded them that Congress wanted to be sure that the "American taxpayer gets his dollars' worth for the tremendous federal investment in the training of medical manpower." Cotton thought the Nixon administration was inclined to "get out of the business of medical training." He warned that Senator Edward Kennedy was "heavily involved with direct federal solutions" regarding physician distribution and had introduced legislation that would set "very strict" limits on what specialties medical graduates could choose and where they could practice. The process would be managed by the "expenditure of federal dollars."[125]

Kennedy and New York Senator Jacob Javits cosponsored a bill (S 3585) in 1974 that included provisions that would influence the number and type of specialty training slots. The ACC warned its members that "Congress is beginning to show concern with the distribution of physicians by medical specialty throughout the country."[126] Concern intensified with passage of the Health Professions Educational Assistance Act of 1976 (PL 94–484). That law charged that "physician specialization has resulted in inadequate numbers of physicians engaged in the delivery of primary care" and provided subsidies to support training general internists and family physicians.[127] Despite real and threatened funding cuts, cardiology program directors were still able to get support from a variety of sources (e.g., government, AHA, hospitals) to train more fellows during the late 1970s.

By this time, America had entered the age of consumerism. Ralph Nader's provocative book *Unsafe at Any Speed* had sounded a call to arms that signaled a new era in relations among Americans, their government, and the producers of goods and services. Patients began to expect more from their doctors and hospitals.[128] Citizens were exhorting government officials to justify their decisions and explain the fiscal impact of their votes. Assistant Secretary of Health, Education and Welfare Theodore Cooper told ACC members in 1975 that the government's expenditures for health care were nearly $125 billion. That meant "the public has bought a large share of the so-called health industry and (as any major stockholder is wont to do) is demanding a greater voice in policy formulation and program development." He noted that the AMA had adopted a resolution encouraging at least 50 percent of medical graduates to go into primary care residencies. That arbitrary number had "been repeated so often that it is now the primary figure for all planning." Cooper acknowledged that recent government policies on specialty and geographical distribution of health professionals had "relied too heavily on the notion that an increase in total supply would solve the distribution problems."[129]

The problem was not just one of supply and distribution; it was also one of definition. In 1976 health policy analyst Eli Ginzberg reminded ACC members that specialists were still mainly self-designated: "At present, anyone who calls himself a specialist, is one." The ACC manpower study had confirmed that this was true for cardiology. Ginzberg also discussed the concept of "functional overlap," noting that "cardiologists [also] practice internal medicine and, in fact, provide general care for many elderly people."[130]

Forrest Adams, a pediatric cardiologist at the University of California at Los Angeles and former ACC president who had headed the college's study, asked rhetorically in 1975, "Who is a cardiologist?" He urged adoption of a narrower definition that required "cardiologists" to complete a fellowship in an approved training program and pass a "nationally administered board examination." He decried the fact that only 10 percent of America's self-designated cardiologists were certified in cardiovascular disease. This was not "in the best interests of the patient," because it was difficult for an individual to "determine that the doctor treating his cardiovascular problem is qualified to do so." Adams closed his editorial with a warning: "Some form of national health insurance is close at hand! Licensure, standards of care and evidence of continuing professional competence will almost certainly be a part of the legislation." He urged college members to "give serious thought to the various ramifications of, 'who is a cardiologist?'"[131]

Specialty credentials were becoming important, because it seemed that hospitals might finally require cardiologists and other specialists to have them. The days of self-designation seemed to be numbered. In 1975 the Inter-Society Commission for Heart Disease Resources proposed that any cardiologist participating in an open-heart surgery program should be board certified in both internal medicine and cardiology.[132] The message was clear: "Get your boards and become a fellow of the American College of Cardiology!" Trainees listened. By the end of the decade, taking board examinations at the completion of fellowship training and applying for membership in the college had become routine. This was true of other specialists as well. A 1978 study of trends in board certification concluded that an increasing number of American medical graduates "recognized the need for complete residency [or fellowship] training and specialty certification to conduct a specialty practice."[133] The career path to cardiology and other specialties was now clearly marked, and board certification was becoming a mandatory stop.

Meanwhile, the process of board certification in cardiology had become less onerous. The ABIM had decided to ease the requirements for board eligibility, beginning with medical residents who began training in 1970. They would have to spend just four years instead of five in postgraduate training to be board eligible in cardiology and other medical specialties, if they had passed their medicine board examinations. A two-year internal medicine residency followed by a two-year cardiology fellowship would suffice. Moreover, the oral examinations in cardiology (which discouraged many trainees from taking board examinations) were discontinued in 1974. This "short-track" system was short-lived, however. For candidates starting their medical training in June 1977, three years of general medical residency would be required for board eligibility. The oral examinations were never reinstated.[134] During the 1970s the number of board certified cardiologists skyrocketed as the number of trainees increased dramatically, and virtually all of them took the board examination upon completion of their training.

In 1975 the ACC held a Bethesda Conference on cardiology manpower that brought together seventy-three persons representing academic and practitioner cardiologists, academic internists, family physicians, critical care nurses, cardiology fellows, medical students, medical educators and deans, health care economists, the AMA, the Department of Health, Education and Welfare, the U.S. Public Health Service, and the NIH. By this time, the college was viewed widely as the organization that represented cardiology. It had sponsored a sophisticated workforce study and was now well represented on the cardiovascular subspecialty board of the ABIM.[135] The Health Resources Administration of the Department of Health, Education and Welfare cosponsored the meeting, which was summarized in a series of reports in the ACC's journal.

As part of the Bethesda Conference, a task force was charged to review and critique the college's two-year-old workforce study. The task force disputed several of the study's conclusions. Their most serious challenge related to whether there was an impending shortage or a surplus of cardiologists. Why the disagreement? It was as much a matter of ideology as of numbers. A team of cardiologists had interpreted the data in 1974 and concluded there would be too few heart specialists. But only one of the eight members of the 1976 Bethesda task force was a cardiologist. This new group predicted there soon would be too many heart specialists and recommended that the number of cardiology trainees be reduced from eight hundred to three hundred annually. Moreover, they suggested that the number of cardiovascular training programs "should be reduced sharply." If implemented, this recommendation would have profound implications for academic cardiologists.[136]

The main criticism the revisionists lodged against the 1974 survey was "its failure to evaluate all physicians who deliver cardiac care." Another problem, according to the 1976 task force participants, was that the original projections failed to take into account "the widespread inefficient use of well trained cardiologists as primary care physicians."[137] General internists and family physicians cared for many heart patients. One board certified "practitioner internist" surveyed his practice in 1973 and found that 30 percent of his patient contacts were for cardiac complaints.[138]

A 1978 study cosponsored by the Robert Wood Johnson Foundation and the Department of Health, Education and Welfare confirmed the ACC survey finding that most heart specialists were not practicing cardiology full-time. Board certified cardiologists spent about one-third of their time dealing with noncardiovascular problems.[139] These conclusions were problematic for the nation's 250 cardiology training program directors, whose annual output of fellows was 267 percent of the 1976 task force's recommendation. Other interested observers joined the chorus claiming there were too many cardiologists. Robert Chase of the National Board of Medical Examiners argued in 1975 that the number of "highly trained" cardiologists and heart surgeons was "beyond the public's demand." He protested that the ongoing "proliferation of new cardiac diagnostic centers and cardiac-surgery teams continues in hospitals where good regional sense deems them unnecessary" when highly trained cardiac teams were "underoccupied" in referral medical centers.[140]

Health policy analyst Eli Ginzberg participated in the 1976 ACC Bethesda manpower conference. In a presentation entitled "Manpower for cardiology: no easy answers," he pointed out the recent spectacular increase in new physicians fueled by government grants to medical schools: "By the late 1970s, the nation will have twice the number of trained physicians that it had in the late 1960s." Many people thought this was good, but Ginzberg worried about the cost. "Health care expenditures have been growing at an unsustainable rate. . . . the American public will eventually limit the share of their income devoted to health care." Still, he thought people would prefer spending those dollars for specialty care. "In spite of government policy, the public will continue to prefer specialists for many of their problems." Ginzberg predicted, "Specialization, perhaps with some modifications, will be around for a long time."[141]

The 1976 Bethesda Conference on manpower was problematic, since participants reached a conclusion diametrically opposed to that based on the college's own manpower study. Several trustees urged the college to take action. Philadelphia cardiologist Leonard Dreifus wanted the ACC to begin defining privileges for cardiologists and heart surgeons. "If we do not," he argued, "the government will." ACC president Charles Fisch thought the workforce issue was an "ideal example" of why the college "whether it likes it or not, will have to be involved, and very much so, in government relationships, relationships with other organizations, and in the economics of cardiology." Conceding the ACC's traditional focus on education, Fisch (who headed one of the nation's largest cardiology training programs at Indiana University) pointed out that the college had assumed the responsibility to represent America's cardiologists.[142]

As the workforce debate intensified, more organizations entered the fray. Academic internist Alvin Tarlov had participated in the college's Bethesda Conference on cardiology manpower as a representative of the Association of Professors of Medicine, an organization consisting of the chairs of medical school departments of internal medicine. Tarlov also chaired the Federated Council for Internal Medicine (FCIM), which included representatives of the ABIM, the ACP, the American Society of Internal Medicine (ASIM), and the Association of Professors of Medicine (APM). The FCIM, according to ACP executive vice president Edward Rosenow Jr., was designed to be a "strong single voice for internal medicine."[143]

Franz Ingelfinger, editor of the *New England Journal of Medicine,* characterized the FCIM as a "league for beleaguered internists" and charged that it was created, in part, to help internists fend off a challenge in the arena of primary care from newly empowered family physicians.[144] Cardiology and the other medical specialties were not represented in the FCIM, which was homogeneous and inbred. Rosenow explains that there was "much overlapping and cross-over representation of the leadership" of the FCIM, the ABIM, and the APM.[145] Robert Moser, Rosenow's successor at the ACP, agreed. He characterized it as "an all-internal medicine organization. We all knew each other."[146] The FCIM was composed mainly of academics who resisted the progressive fragmentation of internal medicine into subspecialties. They wanted to maintain control over their subspecialty divisions and embraced the traditional paradigm of internist first, medical specialist second.[147]

In 1978 the FCIM urged the medicine department chairs and program directors to "modify, limit, or reduce the number of clinical subspecialty training slots available in accord with the needs of the specialty." The council members also advocated changing reimbursement formulas "to achieve a better balance between payment for technical procedures and payment for cognitive clinical skills." This would encourage more doctors to enter primary care and narrow the earnings gap between internists and surgeons. It would also limit the growing income differential between internists and procedurally oriented medical specialists such as cardiologists and gastroenterologists.[148]

ACC president Borys Surawicz challenged the FCIM's recommendations. Why is the "increased knowledge, experience, and competence" of the subspecialist "not in the public interest? Why is it wrong to be motivated by the prospect of higher reimbursement levels?" Rather than a bureaucracy, Surawicz preferred "self-regulation" of specialty growth "based on the laws of supply and demand." He cited a recent AMA report that concluded "the public can best be served under an educational system which maximizes the freedom of individuals to choose and develop their career interests and opportunities under normal competitive conditions. This applies to both the selection of medicine as a career and the choice in specialty."[149]

Tarlov, who had become internal medicine's manpower maven, also chaired the influential Graduate Medical Education National Advisory Committee (GMENAC), charged by the Secretary of Health, Education and Welfare to assess the specialty distribution of physicians and project future needs. Active between 1976 and 1980, GMENAC had a full-time staff of twenty and a budget of more than $5 million and published a seven-volume report with 107 recommendations in 1981 (Table 8-7).[150]

GMENAC predicted surpluses for all adult medical and surgical specialties except hematology-oncology, emergency medicine, and preventive medicine. The report, which health policy analyst Uwe Reinhardt characterized as so ambitious that "it steamed into the station like a heavily laden freight train," brought forth a chorus of lamentations.[151] An academic neurologist urged his colleagues "to work together through our national organizations to explore policy alternatives [and] implement needed restructuring." If academic departments responded, neurologists would "not be tyrannized by numbers, nor swept along by external tides."[152] An academic plastic surgeon worried that Congress would view GMENAC data as "absolute" and use them "for regulatory purposes." Citing recent health manpower legislation, he protested, "Additional legislatively induced confusion should not be imposed, at least until the results of the previous meddling have been observed."[153]

Cardiology stood out as the specialty with the greatest projected supply-demand mismatch. GMENAC predicted that in 1990 there would be nearly twice the number of heart specialists as needed.[154] At the time (1980), there were 1,492 cardiology fellows in 239 cardiology training programs in the United States (Table A9). The issue that confronted academics and the ACC, which represented them and practitioner cardiologists, was whether GMENAC was right. If it was, the harder

TABLE 8-7

GMENAC *Summary of Specialist Physician Supply and Need Estimates (1978–1990)*

	SUPPLY 1978	ESTIMATES 1990	PERCENT CHANGE 1978–1990	GMENAC MIDPOINT 1990	PERCENT EXCESS 1990
All physicians	374,800	535,750	+ 43	466,000	+15
Family practice	54,350	64,400	+ 18	61,300	+ 5
General internal medicine	48,950	73,800	+ 51	70,250	+ 5
Cardiology	7,700	14,900	+ 94	7,750	+92
Gastroenterology	2,900	6,900	+138	6,500	+ 6
Hematology/oncology	3,000	8,300	+177	9,000	− 8
Nephrology	1,450	4,850	+235	2,750	+76
Neurology	4,850	8,650	+ 78	5,500	+57
Rheumatology	1,000	3,000	+200	1,700	+76
Orthopedic surgery	12,350	20,100	+ 63	15,100	+33
Cardiothoracic surgery	2,100	2,900	+ 38	2,050	+41
Emergency medicine	5,000	9,250	+ 85	13,500	−31
Preventive medicine	6,100	5,550	− 9	7,300	−24

SOURCE: *Report of the Graduate Medical Education National Advisory Committee. Vol. 1.* GMENAC *Summary Report* (Washington, D.C.: U.S. Dept. of Health and Human Services, 1981), table 3, p. 11 and table 5, p. 14.
NOTES: "GMENAC Midpoint" is the GMENAC estimate of the number of specialists "required." "Percent Excess 1990" is the percentage by which the projected 1990 number exceeds the GMENAC recommended 1990 number. A minus in the "excess" column represents a predicted shortfall. The original paper includes 33 specialties.

questions were how (and whether) to reduce the output of heart specialists. The ACC concluded that the GMENAC recommendation to reduce cardiology fellowship positions by 20 percent was unwarranted. College leaders thought the study failed to consider adequately several factors that would increase demand for cardiologists: an aging population, new diagnostic and therapeutic developments, and the need for specialists in "cardiologically underserved" areas.[155]

Cardiology ignored the GMENAC recommendations, which carried no legislative authority and were unenforceable. The number of cardiology fellows increased by 27 percent from 1,492 in 1980 to 1,894 in 1985, despite GMENAC's prediction and the FCIM's directive.[156] The increasing output reflected continued strong demand for practitioner cardiologists and the introduction of new technologies and procedures, such as invasive electrophysiology testing and percutaneous transluminal coronary angioplasty (PTCA) (which will be discussed in Chapter 9). But the diffusion of more specialists and these new technologies only intensified concerns about costs. And GMENAC was "concerned about costs," according to health policy analyst Rashi Fein.[157] For cardiology the 1980s would witness steady growth despite increasing tensions in academic and private medicine regarding resources.

CHAPTER 9

*The Price of Success:
Tensions in and around
Cardiology*

Money has influenced virtually every facet of American medicine in recent decades, a phenomenon health policy analyst Eli Ginzberg terms the "monetarization" of medical care.[1] Following World War II, federal grants transformed medical schools and teaching hospitals into academic centers that produced hundreds of thousands of specialists trained to value science and rely on technology. The prevalence of heart disease, a series of technological and procedural innovations, and reimbursement policies placed cardiology squarely in the center of this phenomenon. American heart specialists were not alone in their infatuation with new diagnostic tools and techniques. British cardiologist John Goodwin writes, "The appeal of technological investigation is irresistible. The young cardiologist, vibrating with passionate desire to analyze the instrumental results, cannot always see the point of laborious clinical examination."[2]

Gradually, some people began to question whether America could afford all the medical specialists and technology the government had helped to create. By the 1980s critics portrayed hospitals, doctors, the pharmaceutical industry, medical equipment manufacturers, insurance companies, voluntary health agencies—virtually everyone involved in medical care—as greedy opportunists.[3] Understandably, these groups protested this characterization, citing their roles in advancing the health of American citizens. Yet for a growing number of people, the issue was no longer what had been accomplished and what was still possible, but what was affordable. The intensity and focus of the debate has been modulated by the ideology of the political party in power, but today there is a consensus that uncontrolled expansion of medical

technology, unrestricted production of specialists, and unlimited hospital-based care cannot continue.[4]

This chapter explores some of the tensions that surround today's
specialists, especially cardiologists, as a result of their success. The
concerns relate to such fundamental matters as income, political and
social ideology, professional autonomy, peer relationships, and the
control and use of specialized procedures and technology. As I have
shown in earlier chapters, each of these issues has a history. Although
this helps us understand the present, it does not necessarily give us a
clear vision of the future, especially when so many new and powerful
forces are operating in health care.

The medical profession has long been the target of criticism. Internist Russell Elkinton editorialized in 1961, "In recent times, the
image of the American physician in the public mind, and especially as
portrayed in the public press, has undergone a deplorable change. He
has been depicted at worst as a reactionary money seeker and at best as
a well-motivated but narrow-minded participant in a changing social
scene—a professional unable to see beyond the immediate problems of
diagnosis and treatment and fee for same."[5]

Two years later, a writer in the *Saturday Evening Post* declared, "For
some time now the generations-old love affair between the American
physician and the American people has been rapidly cooling." The
strain reflected the changing context, content, and cost of medical care.
"With the immense growth of specialization coupled to the phenomenon of the vanishing family doctor, the patient finds it somewhat
unrewarding to love a scientific instrument." The author admitted this
was ironic, because never before had patients received "such good
care" from "such carefully selected, highly trained" doctors. Americans
had never "lived so long, enjoyed such good health and been so free of
crippling diseases."[6]

Reflecting on American medicine a quarter of a century ago, historian George Rosen predicted that specialization would continue to
flourish. "Nostalgia for the general practitioner, the Mr. Chips of medicine, will not change the current situation and its impacts, or reverse
the trends which led to it and which are continuing."[7] Some politicians
looked well beyond nostalgia; they argued that the federal government
should intervene and coordinate medical care in the United States.
When Democratic Senator Edward Kennedy examined "the crisis in
America's health care" in 1972, he identified doctors (specialists in

particular) as one part of the problem.[8] Yet for every writer or speaker who mourned the passing of the general practitioner and the unrelenting trend toward specialization a generation ago, a score celebrated innovations and "breakthroughs" and the specialists responsible for them.

Some of the most dramatic and widely publicized advances were in heart care—coronary care units, coronary angiography, bypass surgery, and cardiac transplants. The media compared transplantation of the human heart, first performed in 1967 by South African surgeon Christiaan Barnard, "to the awesome daring and danger of mankind's attempts to reach the moon," according to medical sociologist Renée Fox.[9] Other researchers regarded technology (rather than transplants) as the key to treating patients with end-stage heart disease. The National Heart Institute (NHI) had launched an ambitious program to develop an artificial implantable heart three years before Barnard performed the first heart transplant.[10] Unexpected obstacles retarded progress on both fronts. Heart transplants were limited initially by serious problems with organ rejection and eventually by an inadequate supply of donors. The artificial heart program was plagued by technical, medical, fiscal, and political problems. Although these two innovative approaches for replacing damaged human hearts were widely publicized, their impact on heart care (up to now) has been trivial.[11]

Politics and the cost of health care

A generation ago, the leaders of the American College of Cardiology (ACC) and other members of the heart lobby were aware of the growing concern on Capitol Hill about health care costs. Cardiology, already seen as a technologically intense specialty, was sure to get special scrutiny. The prevalence of cardiovascular disease meant the potential market for new heart tests and therapies was huge—and lucrative.[12] Although the goal of preventing heart disease remained elusive, doctors did have better treatments for several congenital and acquired cardiac disorders. Research funded by the government, the American Heart Association (AHA), and industry had transformed the outlook for many heart patients, but at a cost. Despite compelling evidence that coronary care units and open-heart operations (and innovations in many other specialties) saved or prolonged lives, calls to

justify the government's massive investment in medical research, training, and technology—and now care—grew more insistent.[13]

Joseph Cooper, professor of government at Howard University, told
a Senate committee in 1967, "Sooner or later an impatient public was
bound to ask for delivery on promises made recurringly that the conquest of the innumerable diseases would be achieved quickly if only
enough were spent in a hurry."[14] Three years later, a science writer for
the *Wall Street Journal* claimed that a cure for cancer was unlikely,
regardless of how much money was spent to achieve that goal. He
warned that "any group of experts" promising this "could raise high
hopes among the public," but "disenchantment" would result if cures
were not forthcoming.[15] James Shannon, National Institutes of Health
(NIH) director between 1955 and 1968, was an effective voice for the
research lobby. He conceded later that the claims about the potential of
research to solve health problems "were doubtless exaggerated" and
that "the estimates of cost and time required for results were low."[16]

The National Heart, Blood Vessel, Lung, and Blood Act of 1972 (PL
92-423) stated that more than half of Americans died from cardiovascular disease and that these illnesses had "a major social and economic
impact on the nation," a point the heart lobby had made for a quarter
of a century. It was estimated that eliminating cardiovascular diseases
would prolong the average American's life by eleven years and save the
country $30 billion annually in health care costs, lost wages, and
reduced productivity. Although that goal was remote, the government
could begin in the meantime to measure more deliberately the yield
from its investment in cardiovascular research and heart care. The 1972
law charged the NIH with evaluating "techniques, drugs, and devices"
used to diagnose and treat heart disease.[17]

By this time, a surge of consumer activism in the United States had
stimulated Congress to pass laws and create agencies to help protect
citizens from a host of real and perceived threats to their well-being.
The Medical Device Amendments to the Federal Food, Drug, and
Cosmetic Act of 1976 (PL 94-295) empowered the Food and Drug
Administration (FDA) to demand that manufacturers prove that new
medical devices were both safe and effective. Health policy analyst
Susan Foote explains, "By the late 1960s, problems associated with
legitimate, therapeutically desirable medical devices that were flooding
the market began to surface." One such product was the Dalkon shield
intrauterine birth control device. In cardiology, the focus was on artifi-

cial heart valves and permanent pacemakers, a few of which were defective and had caused deaths.[18]

The unifying theme would be value. Was the patient (or the insurer) getting a quality product at a reasonable price? Although the initial focus was on medical devices, some observers worried that physician services would be the next target—with implications for professional autonomy. National Heart, Lung, and Blood Institute (NHLBI) director Robert Levy informed the ACC trustees in 1977 that Jimmy Carter's administration was committed to "cost containment and quality assurance."[19] The following year, the NIH established an Office for Medical Applications of Research and charged it with evaluating the appropriate use, efficacy, and safety of medical procedures, devices, and drugs. Meanwhile, the newly created National Center for Health Care Technology of the Department of Health and Human Services was given a broad mandate to consider the scientific, clinical, social, ethical, legal, and cost implications of medical innovations. These agencies were also ordered to develop "consensus statements" to help the public and health care professionals make informed choices regarding drugs, therapeutic devices, and procedures.[20]

Although new biomedical devices might offer advantages over existing products or traditional approaches, they also carried the risk of unforseen design and manufacturing defects. Conceding the need for quality control, some heart specialists feared that the flood of government regulations would inhibit the development and diffusion of promising medical devices. ACC president Leonard Dreifus was especially concerned about the impact on cardiac patients. Calling the 1976 Medical Device Act a "crippling bit of legislation," he warned that patients would be "getting the short end of the stick." In 1978 Dreifus created an ACC committee for medical devices, because he thought the college "must assume its proper position as spokesman for cardiology."[21]

Cardiologists and cardiac surgeons were not the only medical specialists whose practices and patients were affected by what sociologist Paul Starr terms a "blizzard of regulation."[22] Gastroenterologists also watched Washington nervously. Their field was being transformed by new flexible fiberoptic endoscopes used to examine the stomach and intestines. This technological innovation catalyzed gastroenterology much as the cardiac catheter and the artificial kidney had changed cardiology and nephrology.[23] Health policy analyst Martin Strosberg discussed the clinical impact, professional implications, and political life of the fiberoptic gastroscope in 1979. His conclusions also applied to cardiologists, their technologies, and their college. "Organizations representing academic physicians and practitioners are . . . expanding their roles in response to increasing emphasis on cost containment and regulation." Strosberg urged societies representing the innovators and users of medical technology to establish contacts with third-party payers, peer review organizations, the FDA, the NIH, and Congress.[24]

The ACC was doing just that; college leaders wanted to be at the table when government agencies and other groups discussed heart-related technology and procedures. During his presidency (1978–1979), Dreifus appointed representatives to the FDA, the Association for the Advancement of Medical Instrumentation, the National Commission for Clinical Engineering Certification, and the Medical Devices Technical Advisory Board. The stakes were high for doctors as well as for patients, manufacturers, and payers. Dreifus told college members that the ACC would now address the "socioeconomic and regulatory affairs of our country in the interest of our membership, as well as patients." There was broad support for the move because of the recent "flurry of government interventions into the health care field."[25]

Dreifus and other ACC leaders who shared his concerns were positioning their organization to be proactive. The college would begin "establishing standards for quality cardiovascular health care delivery" and be "a principal source of advice to government" on these issues.[26] Washington's interest in cardiac technologies and procedures reflected the huge direct and indirect cost of heart care. It was estimated in 1980 that cardiovascular diseases resulted in $33 billion in health care expenditures and $1.6 trillion in lost productivity, far more than any other disease category. Cardiovascular conditions accounted for approximately one-third of all ambulatory visits, hospital days, and health care charges.[27]

In 1981 Raymond Cotton, the ACC's part-time government relations counsel, warned members, "Amid the talk of Kemp-Roth, supply-side economics, 'Stockmania,' El Salvador, and a host of other issues, one could easily be unaware that the [Reagan] administration has proposed a multitude of changes in federal health programs that could have a significant impact on the delivery of health care by cardiologists in particular, and medical practitioners in general."[28] Later that year the college created a full-time government relations department to better evaluate and respond to Washington's increasing involvement in medicine.

When she became president of the ACC in 1982, Suzanne Knoebel, an academic cardiologist at Indiana University, encouraged the college to develop "consensus statements" on cardiovascular technologies, procedures, and practices. She told members that these publications would help to assure quality care and could be sent out in response to the many requests the college received "almost daily" for information about "some specific technique, practice, or training requirement."[29] Initially, some members were wary of having their professional society develop practice guidelines. They were reminded that the alternative was accepting government guidelines or regulations that might be formulated with little or no input from heart specialists.[30] During the next decade, the ACC issued guidelines on most of the procedures heart specialists performed.

Transformation of the cardiac catheter into a therapeutic tool

Despite fears that government regulations would suppress the invention and diffusion of technologies and procedures, the 1980s witnessed several notable innovations in heart care. Scientists and biomedical engineers collaborated with academic and practitioner cardiologists to develop new tools and techniques to treat common cardiac conditions such as arrhythmias and angina pectoris. These innovations also contributed to the fragmentation of cardiology into subspecialties.[31] Today, heart specialists are often defined by the technologies they emphasize in their practices, a phenomenon inherent in professionalization. Most cardiologists combine two or more of the areas listed in Table 9-1, and nearly all perform the traditional clinical functions of providing consultations and routine followup of some patients with chronic heart disease.

Cardiology entered a new era in the late 1970s when medical heart specialists began to perform *therapeutic* catheterization procedures in adult patients. German cardiologist Andreas Grüntzig performed the first percutaneous transluminal coronary angioplasty (PTCA) for the treatment of angina pectoris in September 1977 in Zurich, Switzerland. He reported his initial experience with the procedure at the annual AHA meeting two months later and published a brief description of it early the following year.[32] As outlined in Chapter 8, coronary artery bypass graft surgery (CABG) was invented to overcome the limitations of medical therapy of angina, but it is a major operation that is expensive, requires several weeks for complete recuperation, and carries risk to life. PTCA, performed in a catheterization laboratory on an awake patient, is a technique in which a catheter with an inflatable balloon tip is advanced into a narrowed coronary artery and inflated in an attempt to reduce the obstruction and enhance blood flow. Most patients leave the hospital in a day or two without a scar.[33]

PTCA migrated to the United States within a few months of Grüntzig's first procedure. Richard Myler of San Francisco and Simon Stertzer of New York performed the first PTCAs in America in March 1978.[34] Three months later, readers of *Time* magazine learned about Robert, a forty-seven-year-old chauffeur "stricken with suffocating spasmodic chest pains of severe angina." An angiogram showed that Robert was a candidate for CABG, but he accepted his doctors' advice and decided to "try a new and highly experimental alternative: a procedure with a tongue-twisting name of 'percutaneous transluminal coronary angioplasty.'" Stertzer performed the PTCA in less than an hour and proved angiographically that the narrowed artery had been successfully dilated. "Two days later, his angina gone, Robert left the hospital and returned to work." The article reported that the procedure might be feasible in 10 to 15 percent of CABG candidates "at about one-tenth the $15,000 average cost of a bypass." Conceding that PTCA

TABLE 9-1
Categories of Clinical Cardiologists (1995)

Invasive cardiologist: performs diagnostic cardiac catheterization and coronary angiography

Noninvasive cardiologist: does not perform catheterization or coronary angiography; focuses on some combination of electrocardiography, echocardiography, nuclear cardiology, and stress testing

Interventional cardiologist: performs therapeutic catheterization procedures such as percutaneous transluminal coronary angioplasty (PTCA) in addition to diagnostic cardiac catheterization and angiography

Electrophysiologist: performs invasive (catheter-based) procedures to diagnose and treat complex heart rhythm disturbances; may insert permanent pacemakers

Preventive (or public health) cardiologist: focuses on some combination of cardiac rehabilitation, risk factor modification (especially cholesterol and lipid abnormalities), disease prevention, and epidemiology

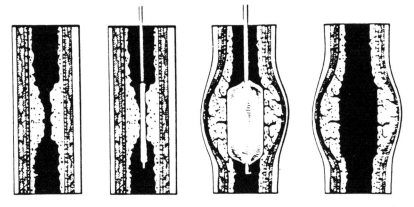

Presumed mechanism of angioplasty (1980) by which the balloon technique relieves obstruction in a narrowed artery.

SOURCE: W. R. Castaneda-Zuniga, A. Formanek, M. Tadavarthy, Z. Vlodaver, J. E. Edwards, C. Zollikofer, et al., "The mechanism of balloon angioplasty," *Radiology* 135 (1980): 565–571, figure 11, p. 570.

was still experimental, Stertzer proclaimed, "We're into a revolution in cardiology" if early positive results were confirmed.[35]

"Ever eager for a 'breakthrough,'" the news media "gave a good bit of space and time" to PTCA in 1978, according to two academic cardiologists from Philadelphia.[36] The potential market was huge; as many as 5 million Americans were thought to suffer from angina when PTCA was invented. It was estimated that 486,000 cardiac catheterizations and 161,000 open-heart operations were performed in the United States in 1980 alone, most of them on patients with angina.[37] The money at stake was even more impressive: that year cardiovascular surgical procedures cost about $4.4 billion in the United States.[38]

PTCA was more dangerous than routine diagnostic coronary angiography; it could cause a heart attack if the narrowed artery became totally blocked as a result of the procedure. Grüntzig warned that "potential complications are both serious and sudden" and cautioned against the premature diffusion of angioplasty. "Prospective randomized [clinical] trials . . . are clearly needed if we are to evaluate the efficacy of this new technic as compared with current medical and surgical treatments" of angina.[39] Conceding that it was impossible to contain PTCA long enough for a prospective randomized clinical trial to be completed, the NHLBI developed a national registry to assess the safety and results of the procedure. Two years later, data from fifteen hundred patients in seventy-three centers showed that the risk and short-term success rates of PTCA were acceptable.[40]

Powerful social and economic forces encouraged the diffusion of angioplasty before its efficacy had been proved. This occurred, in part, because new procedures such as PTCA were not subject to the strict regulations that applied to new medical devices or drugs. Patient demand was a major factor. Understandably, many angina patients chose PTCA over CABG because it seemed to work and meant they could avoid the discomfort and risks of open-heart surgery. Although the desire to provide state-of-the-art care to heart patients was the most common justification for learning (or introducing) angioplasty, individual and institutional economic incentives were also operative. Academic medical centers and community hospitals encouraged some of their invasive cardiologists to learn to perform PTCA because it would expand their services and attract patients from competitors. Cardiologists could not only augment their therapeutic armamentarium by learning to do PTCA, they could also increase their incomes because the procedure was reimbursed separately from a standard coronary angiogram.

Angioplasty revolutionized cardiology, much as open-heart surgery and the electrocardiograph had done one and two generations earlier, respectively. But there were important differences. Open-heart operations were performed by surgeons, and the electrocardiograph was not the exclusive property of heart specialists. Although cardiologists controlled the cardiac catheter, they had used it as a *diagnostic* tool to help channel patients to surgeons. Now, a new type of medical heart specialist, the interventional cardiologist, could perform *therapeutic* procedures on patients with angina. This changed the traditional relationship between medical and surgical heart specialists; collaborators suddenly became competitors who offered angina patients dramatically different treatment approaches.

By the 1970s cardiologists controlled the path to bypass surgery because they performed the compulsory preoperative angiogram. With the invention of PTCA, medical heart specialists could set up a detour that led back to the catheterization laboratory where an interventional cardiologist performed a procedure that was portrayed as a simpler, equally effective, and less expensive alternative to the surgeon's bypass operation for certain patients. Understandably, some surgeons (and others) raised the thorny issues of self-referral and economic self-interest. In most cases, however, patient preference was the deciding factor.

By the time the NHLBI published guidelines for performing PTCA in 1982, hundreds of aspiring interventionalists had already attended continuing medical education programs devoted to the technique that Grüntzig had organized in Zurich and later at Emory University in Atlanta where he moved in 1980.[41] The NHLBI document emphasized that cardiologists planning to perform PTCA needed "specialized training beyond that necessary for routine diagnostic cardiac catheterization and angiography." Assuming that safety and success were partly volume-dependent, interventional cardiologists were urged to do "about one case per week" to maintain their skills. In order to confine angioplasty to centers with active open-heart surgery programs, the NHLBI recommended that it be undertaken only at institutions where a "skilled surgical team" was immediately available to perform emergency bypass surgery if major complications arose.[42]

Angioplasty spread rapidly during the 1980s as many practitioner cardiologists learned the technique by attending "demonstration" courses and hundreds of fellows trained to perform PTCA entered practice. Meanwhile, clinical investigators and equipment manufacturers collaborated to develop new balloon catheters to simplify the procedure, and innovators showed that multiple coronary lesions and multiple vessels could be safely dilated in a sequential fashion. By the end of the decade, the number of angioplasties nearly equaled the number of bypass operations performed in the United States.[43] Soon, several new interventional cardiology procedures were introduced into clinical practice, including laser-assisted angioplasty, atherectomy (a procedure designed to physically remove the material narrowing the affected coronary vessel), and stents (devices inserted into a coronary artery to keep it open).[44]

Concurrent with the development of PTCA, other medical scientists and heart specialists were inventing new techniques and refining old ones to study and treat arrhythmias (disorders of the heartbeat). Physiological cardiologists fostered the development of the subspecialty of clinical electrophysiology in the 1960s. Beginning with the efforts of Benjamin Scherlag and his colleagues at the Staten Island Public Health Service Hospital, the field of invasive clinical electrophysiology had evolved into a formal subspecialty of cardiology by the mid-1970s. The cardiac electrophysiologist's unique tool was an electrode attached to a catheter that made it possible to record and study the origin and spread of electrical impulses inside the heart.[45]

As the clinical value of new techniques to study the heartbeat became more apparent during the 1980s the demand for electrophysiologists grew. Leonard Dreifus remarked in 1992 that until very recently "an electrophysiologist was a rarity. Today, almost every major hospital has to have" one.[46] These specialists also participated in the creation and diffusion of new therapeutic procedures to treat rapid heartbeat, such as automatic implantable cardiac defibrillators for ventricular tachycardia and catheter "ablation" techniques for supraventricular tachycardia.[47]

Cardiology's prosperity inflames chronic interspecialty tensions

Innovations in diagnosis (e.g., echocardiography, coronary angiography, and invasive electrophysiology testing) and therapeutics (e.g., pacemakers, bypass surgery, angioplasty, and implantable defibrillators) greatly stimulated the growth of cardiology during the 1980s. Heart specialists now had several powerful tools to help them care for patients with a wide range of cardiac problems. These new approaches contributed to changes in the content and duration of cardiology training. Hospitals, group practices, and cardiologists across the country wanted to offer advanced interventional and electrophysiological techniques to their patients. The job market expanded as demand surged for newly trained fellows and academic cardiologists who possessed these special skills. ACC leaders and others who had rejected GMENAC's prediction of a surplus of cardiologists by 1990 felt vindicated.

Academic cardiology programs grew larger and wealthier during the 1980s as clinical activity increased in volume and scope, the NHI budget doubled, and equipment manufacturers and pharmaceutical companies sponsored a growing number of clinical trials of their products. The most compelling reason to increase the number of full-time cardiology faculty members and fellows was the steady escalation of workload as more cardiac patients were referred for specialized diagnostic tests and procedures. Academic cardiologists welcomed the help that allowed them to devote more time to research. For most of them, salary and promotions were linked to their research productivity and their ability to get grants. Academic medical centers had another incentive to expand their cardiology training programs: they were profitable. Two Harvard physicians pointed out in 1980 that medical department chairs and hospital administrators maintained fellowship programs in spite of growing concerns about an oversupply of some types of specialists because "subspecialty fellows provide some of the highest revenue-yielding services to the hospital for very low salaries."[48]

Public Health Service cardiologist Thomas Preston and academic internist Robert Petersdorf agreed. Declaring in 1980 that the nation did not need 350 cardiology training programs (actually there were fewer than 250), they argued that the size of each one reflected the institution's short-term requirements rather than the nation's long-term needs. They repeated the familiar charge that government grants designed to produce researchers and academic cardiologists had been subverted to train practitioner (especially invasive) cardiologists. As government support of clinical training expired, program directors showed "remarkable ingenuity in obtaining support from other sources," according to Preston and Petersdorf.[49] Federal research grants accounted for less than 5 percent of cardiology fellowship stipends by this time; hospital revenues were used to cover nearly half of the $41 million paid to cardiology fellows in 1984.[50]

Tensions in academic medical centers increased as full-time physicians were encouraged to devote more time to clinical work in order to help their institutions compete with private practitioners and generate more money for their departments. Petersdorf claimed that "academic life is no longer genteel" and "no longer fulfills the academician's expectations."[51] Robert Wood Johnson Foundation president David Rogers agreed. This former Johns Hopkins dean characterized academic medical centers as "stressed American institutions" whose relations with the government had become "increasingly adversarial."[52] During the 1980s, many academics expressed concern about the future of clinical research. James Wyngaarden, chair of the department of medicine at Duke, warning that the clinical investigator was an "endangered species," listed a dozen reasons for the declining interest in research careers among trainees and young academic physicians, including the "seductive lure of lucrative practice and the extraordinary incomes that can be made in procedure-based specialty medicine."[53]

More defections from research careers and more cardiology fellows meant more practitioner cardiologists. Academics found themselves competing with an increasingly large and sophisticated cardiological community that had sprung up around them. They had trained thousands of practitioners, many of whom had settled in nearby community

TABLE 9-2

Hospitals with Specialized Cardiovascular Facilities (1960–1991)

YEAR	TOTAL NUMBER OF HOSPITALS	CATHETERIZATION LABORATORY	PTCA	OPEN-HEART SURGERY
1960	6,876	513 (7%)	–	327 (5%)[a]
1980	6,965	913 (13%)	–	605 (9%)[b]
1991	6,634	1,537 (25%)	1,076 (18%)	919 (15%)[c]

SOURCES: The total number of hospitals is taken from American Hospital Association, *Hospital Statistics*. 1993–1994 ed. (Chicago: AHA, 1993), table 1, p. 2. [a] A. F. Crocetti, "Cardiac diagnostic and surgical facilities in the United States," *Public Health Rep.* 80 (1965) 1035–1053. [b] R. H. Kennedy, M. A. Kennedy, R. L. Frye, E. R. Giuliani, D. C. McGoon, J. R. Pluth, et al. "Cardiac-catheterization and cardiac-surgical facilities: Use, trends, and future requirements," *N. Engl. J. Med.* 307 (1982): 986–993, table 5, p. 989. [c] Data from a 1991 national survey by the American Hospital Association, summarized in J. L. Ritchie, M. D. Cheitlin, M. A. Hlatky, T. J. Ryan, and R. G. Williams, "Task force 5: Profile of the cardiovascular specialist: Trends in needs and supply and implications for the future," *J. Am. Coll. Cardiol.* 24 (1994): 275–328, p. 314.

hospitals, taking with them the latest innovations in diagnosis and treatment (Table 9-2). Even though academics had been warned, the incentives to maintain or expand cardiology fellowship programs outweighed the threat of creating even more competition. David Rogers listed several problems facing academic medical centers a decade ago. One of the most serious: "Young subspecialist physicians [are] moving to well-financed suburban hospitals and taking paying patients with them." By fulfilling their educational mission, academics had contributed to their potential downfall. "Thanks to their own training programs, academic medical centers received far less referrals than they had in times past."[54]

Petersdorf claimed in 1985 that several community hospitals had eliminated their subspecialty training programs because the medical staff knew that "today's fellow will . . . become tomorrow's competitor." Although there was a 20 percent decrease in the number of cardiology training programs between 1972 and 1990, the total number of fellows nearly doubled. It was not simply a matter of closing marginal and low-volume training programs (Table A9). Petersdorf declared that "the only ones foolish enough to continue training surgical and medical specialists and subspecialists are residency and fellowship training program directors in academic medical centers." This acerbic observer of the academic scene concluded, "Somehow they are under the delusion that they are immune to the competition created by the physician manpower glut."[55] Ironically, Petersdorf's own department of medicine at the University of Washington expanded dramatically during his tenure as chair (Table 9-3).

Although the problem of competition was real, it was not new. In 1975 readers of the *American Journal of Cardiology* learned that of the twenty-four recent graduates of the Indiana University Medical Center's cardiology training program who had remained in the state, twenty-two practiced in Indianapolis.[56] Fifteen years later the two largest private hospitals in Indianapolis (combined) performed more than three times as many cardiac catheterizations, seven times as many CABG operations, and nearly thirty times as many PTCAs as Indiana University Medical Center, which had trained most of the specialists who performed those procedures. The same phenomenon occurred in Minneapolis and other large cities.[57] Richard Ross headed the cardiology division at Johns Hopkins from 1960 to 1975, when he became dean of the medical school. Asked when deans and cardiology division chiefs began worrying about training their competition, he laughed and responded, "Not soon enough."[58]

TABLE 9-3
Faculty in the University of Washington Department of Medicine (1964–1979)

	NUMBER OF FACULTY MEMBERS			% INCREASE
SPECIALTY	*1964*	*1970*	*1979*	1964–1979
Cardiology	7	12	19	171
Endocrinology	14	26	44	214[a]
Gastroenterology	5	7	12	140
General medicine	0	6	33	–
Hematology	9	13	20	122
Infectious disease	3	8	16	433[b]
Medical genetics	5	8	14	180
Nephrology	4	9	17	325
Oncology	1	8	26	2,500[c]
Pulmonary medicine	1	6	15	1,400
Rheumatology	2	4	7	250
Other	18	41	99	465
TOTAL	69	148	322	367

SOURCE: Adapted from R. G. Petersdorf, "Departments of medicine: Examples of academic hypertrophy," in *Academic Medicine: Present and Future*, ed. J. Z. Bowers and E. E. King (North Tarrytown, N.Y.: Rockefeller Archive Center, 1983), pp. 95–105, table 1, p. 98.
NOTES: Local circumstances influenced recruiting, so these numbers are only suggestive of national trends. [a]Petersdorf's predecessor as chair was an endocrinologist, which explains the disproportionate number of faculty in that field in 1964. [b]Petersdorf was an infectious disease subspecialist. [c]Medical oncology was considered a "new subspecialty" in 1970; see B. J. Kennedy, "Oncology in medicine," *Ann. Intern. Med.* 73 (1970): 637–639.

People also failed to appreciate that technology and trainees were equally important (and critically interdependent) in cardiology's growth equation. After studying the use, trends, and future requirements of catheterization laboratories and open-heart surgery programs in the United States, a group of Mayo Clinic researchers concluded in 1982 that "further growth in the number of cardiac centers should be avoided."[59] But market forces prevailed. A decade later, while there were 127 medical schools and 221 cardiology training programs in America, there were 1,452 cardiac catheterization laboratories and more than ten times that many cardiologists.[60] There was no national strategy or mechanism to control either the diffusion of technology or the production of cardiology fellows—let alone both. Market forces (e.g., patient demand, economic incentives) favored the status quo, which meant steady expansion. Academics largely ignored the implications of their fecundity, and the ACC and the American Board of Internal Medicine (ABIM) had no mandate or means to control cardiology's growth.

Meanwhile, the relations between cardiology and internal medicine became progressively strained. In academic medical centers, the tensions related to ideology, autonomy, power, prestige, and money. The main issue in the practice setting was who controlled the patient, with its financial implications. Specialists protested that generalists referred patients "too little or too late," while generalists resented specialists who "stole" their patients rather than returning them for ongoing care. For decades most cardiologists were content to be viewed as internists with a special interest in heart disease. Gradually, however, faint calls for independence grew louder as new technologies and procedures, and the income they produced, began to differentiate cardiologists more clearly from other medical specialists.

Tensions escalated as money fueled academic cardiology programs and the production and diffusion of heart specialists with their modern tools and techniques. The prevalence of cardiac disease, the advent of potent diagnostic technologies and therapeutic procedures, and favorable reimbursement formulas had transformed cardiology into a large, influential, and impatient discipline. The subtle fault line between internal medicine and cardiology gradually developed into a crevasse that grew wider and deeper over time. But stresses were apparent even before money was a significant factor in the equation, and they were not limited to American cardiology. Swedish surgeon Gunnar Bjork declared in 1952 that there was "no doubt" that cardiology already was "a specialty . . . based chiefly on diagnostic procedures and certain technical equipment." He predicted that "the problem of the separation of cardiology from internal medicine" would not "be solved without pain."[61]

In America, federal research funding policies and reimbursement strategies contributed to the disequilibrium. James Warren, an academic cardiologist who chaired the department of medicine at Ohio State, warned more than three decades ago that internal medicine "may be crumbling" because of the NIH's emphasis on organ- or disease-specific research and the growth of specialized diagnostic techniques.[62] Warren made this observation on the eve of the advent of the coronary care unit, an innovation that threatened the traditional organization of inpatient internal medical services as units where adult patients with all types of nonsurgical problems were hospitalized together rather than separated on the basis of organ-specific diseases.

The coronary care unit was a tangible symbol of cardiology's growing independence. Some chairs of academic internal medicine departments resisted the coronary care unit movement because they opposed the segregation of hospitalized patients by organ system. Richard Ross thinks they saw the coronary care unit as the "first wedge" that would ultimately result in "splitting the department of medicine apart. You get a coronary care unit, then you'll want a cardiac unit, then you'll want to be a separate department." Although most academic internal medicine department chairs were subspecialists, when they assumed control of the medical *department* they sought to maintain its integrity.[63]

A few academics ignored or denied the growing popularity and importance of medical specialties such as cardiology. Arguing that the ABIM sub-boards (cardiology, gastroenterology, allergy, and pulmonary disease) "serve no purpose," the chief of the medical department at Marquette School of Medicine declared in 1969 that "subspecialty interest is merely a professional hobby in internal medicine."[64] Rhetoric like this, denigrating the significance of a major career decision, offended the formally trained, board certified cardiologists who were rapidly replacing part-time, self-designated heart specialists in academic medical centers and community hospitals across the country.

A social scientist warned America's internists in 1970 that specialization was "probably the major factor disturbing traditional ethical and economic patterns in medicine" and was triggering "jurisdictional disputes within the profession."[65] Two years later, Eugene Braunwald, then chair of the medical department at the University of California at San Diego, noted that "the current social revolution clearly influences patterns of academic medicine" and warned that medical school departments were "in line for major shake-ups." He predicted the traditional model would evolve gradually into a new system with a primary care division and specialty divisions that would be "divided along organ-system lines."[66]

John Beck, professor of medicine at the University of California at San Francisco and an ABIM board member between 1964 and 1973, recalls that he and his peers "often decried the impact of subspecialty divisions within our departments." Fragmentation threatened the paradigm that every internal medicine subspecialist was first and foremost a general internist. "We worried that the subspecialties would go off as independent factions without commitment to the other subspecialties or to internal medicine as a whole." Moreover, academic medicine department chairs would lose control over the income that subspecialty divisions generated from research grants and patient care.[67]

In many academic institutions, cardiologists led the charge for independence. "Cardiology was clearly the *bête noir* in this group," according to Beck, "but it was rapidly followed by other subspecialties." These secessionists felt empowered by liberal "extramural research funding" and increasing income generated as a result of specialty procedures. In Beck's opinion, one reason the ABIM decided to develop subspecialty examinations in five additional medical specialties (endocrinology, hematology, infectious diseases, nephrology, and rheumatology) was that medical department chairs had urged the board's leaders to develop "strategies . . . on a national scene which would help them at their local department level."[68]

Few of the individuals who either argue for independence or champion the status quo have any sense of how internal medicine and its specialties evolved in the United States. Academic internist Edmund Pellegrino proposed in 1974 that the internist's "persona" represented the fusion of two late nineteenth-century models: the scholar-consultant (embodied in William Osler) and the German physician-scientist. But Pellegrino thought this "pastiche" was undergoing "fragmentation and polarization" because "interest in an organ system is a more powerful organizing principle than identification with internal medicine *per se*." In his opinion, "physicians, surgeons, physiologists, pathologists, and radiologists interested in the cardiovascular system" have more in common and work more closely together than do cardiologists and other medical specialists. Pellegrino predicted that identification with an organ system rather than with the department of medicine "is a centrifugal force that will have increasing impact on the future development of departments of medicine."[69]

ACC president Dean Mason argued in 1977 for the adoption of a new organizational model that reflected cardiology's growing functional independence from internal medicine. Mason, chair of the cardiology division at the University of California at Davis Medical Center in Sacramento, told college members that the "Department of Cardiovascular Diseases" was "a functional concept that has come of age." The "tremendous accomplishments in cardiovascular patient care" and the prevalence of heart disease justified the reformation. Mason explained that he had discussed this "new rational approach . . . with several members of the college from different institutions," and they were supportive of it. The conventional arrangement (cardiology as a division of the department of medicine) was "outmoded," in Mason's opinion, because it hampered the "essential cooperation" between adult cardiologists and members of parallel disciplines such as "cardiovascular surgery, pediatric cardiology, cardiovascular radiology, nuclear cardiology, cardiovascular epidemiology, cardiac pathology, [and] cardiac physiology."[70]

Ongoing professionalization, technological innovations, and powerful market forces were straining the traditional order. Institutional and external pressures on full-time clinicians were especially intense in cardiology, with its large and expanding patient load. Mason conceded that some frustrations were common to all academics: teaching demands, the "pressures of clinical and basic research, escalating committee assignments, and ever-increasing paperwork." From his perspective, the whole situation was confounded by "federal, state and institutional fiscal ischemia (often infarction)." But these fiscal strains related more to increasing demand than to decreasing supply: the NHI appropriation had risen 32 percent between 1973 and 1977. Academic cardiology in the United States had become an enormous enterprise in human and economic terms.[71]

Mason brought up a contentious issue that was rarely discussed openly—money. Academic cardiologists were delivering (or at least supervising) a significant amount of heart care that was now liberally reimbursed by Medicare and other third-party payers. But this income usually went to the department of medicine, which then returned salaries to the full-time cardiologists based on an institutional formula. Money was not the only issue; power was also at stake. Cardiology chiefs wanted a stronger voice within their institutions; they were tired of being in the "unfavorable position of having to effect solutions with less than departmental status."[72]

Mason knew the issues he was raising were "highly charged emotionally." He attributed the reluctance of medical department chairs to consider the model to "economic and related reasons although their resistance is usually expressed in different terms." Although Mason did not anticipate a "spontaneous rush by institutional authorities to formulate Departments of Cardiovascular Diseases," he noted that a few "forward-looking" centers had established them. Subspecialty faculty defections potentially threatened the integrity and financial stability of academic medical centers. "It is little wonder that many dedicated and productive cardiology faculty members eventually turn to private practice for relief of [the] insurmountable problems of academia."[73]

Mason's proposal reverberated in academic medical circles, but to little avail. In 1982 Eugene Braunwald, now chair of the department of medicine at two Harvard teaching hospitals, told members of the AHA Council on Clinical Cardiology that he had "heard disgruntled chiefs of cardiology fantasize that they will secede from their departments of medicine." His response: "Forget it." Why? Because "no dean in his right mind will simultaneously approve the costs involved in setting up another department while accepting the responsibility for supporting poor revenue earners who would remain in the department of medicine if cardiology left." Money was a critical factor; cardiology was "much wealthier" than the other medical specialties. But Braunwald (who had completed his training a decade before Medicare) knew cardiology's strong financial position was not inevitable—it reflected the "peculiarity of our reimbursement system, which is based on 'piecework,' and rewards procedures more than 'hands on' patient care."[74]

Braunwald had pointed out something that many general internists and noncardiology medical specialists resented: the increasing discrepancy between their income-generating capacity and that of cardiologists based on an arbitrary but entrenched reimbursement strategy. He claimed that by interpreting electrocardiograms and echocardiograms, "a cardiologist can earn as much in 30 minutes as an equally well-trained diabetologist who supervises the care of a patient in diabetic coma can in 10 hours!" Braunwald continued, "Such gross inequalities inevitably lead to jealousy and friction, and it is fair to say that in most of our academic medical centers today there is at best an uneasy truce and at worst an outright war between departments of medicine and their divisions of cardiology."[75] Outside observers sensed the stresses. Sociologist Sydney Halpern writes, "Conflict is endemic within hospitals and medical schools where specialties compete for prerogatives and institutional resources."[76]

Cardiologists became increasingly isolated from generalists and other medical specialists as a result of their incomes and technologies. Academic heart specialists are also separated scientifically from their peers in other medical fields. Although molecular cardiologists are beginning to emerge in some academic centers, cardiology research and practice is still based largely on physiology. Other medical specialties are more firmly grounded in molecular biology. Braunwald notes that "academic hematologists, virologists, oncologists, endocrinologists, immunologists, and rheumatologists now all speak the same scientific language, use the same research techniques and the same instruments, attend the same meetings, and read and publish in the same journals." Cardiologists have not been part of this culture.[77]

Clinical cardiology still relies mainly on gross, visual diagnostic technologies like echocardiography and angiography rather than the techniques of immunology and molecular biology. Most of the unique therapy dispensed by medical and surgical heart specialists is at the "macro" level (e.g., angioplasty, bypass surgery, valve replacement, and cardiac transplant). It is true that drug therapies for congestive heart failure, arrhythmias, heart attacks, and other cardiovascular conditions are not macrotherapies. The current treatment of a heart attack includes the administration of "thrombolytic" therapy designed to dissolve the blood clot that usually triggers the event. Tissue plasminogen activator (t-PA), the most popular thrombolytic agent, is a naturally occurring enzyme produced commercially using recombinant DNA technology. Members of the NHLBI advisory council were told recently, "molecular genetics . . . could have a profound impact on the diagnosis, treatment, prevention, and management" of heart disease.[78] Acknowledging the growing clinical relevance of molecular biology to cardiology, the ACC has begun to produce continuing medical education programs and products to help practitioners learn about this dynamic area.[79]

The increasing intellectual, technological, financial, and physical isolation of academic cardiologists from their peers in other medical specialties (and specific tensions between some cardiology division chiefs and medicine department chairs) led to the creation of the Association of Professors of Cardiology (APC) in 1990.[80] Three APC leaders declared recently that departments of internal medicine and divisions of cardiology "stand at major, diverging roads" because of "conflicting social, intellectual and administrative forces and pressures." They reported that 60 percent of APC members supported the creation of separate cardiology departments. Money is a major issue; many academic cardiologists believe their institutions (especially the department of medicine) "tax" them excessively. The APC estimates that cardiology divisions generate more than 40 percent of the clinical income in departments of medicine. APC members are also frustrated by their "lack of control of necessary clinical and research resources, and lack of representation in governance at both the hospital and university levels."[81]

Responding to the APC's position paper, Braunwald reiterated points he had made ten and twenty years earlier. He used a compelling analogy to illustrate why the "secessionist movement" was causing such "consternation" in academic circles. Medical department chairs viewed the threatened loss of their cardiology divisions "as the mayor of New York City might view the secession of Manhattan." He conceded the taxation issue: "With financial support from all sources dwindling . . . many cardiologists feel that a disproportionately large percentage of their clinical income is being used to subsidize other divisions within the department of medicine whose clinical services are in less demand and whose revenues often fail to match their expenses."[82]

Discussing the conflict, a British observer remarked that it was unrealistic to "enforce a historical solution on a changing medical community" in order to keep "the escaping subspecialty groups under control."[83] Although the traditional academic paradigm is still intact in most university centers despite decades of conflict, the structure of cardiology practice has changed dramatically in recent years. In 1972 solo office-based practice was the most common arrangement for America's heart specialists, but by 1992 almost half of practitioner cardiologists belonged to cardiovascular group practices (Table 9-4).

TABLE 9-4

Practice Arrangement of Cardiologists (percentage) (1972–1992)

	1972	1992	% CHANGE
Solo	39.1	22.0	– 44%
Cardiovascular group	15.3	46.0	+201%
Multispecialty group	14.2	11.0	– 23%
Hospital	11.0	4.0	– 64%
Medical school	8.5	15.0	+ 76%
Combination or other	11.9	2.0	–830%

SOURCES: W. H. Pritchard and W. H. Abelmann, "Current status of manpower in cardiology," *Am. J. Cardiol.* 34 (1974): 408–416, table 6, p. 411, and *Cardiovascular Specialists and the Economics of Medicine* (Bethesda, Md.: ACC, 1994), figure 7.2, p. 38.

The economics of cardiology practice

Single-specialty cardiology groups have thrived in America for several reasons: (1) growing procedural and patient care demands stimulated practitioners to add partners to share the workload; (2) reimbursement patterns encouraged heart specialists and community hospitals to acquire and use diagnostic equipment; (3) the desire to be on the "cutting edge" and to gain a competitive advantage led practitioners to add partners who could introduce innovations such as PTCA and electrophysiology into their group or community; (4) the lack of restrictions (before the recent rise of managed care) on self-referrals and doctor-generated consults permitted free flow of patients to heart specialists who provided cardiology-specific (noncompetitive) services; (5) they offered functional autonomy that did not exist in most academic cardiology divisions or multispecialty groups; (6) they offered financial autonomy, which meant greater income potential for partners; (7) a critical mass of practitioners made it easier to keep up with new advances and purchase equipment.[84]

Income potential was the most powerful incentive to form and join single-specialty cardiology groups. The cardiologists who associated with these groups knew they would not have to subsidize some other specialists, services, and programs, as did their peers in academics and in multispecialty groups. Not only were their incomes higher, they did not have to justify them (or their practice style) to other medical specialists. They could practice consultative cardiology without institutional or organizational requirements to deliver primary care or share

TABLE 9-5

Median Compensation of Heart Specialists ($) (1992–1993)

	INVASIVE CARDIOLOGY	NONINVASIVE CARDIOLOGY	CARDIOVASCULAR SURGERY
Multispecialty group	280,499	209,414	391,899
Cardiology group	385,037	314,482	598,950

SOURCE: "Update on physician compensation in different practice settings," *[ACC] Affiliates in Training* 11 no. 3 (1994), table 2, p. 3.

in general medical duties. If they hoped to prosper during the 1970s and 1980s, cardiologists in single-specialty groups had only to focus on being accessible, providing quality state-of-the-art heart care, and returning referred patients to their primary physicians for ongoing care.

A professional recruiter observed recently, "There is no doubt that fellows looking for a private practice are more interested in joining a single specialty group of cardiologists, as opposed to a multispecialty group." He explained that "cardiologists (especially procedurally oriented) in single specialty groups earn more money than their counterparts in multispecialty groups" (Table 9-5). There are few secrets in today's medical marketplace, where salary surveys and recruiters abound. "Fellows are aware of the revenues invasive procedures generate, and they see the multispecialty setting as one in which invasive cardiologists support and subsidize the lower generating specialties—family practice, pediatrics, etc. This is the major reason why more fellows are drawn to single specialty groups."[85]

There have been powerful economic incentives to enter cardiology for a generation—ever since Medicare, procedures such as coronary angiography and bypass surgery, and powerful technology such as echocardiography appeared on the scene simultaneously.[86] Summarizing a 1980 earnings survey, a writer in *Medical Economics* proclaimed, "Cardiologists have the most to cheer about." They were in first place among the five surveyed nonsurgical specialists and "netted substantially more" than general surgeons. Moreover, the "economic position" of cardiologists relative to all doctors "improved considerably" during the 1970s (Table 9-6).[87] This favorable earnings picture continued throughout the 1980s and early 1990s. Between 1983 and 1988, the real net income of self-employed cardiologists increased more than that of any other specialists except orthopedic surgeons.[88] The ACC summarized several salary surveys in 1994 and found that the median salaries of invasive cardiologists ranked third among forty-eight medical and surgical specialties (cardiovascular surgery and neurosurgery were first and second).[89]

By this time, many academic medical centers were actively competing with single-specialty cardiology groups for both patients and heart specialists. Market forces pushed salaries upward. Braunwald acknowledged that "it only appears fair to academic cardiologists that their salaries bear a close relationship to their income generation within the medical center and their potential income in the community."[90] In 1991–1992, the mean salary of all academic cardiologists (assistant professor through division chair) was $154,000, while the mean *starting* salary for experienced cardiologists joining private groups (single-specialty and multispecialty groups combined) was $193,000. Thus a significant salary gradient existed between academic and practitioner cardiologists. But most academics got some protected time for research and teaching, and in general they produced less revenue than their peers in private practice.[91]

Aspiring academic cardiologists recognize their value in the marketplace. Former ACC president William Parmley remarked recently that he was "struck by the importance of salary, incentive, and security" in candidates applying for full-time positions in cardiology.[92] The pressure to offer higher salaries to recruit and retain cardiologists in academic centers and multispecialty groups intensified the interdisciplinary stresses that already existed in those settings.[93] Although many primary

TABLE 9-6
Growth in Median Net Incomes of Incorporated Doctors ($) (1973–1979)

SPECIALTY	1973	1979	PERCENTAGE GAIN
Cardiology	67,500	104,440	55
Internal medicine	58,750	79,790	36
All M.D.s	67,500	86,260	28
Family practice	55,000	68,040	24
Neurology	62,500	80,000	23
Pediatrics	55,000	67,040	22

SOURCE: M. Kirchner, "Non-surgical practice: What's the key to higher earnings?" *Med. Econ.* 58 (1981): 182–197, p. 185.

TABLE 9-7

Mean Compensation and Productivity—Group Practices (1991)

SPECIALTY	COMPENSATION ($)	PRODUCTION ($)	COMPENSATION AS A PERCENTAGE OF PRODUCTION
Cardiology	225,347	706,181	32
Cardiovascular surgery	372,244	1,067,256	35
Family practice	116,016	286,712	40
Gastroenterology	194,457	599,692	32
General surgery	204,739	580,666	35
Internal medicine	128,571	297,084	43
Neurology	148,089	373,274	40
OB-GYN	210,358	602,507	35
Oncology	200,775	646,995	31
Ophthalmology	199,396	642,516	31
Orthopedics	285,727	803,047	36
Pediatrics	124,315	307,548	40
Psychiatry	127,890	235,400	54
Pulmonary medicine	155,800	376,406	41
Radiology	228,279	766,579	30
Rheumatology	131,563	281,005	47

SOURCE: "What's new in physician compensation," *Group Practice Journal* 41 (1992): 18–25, table 2, p. 21.
NOTE: Single-specialty groups and multispecialty groups combined.

care physicians resented the spiraling salaries of heart specialists, they reluctantly conceded that their institutions "taxed" cardiologists and some other specialists at higher rates (Table 9-7). But the focus was on salary rather than the financial or physical contribution cardiologists (or other high revenue-producing specialists such as orthopedic surgeons) made to the institution. "From those to whom much is given, much is required" was the way one medical department chair put it.[94]

Traditional Medicare physician reimbursement formulas and fee schedules are being revised, in part, to change the ratio of specialists and primary care doctors. Senator Edward Kennedy suggested a quarter of a century ago that the federal government should offer incentives to encourage physicians "to practice in a manner, in a specialty, and in a place where the people's need is the greatest."[95] The movement to use financial inducements to stimulate more medical graduates to enter primary care specialties (such as family practice and general internal medicine) gained momentum as health care costs continued to outpace inflation.[96] A vocal coalition supporting this strategy has emerged that includes influential people in academics, government, health policy, and philanthropic foundations, in addition to most primary care physicians and their professional societies. The voices of patients are generally muted in the debate, because most of them no longer pay directly for medical services. Specialists are often labeled as being biased by economic self-interest, a charge that is hard to dispute.

Rheumatologist Daniel McCarty, chief of medicine at the Medical College of Wisconsin, claimed in 1987 that the "sudden shift in student preference toward the technology-oriented specialties is largely attributed to the marked difference in both lifestyle and income of the physicians in those specialties as compared with primary care." Acknowledging that "modern technological advances have made these specialties much more exciting than before," McCarty argued that fees for procedures should be "reduced below their current inflated value." He urged that the money "saved" should be "redistributed" to primary care physicians."[97]

Internists have complained about the income differential between themselves and other specialists for decades. When the American College of Physicians (ACP) board of regents discussed the issue in 1953, one member protested that "the entire setup for hospital and health insurance is controlled, so far as the medical profession is concerned, by the surgeons." Conceding that "we internists do a lot of griping about surgical fees," he asked what the ACP "has done with respect to hospital and medical insurance." Nothing—it was not yet part of the college's agenda, although the organization was receiving "constant inquiries concerning this particular problem."[98] The ACP and ACC entered the field of medical economics recently on behalf of their members. In 1984 ACC president John Williams Jr. told members that most of the letters he received urged the college to pay more attention to the socioeconomic aspects of cardiology practice.[99]

Acknowledging members' concerns about their government's increasing involvement in health care, the ACC developed a "key contact" program in 1986 to familiarize interested college members with federal policies on such things as NIH funding, health care delivery, and physician reimbursement and to give heart specialists a stronger voice on Capitol Hill. The ACC's government relations department organized meetings between college representatives and key senators and congressmen in order to present the profession's views on matters pertaining to cardiovascular research and practice. While the "immediate goal" was to identify a key contact for each Congress member who served on a health subcommittee, the long-term strategy was to have a key contact in every congressional district.[100]

The ACC inaugurated an annual "health policy retreat" in Washington in 1989 where college members met with "prominent and influential representatives of both the government and private sector." That year, participants heard Republican Senator Robert Dole predict that "Congress must consider dramatic reforms in the health care budget."[101] The ACC was positioning itself to participate in the debate. Marie Michnich, a nurse with postgraduate education and experience in health care policy and a former staffer for Dole's Senate Finance Committee, had been hired recently to head the ACC's health policy division.[102]

The government moved aggressively to attempt to control health care costs during the 1980s. President Ronald Reagan signed legislation in 1983 that established the "Diagnosis-Related Groups" method of hospital reimbursement for Medicare patients.[103] Although this system gave Washington a means to begin managing hospital costs, it did not address physicians' charges. That was coming. Three years later, Congress created the Physician Payment Review Commission and charged it with developing a "relative value scale for physicians' services." Health policy analyst William Hsiao and his associates at the Harvard School of Public Health had been creating a conceptual framework for defining the resource costs of physicians' services and for measuring relative work since the late 1970s. Washington liked Hsiao's approach, and Congress passed legislation in 1989 mandating physician payment reform based upon the comprehensive "resource-based relative-value scale" (RBRVS) he was developing.[104]

ACC president Richard Conti, an academic cardiologist at the University of Florida, invited Hsiao to participate in a health policy symposium held during the college's 1990 annual meeting. "We weren't quite sure how this would go over," Conti recalled, but "it went over quite well. Hsiao presented his views, and the discussion was rational." But Conti added, "If he showed up now [1992] we probably would tar and feather him."[105] This assessment reflected the profound (and progres-

TABLE 9-8

Decreases in Medicare Reimbursement for Cardiology Services:
1989 Average Allowed Charges versus 1992 Medicare Fee Schedule (MFS)

PROCEDURE	1989 ALLOWED CHARGES ($)	1993 MFS RATES ($)	1989–1993 PERCENTAGE CHANGE
Electrocardiogram	36	25	–30.8
Two-dimensional echo	240	192	–20.0
Left heart catheterization and angiogram	718	430	–40.1
Single-vessel PTCA	1487	875	–41.2

SOURCE: W. J. Unger, "Implications of healthcare reform for cardiologists," *J. Invasive Cardiol.* 6 (1994): 36–41.
NOTE: The 1992 Medicare Fee Schedule applied to 1993 rates.

sive) negative impact RBRVS and other government reimbursement policies were having on the incomes of cardiologists and several other types of specialists. The first shock wave hit heart specialists when Medicare cuts for "overpriced" procedures were implemented in 1990. This reduced the reimbursement for cardiac catheterization, pacemaker insertion, and bypass surgery performed on Medicare patients. Heart care was an area that attracted the government's attention, because 10 percent of Medicare payments to physicians went to cardiologists and cardiovascular surgeons.[106]

These fee reductions for cardiovascular procedures were partly the result of efforts by Hsiao's group to rationalize physician payments. The implementation of the "Medicare Fee Schedule" in 1992 had a major impact on cardiology (Table 9-8). Hsiao commented recently that the Health Care Financing Administration "created a firestorm" when it released the new fee schedule.[107] Understandably, economic self-interest influenced the attitudes and rhetoric of individual doctors and their professional societies regarding RBRVS and the Medicare Fee Schedule. These two reimbursement innovations were the "main agenda items" when the ACC governors met in November 1991, as rumors about fee cuts filled the air.[108] The college tried to filter the noise and launched a monthly newsletter *Washington Update on Legislation and Regulation* in 1990 that contained a detailed summary of the status of health care legislation.

Cardiologists and other specialists were alarmed by the proposed fee reductions, but many people were unsympathetic because they

TABLE 9-9
Median Earnings for Selected Employment Categories ($) (1994)

Airline pilot	95,794
Computer engineer	70,000
Drywall installer	25,459
General surgeon	200,000
Lawyer	58,500
Pharmacist	49,608
Physical therapist	49,000
Physician	156,000
Physician assistant	53,225
Registered nurse	35,620
Secondary school teacher	35,880
Stockbroker	90,000

SOURCE: L. M. Marable, "The fifty hottest jobs in America," *Money* 24, no. 3 (March 1995): 114–117. Reprinted from the March 1995 issue of *Money* by special permission; copyright 1995, Time Inc.
NOTE: The salary figures are from the Bureau of Labor Statistics or "industry sources." See article for details.

perceived that doctors were well paid (Table 9-9). Readers of *Money* magazine read in 1990 that "the doctors who designed and control the near-bankrupt system are up to their stethoscopes in positive cash flow." The writer proclaimed that "doctors are coming to realize that their future will be very different from their past," in part because RBRVS would "level the playing field" by rewarding "[clinical] diagnostic skills more and technical skills less."[109]

Tensions between primary care physicians and specialists became more evident as the government tightened its purse strings—and made it clear that part of the agenda was to redistribute income among various types of doctors. Responding to an article on occupational hazards (radiation exposure and back problems) faced by invasive and interventional cardiologists, a general internist from Florida wrote, "I can now begin to understand the basis for the exorbitant fees charged by our elite heart specialists for their services." He continued, "It wasn't clear that all that high-tech medicine was causing our medical saviors to suffer from sore backs and hard lenses. I'm certain that perceived risk will only serve to further increase fees, but wouldn't it be great if the result were a decrease in unnecessary invasive procedures that arguably produce no significant benefits." He closed, "I am a general internist in primary care, my back hurts too."[110]

Michael LaCombe, an articulate voice for generalists, complained about "subspecialists with half the responsibility earning twice as much as general internists." This physician essayist told a story that revealed his frustration, shared by many generalists. A cardiologist friend called LaCombe to help a man who got a fishhook stuck in his eyelid. The narrative begins with the cardiologist: "'I had them go and get you, Mike,' he said with some agitating rocking of his chair. 'I figured you were a lot closer to this than I am.' 'Yeah' said one of my sons, 'My dad's a doctor.'"[111]

Meanwhile, Congress passed legislation that united generalists and heart specialists on one issue, payment for interpreting electrocardiograms. Congressman Fortney "Pete" Stark, a California Democrat, sponsored an amendment to the Omnibus Budget Reconciliation Act of 1990 designed to end separate reimbursement for electrocardiogram interpretation for Medicare patients beginning in 1992. Proponents of the amendment argued that the electrocardiogram was a "simple diagnostic test" that could be evaluated by a computer and claimed that the new policy would save Medicare more than $100 million a year.[112] Passage of the legislation energized the ACC's key contact program. Between 1990 and 1993, the "electrocardiogram issue" was discussed constantly in the college's newsletters *Washington Update* and *Cardiology*, and ACC members were urged to contact their legislators to explain the justification for separate reimbursement for electrocardiogram interpretation.

In fall 1991 members of the college's key contact program visited more than seventy senators and representatives to express their concerns about the new electrocardiogram nonreimbursement policy. The challenge was to frame the discussion so legislators and their staffers did not conclude that economic self-interest was the cardiologists' sole motive. Because heart specialists do not control the electrocardiograph, other doctors (such as family physicians and general internists) also interpret the tracings, and their professional societies joined the ACC in calling for the restoration of separate payment for electrocardiogram interpretation. Groups representing academics, the Association of American Medical Colleges (AAMC), and the Association of Professors of Medicine (APM), also joined the coalition. The profession's argument was framed in terms of access and quality of care. Writing "on behalf of the millions of Medicare patients," the coalition explained that electrocardiograms "are an essential diagnostic tool for detecting

heart abnormalities. In the absence of expert interpretation by a qualified physician, however, the results of an electrocardiogram test are
meaningless."[113] The coalition prevailed in 1993 when President Bill
Clinton signed a bill that restored separate payment for electrocardiogram interpretation.

The ACC also raised the issues of access and quality of care when it
responded to the Medicare Fee Schedule. College president Robert
Frye, chief of cardiology at the Mayo Clinic, sent a lengthy letter to
Health Care Financing Administration administrator Gail Wilensky detailing the ACC's concerns in 1991. "What was put forth as an attempt
to reallocate and equalize payments to physicians has become a maneuver to reduce the federal budget without thought to the potentially
devastating effects on the future of American medical practice."[114] Frye
told college members that RBRVS had "resulted in a serious fraction-
ation of the medical profession" but it did not address the "fundamental" issue of "access to care."[115]

Health care reform was advancing rapidly on several fronts. Although federal initiatives attracted the most attention, state and local
developments also concerned physicians and hospital administrators. A
decade ago, an ACC trustee complained that "state mandates and laws"
were "ever-increasing . . . and their regulatory commissions are going
to drown our fellows."[116] The ACC now had a full-time health policy
staff, but they focused on the national scene. Moreover, the organization had no system for tracking legislative, regulatory, or practice issues
at the state level. Some members urged the college to develop state
chapters to help them address local issues.[117] The ACC moved quickly
when president Bill Parmley, an academic cardiologist from San Francisco, learned that a group of Florida heart specialists planned to form a
state cardiovascular society in order to be represented in the Florida
Medical Association. Parmley and ACC executive vice president Bill
Nelligan urged the Florida doctors to let the college help them solve
their problem by forming a chapter in the state.[118]

ACC leaders worried that if Florida cardiologists created their own
organization, heart specialists in other states would follow suit, with
major implications for the college. Nelligan explained, "It doesn't take
a rocket scientist to figure out that they are going to form an association
[of state cardiovascular societies]. And they're going to have a staff and
suddenly the college . . . has a major competitor in the arena of the
clinician and practitioner."[119] The ACC lost no time in filling the void at

the state level: Arizona and Florida became the college's first chapters in 1986. Most ACC governors expressed "overwhelming support" for the concept.[120] With the assistance of staff in Bethesda, college members formed thirty-five state chapters in less than a decade.

During the 1990s "managed care" became a popular organizing principle to help control costs. Managed care organizations (many of them for-profit) gained momentum in many areas of the nation as employers embraced the model as a means to reduce their costs for insuring employees against illness. The spokespersons of these organizations joined the growing chorus of critics who portrayed specialists as overpaid "providers" inclined to use too much technology and perform too many procedures. Some managed care firms contracted with primary care physicians to serve as "gatekeepers" to limit access to specialists in an attempt to reduce costs. This practice prompted warnings that some patients would suffer under a system designed, in part, to redirect profits from doctors and hospitals to insurers.

As managed care plans proliferated, many people questioned the wisdom of such an abrupt and dramatic transformation in the conventional relationships between patients, providers, and payers. Marcia Angell, executive editor of the *New England Journal of Medicine,* decried the implications of "asking doctors to withhold beneficial care to save money for third-party payers. Doing so serves a largely political agenda and endangers the patient-centered ethic that is central to medicine." She protested the fact that doctors were being forced to function as "double agents" who "are supposed to tailor their care of patients to save money for third parties."[121]

Limiting access to specialty care is a critical factor in managed care's cost-savings equation. But *New England Journal of Medicine* editor Jerome Kassirer reminded readers that Americans "have traditionally valued their unrestrained access to care by cardiologists, dermatologists, and other specialists." Noting the explosive growth of managed care plans that limit referrals to specialists, Kassirer warned that "if we are not smart enough to protect patients' access to some of our best physicians, we will all be losers."[122] These were not the voices of cardiologists or other highly paid specialists; Angell and Kassirer were addressing fundamental aspects of the traditional doctor-patient relationship in American society.

Academics and practitioners have come to depend on their professional societies to help them cope with an unpredictable practice environment.[123] Cardiologists welcomed the ACC's stepped-up involvement in the socioeconomic aspects of medicine and health policy. College president Anthony DeMaria, an academic cardiologist at the University of Kentucky, established a private sector relations committee in 1989 to begin to track developments with "employers, insurers, managed care organizations, medical industry, and consumer groups" that might affect cardiovascular specialists. Two years later, the college created a formal private sector relations department to help members deal more effectively with changes in the cardiology marketplace.[124]

Patient demand, free access to specialists, and liberal reimbursement had supercharged cardiology during the 1970s and 1980s. When access and reimbursement were threatened simultaneously in the early 1990s, heart specialists and their college reacted. The ACC assumed a more active advocacy role on behalf of heart specialists and their patients during the presidential terms of academic cardiologist Adolph Hutter Jr., practitioner cardiologist Sylvan Weinberg, and heart surgeon Daniel Ullyot. Access to specialty care was the centerpiece of the college's 1994 "campaign" to inform citizens and politicians about cardiovascular specialists' concerns about managed care and the Clinton administration's ambitious proposal to reform health care. Congress eventually rejected the Clinton plan, but Republican leaders (who controlled the House and Senate after the 1994 elections) focused on Medicare spending as they sought to balance the federal budget.[125]

Meanwhile, managed care firms and third-party payers were now competing aggressively to "sign up" employers, patients, hospitals, and doctors in an expanding array of delivery models such as preferred provider organizations and health maintenance organizations (HMOs). Like other specialists, most cardiologists (accustomed to self-referrals and free flow of physician-consults) were caught off guard. Many heart specialists scrambled to forge links with managed care organizations and other cardiology groups to ensure a steady supply of cardiac patients. Seeing that most cardiologists were unprepared to deal with this new and often hostile environment, the ACC developed a series of educational programs and products to help them adapt.[126]

In our society, market forces are powerful and inexorable. Doctor-patient relationships and physician referral patterns built up over many years were interrupted or redefined overnight. The new paradigm of controlled access to specialists had profound implications for professional autonomy as well as income. Cardiologists began to see articles with titles like "HMO trend squeezes big-fee medical specialists."[127] Extrapolating from HMO staffing patterns, a health policy analyst concluded in 1994 that there would be an excess of 165,000 patient care physicians in the United States by the turn of the century—just six years away. If his assumptions were correct, cardiologists would be one of the most oversupplied specialists in the year 2000, with an excess of 92 percent.[128]

For the past ten years most practitioner cardiologists have felt that there were enough heart specialists. A 1986 survey showed that a majority of ACC members thought too many cardiologists were being trained. Joe Noble, the college governor for Indiana, told the trustees that year that the governors also believed there were too many cardiologists. He urged the ACC to "do something about it. . . . not in a self-serving way, but in a general way."[129] Most academic cardiologists dismissed these rumblings from practitioners (who were more sensitive to competition) as they had GMENAC's predictions a few years earlier. Their fellows were all finding jobs, and cardiology was one of the most popular specialty choices. William Nelligan recalls that in the early 1980s the college leaders "did all we could to disprove the notion that there were too many cardiologists."[130]

But the workforce issue would not go away. In 1987 the college sponsored a Bethesda Conference on "Trends in the Practice of Adult Cardiology: Implications for Manpower." The participants considered the impact of political and demographic trends, innovations in cardiac diagnosis and treatment, and federal policies on research, training, and health care funding. Concluding that there might be a surplus of cardiologists "in the future," the conference participants (a significant majority of whom were academics) did not urge training programs to reduce their output of heart specialists.[131] Six years later the ACC held another Bethesda Conference on cardiology workforce. Now, conceding that "American medicine is in a period of rapid transition," the participants agreed that academics must accept "the inevitability of reducing the number of cardiologists who will be trained in the next decade." They urged that "cuts" in training positions "be made on the basis of program quality."[132]

Arguing for reducing the cardiology workforce, the authors of a recent essay used cross-cultural statistics to support their case. They reported that there are 6.5 cardiologists per hundred thousand people in the United States, compared with 2.9 for Germany, 2.5 for Canada, and 0.4 for Great Britain.[133] But these differences (and equally dramatic variations in the rates of cardiac catheterization, PTCA, and CABG) among nations exist for a variety of historical, social, and economic reasons. Unlike citizens of other nations, Americans have come to expect to be able to see specialists and have access to the technology and procedures they control in a timely fashion. "Americans use more health services by choice," according to Steven Schroeder, president of the Robert Wood Johnson Foundation. This former academic general internist attributes the nation's high per capita health care expenditures and rate of technology utilization compared to other countries partly to a surplus of specialists, who have "professional and economic incentives to perform their special procedures unnecessarily."[134]

William Parmley, an academic cardiologist and editor of the ACC's official journal, warned in 1994, "Although graduating cardiology fellows are still getting jobs, it appears that this may not be true in the future." A growing number of observers agree that the future is now.[135] The ACC alerted trainees in 1995 that "managed care [is] reducing opportunities for cardiovascular specialists in some markets." Highlighting the power of market forces, the writer explained, "While policy makers and academics debate the existence of an oversupply of specialists, private sector forces in some competitive areas of the country already are influencing the demand for cardiovascular services."[136] This pragmatic assessment is supported by a 50 percent decline in the number of cardiology jobs advertised in the *New England Journal of Medicine* between September 1993 and September 1994.[137]

The ACC's executive committee issued a statement on physician workforce in late 1994 that acknowledged an oversupply of invasive cardiologists and supported a reduction in the number of adult cardiology fellowship positions. Some practitioners had hoped the college would take a stronger stand. They worried that many cardiology division chiefs would resist downsizing their training programs, citing the ACC's recommendation that cuts be achieved by "the elimination of marginal programs rather than across-the-board reductions in fellowship positions."[138]

Recently, concerns have been raised about the legal implications of attempting to decrease the cardiology workforce. Cardiology division chiefs and training directors can downsize their own institution's fellowship program voluntarily, but any coordinated effort (at a local, regional, or national level) to reduce the number of fellowship positions might be interpreted as restraint of trade and as a violation of antitrust laws.[139] Although these concerns have retarded the efforts of academic cardiologists to address the workforce issue, the total number of cardiology fellows declined for the first time last year. Between 1994 and 1995 the number of adult cardiology training programs in the United States declined by 2 percent, from 214 to 210, and the total number of fellows declined by 5.6 percent, from 2,791 to 2,633 (Table A9).

The cardiology workforce is also changing in response to larger trends in American society. In 1989 *New England Journal of Medicine* editor Arnold Relman proclaimed, "We seem to be witnessing the beginnings of a demographic revolution of major proportions, which is bound to have great importance for the future of our health care system." He was referring to a 322 percent increase in the percentage of women first-year medical students between 1979 (9 percent) and 1989 (38 percent).[140] This does not ensure a proportional increase in the number of women cardiologists in the future. Based on a demographic analysis of 19,151 physicians (including 3,569 women) trained in internal medicine between 1977 and 1985, a recent study concluded that a greater proportion of women than men became general internists rather than medical subspecialists. The authors concluded that women "placed a higher value on patient contact than did men," and "they continued to choose primary-care-oriented specialties regardless of recent trends away from these areas."[141]

Marian Limacher, an academic cardiologist and member of the ACC's strategic planning committee, reported on the "status of women in cardiology and in the American College of Cardiology" at a meeting of the Society for the Advancement of Women's Health Research in 1992. She explained that although 19 percent of all internists were women in 1990, only 5 percent of cardiologists were women. There appeared to be a trend, however, with women making up 9 percent of heart specialists aged 35 or younger (Table 9-10). The gender of ACC members reflected this trend. In 1992 only 4 percent of fellows were women, but 10 percent of ACC affiliates-in-training were women. Women held 6.4 percent of leadership positions (boards, task forces, and committees) in the college. The college's strategic planning committee passed a motion supporting "the principle of diversity in its committees and leadership roles. This includes encouragement of participation of qualified women and minorities in the college."[142]

TABLE 9-10

U.S. Cardiologists by Age and Gender: Number and Percentage in Various
Age Groups (1990)

	AGE (YEARS)				
	<35	35–44	45–54	55–64	>65
Male	2,421 (91)	5,968 (94)	3,593 (97)	1,929 (98)	1,112 (98)
Female	250 (9)	392 (6)	129 (3)	45 (2)	23 (2)

SOURCE: American Medical Association, *Physician Characteristics and Distribution in the U.S.*, 1992
ed. (Chicago: AMA, 1992), table B-3, pp. 52–53.

During its first century, cardiology emerged as one of American
medicine's most significant specialties. Cardiology's growth was fueled
by the prevalence of cardiovascular disease, the federal government's
desire to blunt the societal and economic impact of these disorders, an
impressive series of procedural and technological innovations, its image
as a dynamic and exciting field, and favorable reimbursement policies.
Despite the dramatic changes occurring in the structure and financing
of medical practice in the United States, cardiologists will likely retain
their key role in the care of people with serious and symptomatic heart
disease.

New health care delivery models, reimbursement strategies, and
societal attitudes are already modulating the growth and focus of the
specialty, however.[143] For a generation, cardiology's "success" has most
often been measured in terms of the quantity of heart specialists produced, research projects funded, the number of procedures performed,
and the dollars generated from clinical services. In a managed care
environment that considers specialists and their tools and techniques as
expensive resources that lower profits, cardiologists will have to
demonstrate their value in terms of enhanced patient outcomes and
satisfaction.[144]

Today, two strong national organizations—the AHA and the ACC—
complement one another. The AHA pursues its program of fund-raising
to support basic research and a variety of public health and education
programs. While heralding a dramatic 25 percent reduction in the
age-adjusted death rate for cardiovascular diseases between 1982 and
1992, both organizations agree that more basic research and greater
emphasis on prevention are crucial if disorders of the heart and circulation
are to be displaced as the leading cause of death in the United States.[145]

Although Washington's increasing involvement in health care and dramatic changes in the marketplace have led the ACC to expand its activities in the areas of government and private sector relations, the organization's main focus reflects its original mission—continuing medical education. Today, the college's educational programs include a broad range of self-study materials, scheduled courses at Heart House and around the country, a journal with 30,000 subscribers, and an annual meeting attended by 25,000 people.[146] With almost 23 thousand members, the ACC is one of medicine's largest professional societies. Reflecting the growing complexity of cardiology (in its scientific and social dimensions), more than 500 people currently serve on nearly sixty college committees.[147]

Driven largely by new procedures and technologies that require time to master, cardiology training continues to expand in both duration and scope. The summary statement of a recent ACC-sponsored symposium on the education of heart specialists is compelling evidence of the transformation of cardiology training during the past half-century from a *laissez faire* system based on apprenticeship to a rigorous three- or four-year program following a standardized internal medicine residency.[148] Despite the present climate of apprehension and uncertainty among academics and practitioners alike, American heart specialists and the leaders of their professional society are justifiably proud of the dramatic achievements in the science and practice of cardiology during the past century. The prototypical heart specialists described in the first chapter would marvel over the evolution of the discipline they helped to create.

Historian John Burnham emphasized recently that it is risky to attempt to predict the future.[149] As we approach a new century and millennium, it is safe to wager that many people will assess the progress and prospects of American medicine in general, and medical specialties such as cardiology in particular. Writing at the dawn of the twentieth century, William Osler, North America's most celebrated internist, applauded the many contributions specialists had made to knowledge and practice. Conceding that specialization was "not without minor evils," he argued that "this custom has yielded some of the great triumphs of the profession."[150] Cardiology emerged as a specialty in the United States shortly after Osler offered this opinion.

Although our society will likely reward the work of physician specialists less in the future than it has in recent years, specialization is an unrelenting cultural force that transcends medical politics. The future of medicine and cardiology in the United States will not be a mere extrapolation of the past, however. Increasingly, complex political, social, and economic forces will determine the agenda of American medicine, direct the activities of doctors and medical scientists, and dictate the options of patients seeking care. America's cardiologists and their college must work constructively in this new cost-sensitive environment to ensure that people benefit from what has already been learned about the diagnosis and treatment of heart disease—and that our nation's commitment to finding and applying new knowledge is maintained.

Appendix

TABLE A1

Original American Heart Association Board Members (1924)

Lewis Conner	♥*	New York City; professor of medicine, Cornell-New York Hospital; former NYHA president
Haven Emerson	♥*	New York City; professor of public health, P & S, 1922–1943; NYHA president-elect
T. Stuart Hart	♥*	New York City; assistant professor of medicine, P & S; former NYHA president
Robert Halsey	♥	New York City; professor of medicine, New York Post-Graduate Medical School
James Herrick	*	Chicago; professor of medicine, Rush Medical College
Henry Jackson	*	Boston; physician
Hugh McCullough		St. Louis; associate professor of pediatrics, Washington University
C. J. McIntyre		Indianapolis; physician
George Norris	*	Philadelphia; professor of medicine, University of Pennsylvania
Robert Preble	*	Chicago; professor of medicine, Northwestern University
William Robey	♥	Boston; assistant professor of medicine, Harvard-Boston City Hospital
Joseph Sailer	♥*	Philadelphia; professor of medicine, University of Pennsylvania
Sidney Strauss		Chicago; professor of medicine, University of Illinois
William Stroud	♥*	Philadelphia; associate instructor of medicine, University of Pennsylvania
Paul White	*	Boston; instructor of medicine, Harvard-Massachusetts General Hosp.

SOURCE: W. Moore, *Fighting for Life* (Dallas: AHA, 1983) and several biographical directories listed in the bibliography.

NOTES: Entries include city and main institutional affiliation * = Member of the Association of American Physicians ♥ = AHA executive committee member. NYHA = New York Heart Association (Association for the Prevention and Relief of Heart Disease) P & S = College of Physicians and Surgeons, Columbia University.

SUMMARY: 10 of the 15 board committee members were from New York, Boston, or Philadelphia; 12 were internists or cardiologists affiliated with medical schools or teaching hospitals; 1 was a pediatrician (McCullough); and 1 was a full-time public health physician (Emerson).

TABLE A2

*Persons Present at the Organizational Meeting of the Sir James Mackenzie
Cardiological Society (1926)*

David R. Alexander	*	New York City
Thomas Atwood	*	Bridgeport, Connecticut
Walter Bensel		New York City; P & S 1890
Herman Besser		New York City; Bellevue Hospital Medical College 1897; radiologist
Louis Bishop, Sr.		New York City; P & S 1889
Russell Burton-Opitz		New York City; University of Chicago 1895
Harry P. Finck	*	Boston
Charles Gottlieb		New York City; University and Bellevue 1907; radiologist
Albert Hyman		New York City; Harvard 1918
Miller E. Kahn	*	New York City (possibly Milton E. Kahn, University of Buffalo 1925)
Paul Kennedy		Leonia, N.J.; P & S 1927
Murray Levine		New York City; P & S 1918; surgeon
Malcolm McPherson	*	New York City (possibly from Sheffield, England)
Aaron Parsonnet		Newark, N.J.; Maryland Medical College 1911
Maurice Protas		Washington, D.C.; George Washington 1925
Jacob Sobel		New York City; P & S 1895; pediatrician
Allen Sussman		Baltimore, Md.; University of Maryland 1923
Joseph Wolffe		Philadelphia; Temple University 1919

SOURCE: Minutes, Sir James Mackenzie Medical Society, 22 October 1926. Copy kindly provided by Arthur Hollman and Paul Kligfield.
NOTES: Entries include the city listed in the minutes as well as medical school and specialty information from contemporary AMA directories. Those without an occupation are practitioner cardiologists. * = Not listed in AMA directories. P & S = College of Physicians and Surgeons, Columbia University.

TABLE A3
"Charter Members" Present at the "[Re]organizational" Meeting of the New York Cardiological Society (1934)

Walter Bensel	♥	P & S 1890
Kurt Berliner		Friedrich-Wilhelms Universität, Berlin, 1922; clinical assistant physician Mt. Sinai Hospital
Barnett Binkowitz		Long Island College Hospital 1923; assistant chief of cardiology Lenox Hill Hospital
Louis Bishop, Sr.	♥	P & S 1889; consulting cardiologist Lincoln Hospital
Louis Bishop, Jr.		P & S 1925; associate physician Bellevue Hospital
Alton Brill		University and Bellevue 1910; associate physician Lebanon Hospital
Russell Burton-Opitz	♥	University of Chicago 1895; cardiologist Lenox Hill Hospital
Simon Frucht		P & S 1905; cardiologist Beth-El Hospital
Bertram Goldstein		University and Bellevue 1923; chief, cardiology clinic Gouverneur Hospital
Maximillian Goldstein		Loyola 1912; chief, cardiology clinic Montefiore Hospital
Albert Hyman	♥	Harvard 1918; cardiologist Beth David Hospital
Paul Kennedy	♥	P & S 1927; internist Englewood, N.J.
Harry Lowen		P & S 1925; chief, cardiology clinic Beth David Hospital
Gilbert Miller		University and Bellevue 1908; cardiologist Jewish Memorial Hospital
Samuel J. Miller		Tennessee 1924; assistant cardiologist Lenox Hill Hospital
Benjamin Segal		P & S 1921; chief, obstetrics and gynecology Lincoln Hospital
Charles Shookhoff		Cornell 1910; chief, cardiology clinic Jewish Hospital (not present—called away for an emergency)

SOURCES: Minutes, NYCS, 30 April 1934, Reichert Papers, NYH. Hospital appointments obtained from *The Medical Directory of New York, New Jersey and Connecticut*, vol. 35 (New York: Medical Society of the State of New York, 1933).

NOTES: Entries include medical schools and primary hospital affiliation. ♥ = Present at the organizational meeting of the James Mackenzie Cardiological Society, 22 October 1926.

TABLE A4
Founders of the American College of Cardiology (1949)

Walter Bensel[a]	♥ *	New York City 1869; P & S 1890; associate clinical professor New York Medical College; 147 East 72nd Street; Protestant
Samuel Blinder		New York City 1903; George Washington 1926; intern Jersey City Hospital, postgraduate training (medicine and pathology) London and Vienna; attending physician New York Postgraduate Hospital outpatient department, assistant attending physician New York University Bellevue Medical Center, associate clinical professor of medicine New York Medical College; ABIM (internal medicine and cardiovascular disease), FACP; 929 Park Avenue, Jewish
Hannibal DeBellis		Italy 1894; United States 1903; University of Alabama 1920; intern St. Vincent's Hospital, New York City; attending physician and cardiologist St. Vincent's Hospital; 20 Fifth Avenue; Catholic
Seymour Fiske		Philadelphia 1895; University of Pennsylvania 1920; intern Peter Bent Brigham Hospital, Boston; associate attending physician New York City Hospital, associate clinical professor of medicine New York Medical College; ABIM (internal medicine), FACP; 150 East 71st Street; Protestant
Gabriel Greco		Italy 1910; United States ?; Creighton University 1936; postgraduate training (cardiology) Long Island College of Medicine, Columbia, Harvard; 114-08 Linden Boulevard, Ozone Park, N.Y.; Catholic
Franz Groedel		Germany 1881; United States 1933; Leipzig 1904; postgraduate training (medicine and cardiology) Munich, etc.; cardiologist Beth David Hospital, St. Anthony's Hospital, Lenox Hill Hospital; 829 Park Avenue; Protestant (Jewish as youth)
Albert Hyman	♥ *	Boston 1893; Harvard 1918; intern Boston City Hospital, resident Long Island College Hospital, postgraduate training (cardiology) London and Vienna, D.Sc. Med. (cardiology) London University; attending cardiologist, Beth David Hospital, Jewish Memorial Hospital, and New York City Hospital, associate professor of clinical medicine New York Medical College; ABIM (internal medicine), FACP; 450 East 63rd Street; Jewish
Bruno Kisch		Prague 1890; United States 1938; Charles University Prague 1913; postgraduate training (physiology and medicine) University of Cologne; professor Yeshiva University; 845 West End Avenue; Jewish
Samuel Korry		New York City 1895; Long Island College Hospital 1917; intern Our Lady of Mercy Medical Center, Bronx; chief of cardiology Stuyvesant Polytechnic Hospital; 77 Park Avenue; Jewish

TABLE A4
Founders of the American College of Cardiology (1949) (continued)

Max Miller	Austria 1911; United States c. 1940; Vienna 1936; postgraduate training Austria; associate in cardiology Beth David Hospital; 1111 Park Avenue; Jewish
Aaron Parsonnet[b]	Russia 1889; United States ?; Loyola, Chicago 1913; intern Newark Beth Israel Hospital; chief of cardiology Newark Beth Israel Hospital; ABIM (internal medicine), FACP, AHA Scientific Council; 3 Madison Avenue, Newark, N.J.; Jewish
Philip Reichert	New York City 1897; Cornell Medical College 1923; intern Willard Parker Hospital, assistant Rockefeller Institute, fellow (pediatrics) Mt. Sinai Hospital, clinical assistant Mt. Sinai outpatient department; associate cardiologist and chief, cardiology clinic, Beth David Hospital; FACP; Jewish
Attilio Robertiello	Italy 1892; United States 1901; P & S 1917; attending physician Post-Graduate Hospital of New York University; 214 East 16th Street; Catholic
Joseph Wolffe	Vilna, Russia [later Poland] 1896; United States ?; Temple University 1919; intern and resident Mt. Sinai Hospital; medical director Valley Forge Heart Institute and Hospital, associate professor of medicine Temple University; ABIM (internal medicine); 1829 Pine Street, Philadelphia; Jewish
Epaminonda Secondari[c]	Italy 1889; United States c. 1925, M.D. Rome; physician Italian Hospital of New York and Columbus Hospital; 1211 Madison Avenue; Catholic

SOURCES: Minutes ACC (NYCS group), 28 November 1949, Reichert Papers, NYH Archives. Religion provided by H. F. K. [Mrs. Philip] Reichert, who knew the founders. Other information was derived from various directories listed in the bibliography.

NOTES: Format is name; place and year of birth; United States arrival if known; medical school and graduation date; additional training (if known); main institutional affiliation(s); ABIM, Fellow of the College of Physicians; member AHA Scientific Council; office address (all New York City unless noted); religion. [a]Although Bensel signed the original draft constitution, he was not considered a formal ACC founder because he withdrew his support. See text. [b]Parsonnet signed the original draft constitution but died before the college began recruiting members. [c]Secondari did not sign the original draft constitution, but his name was later added to the list of official founders. See Philip Reichert, *Cardiology* vol. 9, no. 1 (February 1980): 2. ♥ = Present at the organizational meeting of the James Mackenzie Cardiological Society, 22 October 1926. * = Present at 1934 NYCS meeting. See Table A3.

Summary of 14 founders (including Secondari but not Bensel): American-born (5): Blinder, Fiske, Hyman, Korry, Reichert. Foreign-born (9): DeBellis (Italy), Greco (Italy), Groedel (Germany), Kisch (Prague), Miller (Austria), Parsonnet (Russia), Robertiello (Italy), Wolffe (Russia), Secondari (Italy). Protestant or Catholic (6): DeBellis, Fiske, Greco, Groedel, Robertiello, Secondari. Jewish (8): Blinder, Hyman, Kisch, Korry, Miller, Parsonnet, Reichert, Wolffe. American-born and Jewish (4): Blinder, Hyman, Korry, Reichert. Foreign-born and Jewish (4): Kisch, Miller, Parsonnet, Wolffe. American-born and Protestant or Catholic (1): Fiske. Foreign-born and Protestant or Catholic (5): DeBellis, Greco, Groedel, Robertiello, Secondari. Foreign-born and American medical school (5): DeBellis, Greco, Parsonnet, Robertiello, Wolffe. Foreign-born and foreign medical school (4): Groedel, Kisch, Miller, Secondari.

TABLE A5

Clinical Cardiology Societies in the United States (1995)

ORGANIZATION	YEAR FOUNDED	MEMBERS 1995
American Heart Association (AHA)[a]	1924	26,300
New York Cardiological Society (NYCS)	1928	529
American College of Cardiology (ACC)	1949	22,240
AHA Council on Clinical Cardiology (CCC)	1952	6,855
Association of University Cardiologists (AUC)	1961	217
Society of Cardiovascular and Interventional Radiology[b]	1974	2,190
American Society of Echocardiography	1975	3,310
Association of Black Cardiologists[c]	1975	500
Society for Cardiac Angiography and Interventions[d]	1977	1,020
North American Society of Pacing and Electrophysiology	1979	1,650
American Society of Hypertension	1985	2,850
Council on Geriatric Cardiology[e]	1986	334
Association of Professors of Cardiology (APC)	1990	114
American Society of Nuclear Cardiology (ASNC)	1993	1,252

SOURCES: C. A. Schwartz and R. L. Turner, eds., *Encyclopedia of Associations* (Detroit: Gale Research, 1995) and ACC Archives.

NOTES: Members hold M.D. or Ph.D. degrees unless otherwise noted. Some numbers rounded off by organizations. [a]Includes some non-physicians; [b]original name was Society for Cardiovascular Radiology; [c]approximate membership, includes some non-physicians; [d]original name was Society for Cardiac Angiography; [e]an independent society with no relationship to the AHA.

TABLE A6

*Presidents of the American Heart Association and the
American College of Cardiology (1924–1996)*

TERM	AHA PRESIDENT	ACC PRESIDENT
1924	Lewis A. Conner	
1925	Joseph Sailer	
1926	Joseph Sailer	
1927	James B. Herrick	
1928	James B. Herrick	
1929	William H. Robey	
1930	William H. Robey	
1931	Robert H. Halsey	
1932	Robert H. Halsey	
1933	Stewart R. Roberts	
1934	Stewart R. Roberts	
1935	John Wyckoff	
1936	John Wyckoff	
1937	William J. Kerr	
1938	William J. Kerr	
1939	William D. Stroud	
1940	Paul D. White	
1941	Paul D. White	
1942	Paul D. White	
1943	Roy W. Scott	
1944	Roy W. Scott	
1945	Annual meeting canceled, officers retained	
1946	Howard F. West	
1947	Arlie R. Barnes	
1948	Tinsley R. Harrison	
1949	H. M. "Jack" Marvin	Franz M. Groedel
1950	Howard B. Sprague	Franz M. Groedel
1951	Louis N. Katz	Bruno Kisch
1952	Irving S. Wright	Bruno Kisch
1953	Robert L. King	Robert P. Glover
1954	E. Cowles Andrus	Ashton Graybiel
1955	Irvine H. Page	Walter S. Priest
1956	Edgar V. Allen	Simon Dack
1957	Robert W. Wilkins	George R. Meneely
1958	Francis L. Chamberlain	George W. Calver
1959	A. Carlton Ernstene	Osler A. Abbott
1960	Ogelsby Paul	Louis F. Bishop
1961	J. Scott Butterworth	E. Grey Dimond

TABLE A6
Presidents of the American Heart Association and the
American College of Cardiology (1924–1996) (continued)

TERM	AHA PRESIDENT	ACC PRESIDENT
1962	James V. Warren	John S. LaDue
1963	John J. Sampson	George C. Griffith
1964	Carleton B. Chapman	Dwight E. Harken
1965	Helen B. Taussig	Eliot Corday
1966	Lewis E. January	C. Walton Lillihei
1967	Jesse E. Edwards	William Likoff
1968	Walter B. Frommeyer Jr.	George E. Burch
1969	W. Proctor Harvey	Bill L. Martz
1970	William W. L. Glenn	William A. Sodeman
1971	J. Willis Hurst	Forrest H. Adams
1972	Paul N. Yu	Samuel M. Fox III
1973	Richard S. Ross	H. J. C. Swan
1974	Elliot Rapaport	Henry D. McIntosh
1975	John T. Shepherd	Charles Fisch
1976	Harriet P. Dustan	Charles Fisch
1977	W. Gerald Austen	Dean T. Mason
1978	John W. Eckstein	Leonard S. Dreifus
1979	Thomas N. James	Borys Surawicz
1980	James A. Schoenberger	Robert O. Brandenburg
1981	Donald C. Harrison	Dan G. McNamara
1982	Mary Jane Jesse	Suzanne B. Knoebel
1983	Antonio M. Gotto	Paul A. Ebert
1984	Thomas J. Ryan	John F. Williams Jr.
1985	Thomas J. Ryan	William W. Parmley
1986	Kenneth I. Shine	John Ross Jr.
1987	Howard E. Morgan	Francis J. Klocke
1988	Bernadine Healy	Anthony N. DeMaria
1989	Myron L. Weisfeldt	C. Richard Conti
1990	Francois M. Abboud	William L. Winters Jr.
1991	W. Virgil Brown	Robert L. Frye
1992	Edward S. Cooper	Adolph M. Hutter Jr.
1993	James H. Moller	Sylvan L. Weinberg
1994	Suzanne Oparil	Daniel J. Ullyot
1995	Sidney C. Smith Jr.	J. Ward Kennedy
1996	Jan L. Breslow	Richard P. Lewis

TABLE A7
Health Care Trends in the United States (Coggeshall, 1965)

Scientific advance. In the past half century, advances in scientific knowledge have had growing influence on health care and continue to be the most powerful force in changing the style of medical practice.

Population change. The population of America is growing and changing in numbers, composition, and distribution. These changes are increasing the number of individuals seeking health care, the amount and kinds of care sought, and health care expectations.

Increasing individual health expectations. Advances in science and health care have stimulated the health expectations of individuals. An attitude of "entitlement" to health care is becoming increasingly prevalent.

Increasing effective demand for health care. The people of America are increasingly able to pay for the health care they want and need. Higher incomes and expanded health insurance coverage are major causes of this increase.

Increasing specialization in medical practice. As medical knowledge has grown, practicing physicians have found it increasingly essential to limit their attention to more specialized areas of activity. This trend continues at the initiative of physicians and patients.

Increasing use of technological advances and equipment. Scientific advances have made vital the development of new skills to apply new knowledge. These advances have spawned a vast armamentarium for the use of the physician and his co-workers.

Increasing institutionalization of health care. Institutionalization of care has manifested itself in expanded use of hospitals, clinics, and nursing homes. The hospital is rapidly becoming the common locus of patient care.

Increasing use of a team approach to health care. The rise of specialization has resulted in an increasing trend toward team practice involving the contribution of a spectrum of specialists. This requires the attending physician to be a "coordinator" or "leader" of a team that collaborates to meet the needs of the patient.

Need for increasing numbers of physicians. The future will see more health care demanded and provided than ever before. More physicians must be trained, and as quickly as possible. Since it is not likely America will ever be able to produce enough physicians to satisfy growing national needs, it is essential that physician productivity be increased through delegation of specific tasks to others.

Need for increasing numbers of health personnel. The need for persons trained in related health fields, to work as members of the team under the leadership and coordination of the physician, is growing even more rapidly than the need for physicians.

Expanding role of government. The expanding role of government in the health field has been manifesting itself in a growing number of ways and with increasing resources and emphasis in recent years. This can be expected to continue and expand.

Rising costs. A clear trend of recent decades—and a virtually certain trend in the future—is the continuous rise in costs. All components of health care costs have risen. The cost of educating physicians has grown.

SOURCE: L. T. Coggeshall, *Planning for Medical Progress through Education* (Washington, D.C.: Association of American Medical Colleges, 1965), pp. 97–98.

TABLE A8
U.S. Medical Schools and Graduates (1900–1994)

YEAR	MEDICAL SCHOOLS	GRADUATES	GRADUATES PER SCHOOL
1900	160	5,214	33
1910	131	4,440	34
1920	85	3,047	36
1930	76	4,565	60
1940	77	5,097	66
1950	79	5,533	70
1955	81	6,977	86
1960	85	7,081	83
1965	88	7,409	84
1970	101	8,367	83
1975	114	12,714	112
1980	126	15,135	120
1985	127	16,319	129
1990	127	15,336	121
1994	126	15,620	124

SOURCES: W. G. Rothstein. *American Medical Schools and the Practice of Medicine, a History* (New York: Oxford Univ. Press, 1987), table 7.2, p. 143 and table 15.1, p. 284, and H. S. Jonas, S. I. Etzel, and B. Barzansky, "Educational programs in U.S. medical schools, 1993–1994," *JAMA* 272 (1994): 694–701, table 6, p. 697.

TABLE A9

Cardiology Training Programs and Cardiology Fellows (1941–1995)

YEAR	PROGRAMS	TOTAL TRAINEES	TRAINEES/ PROGRAM
1941[a]	—	6	
1949[a]	7	15	2.1
1950[b]	19	37	2.0
1955[b]	30	53	1.8
1960[b]	72	142	2.0
1972[c]	280	1260	4.5
1976[d]	253	1409	5.6
1980[e]	239	1492	6.2
1985[e]	243	1894	7.8
1990[e]	221	2310	10.5
1994[e]	214	2791	13.0
1995[f]	210	2633	12.5

SOURCES: [a]V. Johnson, "Implications of current trends toward specialization," in *Trends in Medical Education,* ed. M. Ashford (New York: Commonwealth Fund, 1949), pp. 173–178. [b]AMA List of Approved Residencies and Fellowships, *JAMA* 142 (1950): 1164, *JAMA* 159 (1955): 294, *JAMA* 174 (1960): 682–683. [c]"Adult cardiovascular training programs," *Am. J. Cardiol.* 34 (1974): 449–456, counting the number of programs with trainees and the number of filled positions for 1972–1973. [d]University of Chicago Center for Health Administration Studies, National Study of Internal Medicine Manpower, Chicago. [e]"Education update: 1994," *J. Am. Coll. Cardiol.* 24 (1994): 1146–1177. [f]"Training Program Survey Summary 1994–1995." ACC, Bethesda, Md.

TABLE A10

Health Insurance in the United States (1940–1990)

YEAR	PERSONS PRIVATELY INSURED (MILLIONS)[a]	PERCENTAGE OF POPULATION PRIVATELY INSUREDa	CLAIMS PAID BY PRIVATE INSURERS ($BILLION)	MEDICARE ENROLLEES (A OR B) (MILLIONS)	MEDICARE PAYMENTS (A OR B) ($BILLION)
1940	12.0	9			
1945	32.0	24			
1950	76.6	50	1.3		
1955	101.4	55	3.1		
1960	122.5	68	5.7		
1965	138.7	71	9.6	0	0
1967	146.4	74		20.1	3.2
1970	158.8	77	17.2	20.5	6.8
1975	178.2	83	32.1	22.8	12.7
1980	187.4	82	76.3	25.5	29.4
1985	181.3	76	117.6	28.2	64.5
1990	181.7	73	208.9	30.9	85.1

SOURCES: *Source Book of Health Insurance Data, 1993* (Washington, D.C.: Health Insurance Association of America, 1994), table 2.5, p. 34, and table 3.1, pp. 56–57. The number of "persons privately insured" includes all forms of insurance (e.g., insurance companies, Blue Cross/Blue Shield, self-insured, and HMOs) but does not include government insurance (e.g., Medicaid and Medicare). [a]These numbers are similar to those which others have reported as the population insured for "hospital expenses." See H. M. Somers and A. R. Somers, *Doctors, Patients, and Health Insurance: The Organization and Financing of Medical Care* (Washington, D.C.: Brookings Institution, 1961), chart 1-3, p. 11. Population figures from *Statistical Abstracts of the United States, 1993. 113th ed. The National Data Book* (Washington, D.C.: GPO, 1993), p. 8.

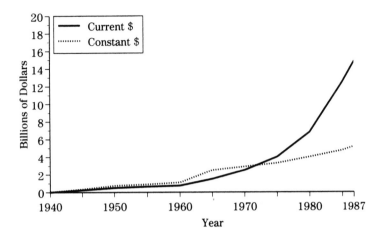

FIGURE A1.   Federal funds for biomedical research and development (1940–1987).

SOURCE: E. Ginzberg and A. B. Dutka, *The Financing of Biomedical Research* (Baltimore: Johns Hopkins Univ. Press, 1989), figure 2.1, p. 11.

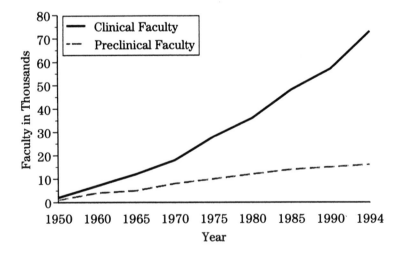

FIGURE A2.   U.S. medical schools: number of full-time faculty (1950–1994).

SOURCES: W. G. Rothstein, *American Medical Schools and the Practice of Medicine: A History* (New York: Oxford Univ. Press, 1987), table 11.3, p. 226, and table 13.1, p. 257, and various annual "Medical Education Issues" of *JAMA*.

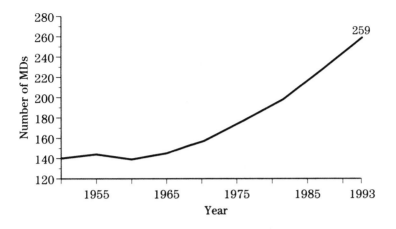

FIGURE A3. Number of U.S. physicians per 100,000 population (1955–1993).
SOURCE: AMA Physician Characteristics, table A-7, 1986, and figure 4, 1994.

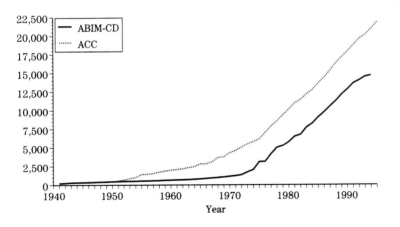

FIGURE A4. ACC membership and ABIM cardiovascular certification (1941–1994).
SOURCE: American College of Cardiology, Bethesda, Md., and American Board of Internal Medicine, Philadelphia.

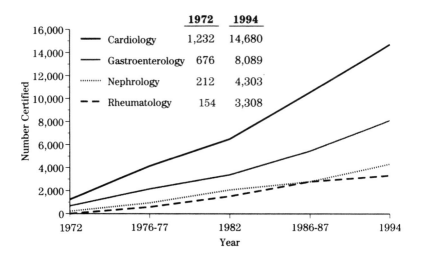

FIGURE A5. Diplomates certified by ABIM (1972–1994).
SOURCE: American Board of Internal Medicine, Phildelphia.

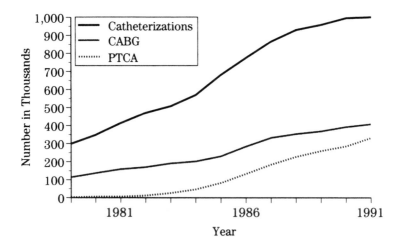

FIGURE A6. Estimated cardiovascular operations and invasive procedures—United States (1979–1991).

SOURCE: Cardiovascular Specialists and Economics of Medicine (Bethesda, Md.: ACC, 1994), figure 8.1, p. 64.

Acronyms and Abbreviations

AAMC	Association of American Medical Colleges
ABIM	American Board of Internal Medicine
ABMS	Advisory Board for Medical Specialties
ACC	American College of Cardiology
ACC AM	American College of Cardiology Annual Meeting
ACC BOG	American College of Cardiology Board of Governors
ACC BOT	American College of Cardiology Board of Trustees
ACC EC	American College of Cardiology Executive Committee
ACCEL	American College of Cardiology Extended Learning
ACCESS	American College of Cardiology Extended Study Services
ACP	American College of Physicians
ACP BOG	American College of Physicians Board of Governors
AHA	American Heart Association
AHA AM	American Heart Association Annual Meeting
AHA BOD	American Heart Assocation Board of Directors
AHA EC	American Heart Association Executive Committee
AMA	American Medical Association
APC	Association of Professors of Cardiology
APM	Association of Professors of Medicine
APS	American Physiological Society
ASIM	American Society of Internal Medicine
ASNC	American Society of Nuclear Cardiology
AUC	Association of University Cardiologists
CABG	Coronary artery bypass graft surgery
CASS	Coronary Artery Surgery Trial

CCC	American Heart Association Council on Clinical Cardiology
DHEW	Department of Health, Education and Welfare (later Department of Health and Human Services)
FASEB	Federation of American Societies for Experimental Biology
FCIM	Federated Council for Internal Medicine
FDA	Food and Drug Administration
GMENAC	Graduate Medical Education National Advisory Committee
MGH	Massachusetts General Hospital
NAHC	National Advisory Heart Council
NASPE	North American Society of Pacing and Electrophysiology
NHI	National Heart Institute (1948)*
NHLBI	National Heart, Lung, and Blood Institute (1976)*
NHLI	National Heart and Lung Institute (1969)*
NIH	National Institutes of Health
NYCS	New York Cardiological Society
NYHA	New York Heart Association
PTCA	Percutaneous transluminal coronary angioplasty
RBRVS	Resource-based relative value scale
SCA	Society for Cardiac Angiography

*The expanding mission of the original National Heart Institute is reflected in its sequential name changes.

NOTES: Standard journal abbreviations are used in the notes and bibliography. See National Library of Medicine, *List of Journals Indexed in Index Medicus* (Bethesda, Md.: National Library of Medicine, 1994), and "Index to journal abbreviations," in National Library of Medicine, *Bibliography of the History of Medicine*, no. 25, 1985–89 (Bethesda, Md.: National Library of Medicine, 1990), pp. 1361–1454.

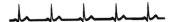

Notes

Introduction

1. See American Heart Association, *Heart and Stroke Facts: 1994 Statistical Supplement* (Dallas: AHA, 1993), and G. Roback, L. Randolph, B. Seidman, and T. Pasko, *Physician Characteristics and Distribution in the U.S. 1994 Edition* (Chicago: American Medical Association, 1994), table A-2, p. 20. There are more family physicians, general internists, and pediatricians than cardiologists, but they are generally classified as primary care specialists.

2. Sources for statistics about heart care and cardiology practice include Agency for Health Care Policy and Research, *The National Bill for Diseases Treated in U.S. Hospitals: 1987. Provider Studies Research Note 19* (Rockville, Md.: U.S. Dept. of Health and Human Services, 1994), esp. table 1, p. 12.; W. R. Harlan, P. E. Parsons, and J. W. Thomas, *Health Care Utilization and Costs of Adult Cardiovascular Conditions, United States, 1980. National Medical Care Utilization and Expenditure Survey. Series C, Analytical Report no. 7* (Washington, D.C.: GPO, 1989); G. M. Anderson, J. P. Newhouse, and L. L. Roos, "Hospital care for elderly patients with diseases of the circulatory system: A comparison of hospital use in the United States and Canada," *N. Engl. J. Med.* 321 (1989): 1443–1448; *National Heart, Lung, and Blood Institute Fact Book. Fiscal Year 1993* (Bethesda, Md.: NHLBI, 1994); and American College of Cardiology, *Cardiovascular Specialists and the Economics of Medicine* (Bethesda, Md.: ACC: 1994). For a nontechnical overview of contemporary approaches to the diagnosis and treatment of cardiovascular diseases, see A. Selzer, *Understanding Heart Disease* (Berkeley: Univ. of California Press, 1992).

3. W. S. Thayer, "The problems of internal medicine," *Am. Med.* (1904): 915–919.

4. [G. Shrady], "Specialism in general medicine," *Med. Rec.* 10 (1875): 255–256.

5. L. D. Bulkley, "On the relation between the general practitioner and the consultant or specialist," *JAMA* 12 (1889): 155–158. See also Bulkley, "Specialties, and their relation to the medical profession," *JAMA* 3 (1884): 651–655.

6. F. C. Shattuck, "Specialism in medicine," *JAMA* 35 (1900): 723–726.

7. G. Rosen, *The Specialization of Medicine with Particular Reference to Ophthalmology* (New York: Froben Press, 1944), quote p. 1. Useful studies of professionalization are E. Freidson, *Medical Work in America: Essays on Health Care* (New Haven: Yale Univ.

Press, 1989), and M. S. Larson, *The Rise of Professionalism: A Sociological Analysis* (Berkeley: Univ. of California Press, 1977).

8. See R. Stevens, *American Medicine and the Public Interest* (New Haven: Yale Univ. Press, 1971); K. M. Ludmerer, *Learning to Heal: The Development of American Medical Education* (New York: Basic Books, 1985); and W. G. Rothstein, *American Medical Schools and the Practice of Medicine, a History* (New York: Oxford Univ. Press, 1987).

9. See C. E. Rosenberg, *The Care of Strangers: The Rise of America's Hospital System* (New York: Basic Books, 1987), and R. Stevens, *In Sickness and in Wealth: American Hospitals in the Twentieth Century* (New York: Basic Books, 1989).

10. P. Starr, *The Social Transformation of American Medicine* (New York: Basic Books, 1982), p. 3.

11. S. M. Farber, "Greatest challenge in medicine today: Continuing education," *JAMA* 193 (1965): 94–97.

12. See S. J. Reiser, *Medicine and the Reign of Technology* (Cambridge: Cambridge Univ. Press, 1978); L. B. Russell, *Technology in Hospitals: Medical Advances and Their Diffusion* (Washington, D.C.: Brookings Institution, 1979); A. B. Davis, *Medicine and Its Technology: An Introduction to the History of Medical Instrumentation* (Westport, Conn.: Greenwood Press, 1981); J. D. Howell, "Diagnostic technologies: X-rays, electrocardiograms, and CAT scans," *S. Calif. Law Rev.* 65 (1991): 529–564; H. M. Marks, "Medical technologies: Social contexts and consequences," in *Companion Encyclopedia of the History of Medicine*, ed. W. F. Bynum and R. Porter (New York: Routledge, 1993), 2: 1592–1618; and M. R. Smith and L. Marx, ed. *Does Technology Drive History?: The Dilemma of Technological Determinism* (Cambridge, Mass.: MIT Press, 1994).

13. R. C. Maulitz, "Grand rounds: An introduction to the history of internal medicine," in *Grand Rounds: One Hundred Years of Internal Medicine*, ed. R. C. Maulitz and D. E. Long (Philadelphia: Univ. of Pennsylvania Press, 1988), pp. 3–13, quote p. 5, emphasis in the original. This useful book also includes chapters on the development of general internal medicine, infectious diseases, gastroenterology, rheumatology, nephrology, cardiology, and clinical trials in America. Recent trends in historiography are described in P. Burke, ed., *New Perspectives on Historical Writing* (University Park: Pennsylvania State Univ. Press, 1991); S. Vaughn, ed., *The Vital Past: Writings on the Uses of History* (Athens: Univ. of Georgia Press, 1985); and M. T. Isenberg, *Puzzles of the Past: An Introduction to Thinking About History* (College Station: Texas A & M Univ. Press, 1985). For an overview of medical historiography, see E. Clarke, *Modern Methods in the History of Medicine* (London: Athlone Press/Univ. of London Press, 1971), and G. H. Brieger, "History of medicine," in *A Guide to the Culture of Science, Technology, and Medicine*, ed. P. T. Durbin (New York: Macmillan, 1980), pp. 121–194.

14. See S. A. Halpern, *American Pediatrics: The Social Dynamics of Professionalism, 1880–1980* (Berkeley: Univ. of California Press, 1988), and G. Gritzer and A. Arluke, *The Making of Rehabilitation: A Political Economy of Medical Specialization, 1890–1980* (Berkeley: Univ. of California Press, 1985).

15. See W. B. Fye, *Bibliography of the History of Cardiovascular Medicine and Surgery* (Bethesda, Md.: National Library of Medicine, 1986); L. J. Acierno, *The History of Cardiology* (Pearl River, N.Y.: Parthenon Publishing Group, 1994); J. D. Howell, "Hearts and minds: The invention and transformation of American cardiology," in *Grand Rounds*, ed. Maulitz and Long, pp. 243–275; J. D. Howell, "The

changing face of twentieth-century American cardiology," *Ann. Intern. Med.* 105 (1986): 772–782; and J. D. Howell, "Cardiac physiology and clinical medicine? Two case studies," in *Physiology in the American Context: 1850–1940.* ed. G. L. Geison (Bethesda, Md.: American Physiological Society, 1987), pp. 279–292.

16. See R. Cooter, *Surgery and Society in Peace and War: Orthopedics and the Organization of Modern Medicine, 1880–1948* (London: Macmillan, 1993), and G. Weisz, "The development of medical specialization in 19th-century Paris," in *French Medical Culture in the 19th Century,* ed. A. La Berge and M. Feingold, *Clio Medica,* vol. 25 (Atlanta: Editions Rodophi B.V., 1994), pp. 149–188.

17. See C. Lawrence, "Moderns and ancients: The 'new cardiology' in Britain 1880–1930," *Med. Hist.* suppl. 5 (1985): 1–33; C. Lawrence, "'Definite and material': Coronary thrombosis and cardiologists in the 1920s," in *Framing Disease,* ed. C. E. Rosenberg and J. Golden (New Brunswick, N.J.: Rutgers Univ. Press, 1992), pp. 50–82; and C. Lawrence, "Incommunicable knowledge: Science, technology and the clinical art in Britain, 1850–1914," *J. Contemp. Hist.* 20 (1985): 503–520.

18. W. B. Fye, "Cardiology in 1885," *Circulation* 72 (1985): 21–26.

19. For a discussion of these issues, see D. M. Fox, *Power and Illness: The Failure and Future of American Health Policy* (Berkeley: Univ. of California Press, 1993), and E. Ginzberg, *The Medical Triangle: Physicians, Politicians, and the Public* (Cambridge: Harvard Univ. Press, 1990).

20. L. T. Coggeshall, *Planning for Medical Progress through Education* (Washington, D.C.: Association of American Medical Colleges, 1965), quote p. 26.

21. M. Cherkasky and M. Pines, "Tomorrow's hospitals," *Harper's Magazine,* October 1960: 158–165.

CHAPTER 1   *Defining a Discipline*

1. See J. D. Howell, "Hearts and minds: The invention and transformation of American cardiology," in *Grand Rounds: One Hundred Years of Internal Medicine,* ed. R. C. Maulitz and D. E. Long (Philadelphia: Univ. of Pennsylvania Press, 1988), pp. 243–275. For European influences (discussed later in this chapter), see the works by Bonner, Faber, Lawrence, Reichert, Rosen (1983), and Stevens (1988) in the bibliography.

2. For role differentiation as part of the process of the professionalization of a discipline, see J. Ben-David, "Roles and innovations in medicine," in *Scientific Growth: Essays on the Social Organization and Ethos of Science,* ed. G. Freudenthal (Berkeley: Univ. of California Press, 1991), pp. 33–48.

3. J. D. Howell, ed., *Medical Lives and Scientific Medicine at Michigan, 1891–1969* (Ann Arbor: Univ. of Michigan Press, 1993), quote p. 11.

4. Two recent works describe the pathological and physiological traditions: R. C. Maulitz, *Morbid Appearances: The Anatomy of Pathology in the Early Nineteenth Century* (Cambridge: Cambridge Univ. Press, 1987); and W. Coleman and F. L. Holmes, ed., *The Investigative Enterprise: Experimental Physiology in Nineteenth-Century Medicine* (Berkeley: Univ. of California Press, 1988). See also K. Faber, *Nosography: The Evolution of Clinical Medicine in Modern Times,* 2d ed. (New York: Paul B. Hoeber, 1930).

5. See R. C. Maulitz, "Pathologists, clinicians, and the role of pathophysiology," in *Physiology in the American Context, 1850–1940,* ed. G. L. Geison (Bethesda, Md.:

American Physiological Society, 1987), pp. 209–235. A contemporary perspective is I. Levin, "Pathological physiology or experimental pathology, its scope and significance in medicine," *Med. Rec.* 58 (1900): 327–336.

6. A physiologist is a scientist whose main interest is the function of whole organs. The physiological cardiologist tradition can be traced to several European physiologists: Claude Bernard and Etienne Marey in France, Carl Ludwig and Hugo Kronecker in Germany, and Michael Foster and Walter Gaskell in England. See K. E. Rothschuh, *History of Physiology,* trans. and ed. G. B. Risse (Huntington, N.Y.: Robert E. Krieger, 1973). See also Faber, *Nosography.*

7. For cardiac research in the nineteenth century, see R. G. Frank Jr., "The telltale heart: Physiological instruments, graphic methods, and clinical hopes, 1854–1914," in *The Investigative Enterprise,* ed. Coleman and Holmes, pp. 211–290, and W. B. Fye, "Acute coronary occlusion always results in death, or does it? The observations of William T. Porter," *Circulation* 71 (1985): 4–10.

8. One writer editorialized, "The dependence of medicine, both as a science and an art, on physiology is everywhere recognized." "The obligations of medicine to physiology, and of physiology to medicine," *Boston Med. Surg. J.* 126 (1892): 345–347. For experimental pharmacology see J. Parascandola, *The Development of American Pharmacology: John J. Abel and the Shaping of a Discipline* (Baltimore: Johns Hopkins Univ. Press, 1992).

9. Krehl also published an important monograph on the myocardium: L. Krehl, *Die Erkrankungen des Herzmuskels und die nervösen Herzkrankheiten* (Vienna: Alfred Hölder, 1901). Translated as L. Krehl, "Diseases of the myocardium and nervous diseases of the heart," in *Diseases of the Heart,* ed. G. Dock (Philadelphia: W. B. Saunders, 1908), pp. 421–763. See also H. Dennig, "Zum gedenken an Ludolf von Krehl," *München Med. Wschr.* 103 (1961): 2489–2503, and H.-H. Eulner, *Die Entwicklung der medizinischen Spezialfächer an den Universitäten des deutschen Sprachgebietes* (Stuttgart: Ferdinand Enke, 1970).

10. For Krehl's European and American pupils, see Dennig, "Krehl," p. 2492. For background on the transfer of European experimental physiology to the United States, see W. B. Fye, *The Development of American Physiology: Scientific Medicine in the Nineteenth Century* (Baltimore: Johns Hopkins Univ. Press, 1987), and H. W. Davenport, "Physiology, 1850–1923: The view from Michigan," *Physiologist* suppl. 24, no. 1 (1982): 1–96.

11. W. B. Fye, "Albion Walter Hewlett: Teacher, clinician, scientist, and missionary for 'pathologic physiology'," in *Medical Lives,* ed. Howell, pp. 45–72, and A. M. Harvey, "Albion Walter Hewlett: Pioneer clinical physiologist," *Johns Hopkins Med. J.* 144 (1979): 202–214. The latter lists most of Hewlett's publications, two-thirds of which related to the cardiovascular system. Hewlett's friend Joseph Erlanger became a pure physiologist; see J. Erlanger, "A physiologist reminisces," in *The Excitement and Fascination of Science* (Palo Alto, Calif.: Annual Reviews, 1965), pp. 93–106.

12. L. Krehl, *The Principles of Clinical Pathology: A Text-Book for Students and Physicians,* trans. A. W. Hewlett (Philadelphia: J. B. Lippincott, 1905). See also A. W. Hewlett, "The relation of pathologic physiology to internal medicine," *JAMA* 61 (1913): 1583–1586.

13. A. M. Harvey, *Science at the Bedside: Clinical Research in American Medicine, 1905–1945* (Baltimore: Johns Hopkins Univ. Press, 1981).

14. Frank Wilson thought Hewlett was among the first academic physicians whose main interest was pathological physiology. F. Wilson, "The Department of Internal Medicine. II. 1908–27," in *The University of Michigan: An Encyclopedic Survey,* ed. W. Shaw (Ann Arbor: Univ. of Michigan Press, 1951), 2: 838–842.

15. L. F. Barker, "The organization of the laboratories in the medical clinic of the Johns Hopkins Hospital," *Bull. Johns Hopkins Hosp.* 18 (1907): 193–198, quote p. 196. The shift from a pathological to a physiological view of disease is explicitly articulated in L. F. Barker, "On some of the clinical methods of investigating cardio-vascular conditions," *Bull. Johns Hopkins Hosp.* 20 (1909): 297–310. See also P. Rous, "The teaching of physiological pathology at the University of Michigan," *Bull. Johns Hopkins Hosp.* 19 (1908): 336–338.

16. A. D. Hirschfelder, *Diseases of the Heart and Aorta* (Philadelphia: J. B. Lippincott, 1910), quote p. vii. Contrast this with R. H. Babcock, *Diseases of the Heart and Arterial System* (New York: D. Appleton, 1903). Babcock's discussion of the role of physiological instruments in cardiac diagnosis is limited to a few passages in the text and a sixteen-page appendix in his 853-page book.

17. See J. D. Howell, "Frank Norman Wilson: Theory, technology, and electrocardiography," in *Medical Lives,* ed. Howell, pp. 101–127; F. D. Johnston and E. Lepeschkin, Selected Papers of Dr. Frank N. Wilson (Ann Arbor: J. W. Edwards, 1954); C. J. Wiggers, *Reminiscences and Adventures in Circulation Research* (New York: Grune & Stratton, 1958); and C. J. Wiggers, *Modern Aspects of the Circulation in Health and Disease* (Philadelphia: Lea & Febiger, 1915).

18. See J. Burnett, "The origins of the electrocardiograph as a clinical instrument," *Med. Hist.* suppl. 5 (1985): 53–76; G. E. Burch and N. P. DePasquale, *A History of Electrocardiography with a New Introduction by Joel D. Howell,* 2d ed. (San Francisco: Jeremy Norman, 1990); W. B. Fye, "A history of the origin, evolution, and impact of electrocardiography," *Am. J. Cardiol.* 73 (1994): 937–949; J. D. Howell, "Early perceptions of the electrocardiogram: From arrhythmia to infarction," *Bull. Hist. Med.* 58 (1984): 83–98; and M. Borell, "Extending the senses: The graphic method," *Medical Heritage* 2 (1986): 114–121.

19. See J. D. Howell, "Cardiac physiology and clinical medicine? Two case studies," in *Physiology in the American Context,* ed. Geison, pp. 279–292, and C. Lawrence, "'Definite and material': Coronary thrombosis and cardiologists in the 1920s," in *Framing Disease,* ed. C. E. Rosenberg and J. Golden (New Brunswick, N.J.: Rutgers Univ. Press, 1992), pp. 50–82, esp. pp. 67–73.

20. Two British physiologists (Edward Schäfer at Edinburgh University and Augustus D. Waller at the University of London) were already using the instrument for basic research. For Lewis, see A. N. Drury and R. T. Grant, "Thomas Lewis," *Obituary Notices of Fellows of the Royal Society* 14 (1945): 179–202 (includes his bibliography). Lewis discusses pathological physiology in T. Lewis, "The Lumleian lectures on medical research," *Lancet* 1 (1917): 1012–1013. For British cardiology, see C. Lawrence, "Moderns and ancients: The 'new cardiology' in Britain 1880–1930," *Med. Hist.* suppl. 5 (1985): 1–33.

21. Americans who coauthored papers with Lewis included Alfred Cohn, H. M. (Jack) Marvin, Arthur Master, Bernard Oppenheimer, William Stroud, and Paul White. See *Heart. A Journal for the Study of the Circulation: Indices of Authors and Subjects. Volumes I to XVI* (London: Shaw & Sons, 1933).

22. L. F. Barker, A. D. Hirschfelder, and G. M. Bond, "Personal experience in electrocardiographic work with the use of the Edelmann string galvanometer (smaller model)," *Trans. Assoc. Am. Physicians* 25 (1910): 648–660. Barker's comments reflected changes at America's hospitals that resulted from the introduction of various technologies. See J. D. Howell, "Diagnostic technologies: X-rays, electrocardiograms, and CAT scans," *S. Calif. Law Rev.* 65 (1991): 529–564. See also A. E. Cohn to G. E. Burch, 26 June 1953, in Burch and DePasquale, *History of Electrocardiography*, pp. 35–39; W. B. James and H. B. Williams, "The electrocardiogram in clinical medicine," *Am. J. Med. Sci.* 140 (1910): 408–421, 644–669; and L. F. Barker, "Electrocardiography and phonocardiography. A collective review," *Bull. Johns Hopkins Hosp.* 21 (1910): 358–389.

23. T. Lewis, *Clinical Electrocardiography* (London: Shaw & Sons, 1913), quotes pp. iii, v, vi. See also E. Shapiro, "The first textbook of electrocardiography, Thomas Lewis: 'Clinical Electrocardiography'," *J. Am. Coll. Cardiol.* 1 (1983): 1160–1161.

24. R. C. Cabot, "The historical development and relative value of laboratory and clinical methods of diagnosis," *Boston Med. Surg. J.* 157 (1907): 150–153, quote p. 151.

25. Wiggers, *Modern Aspects of the Circulation*, quote p. v. See also L. F. Barker, "On some of the clinical methods of investigating cardio-vascular conditions," esp. p. 297. For tensions between traditional clinical methods and laboratory approaches, see G. L. Geison, "Divided we stand: Physiologists and clinicians in the American context," in *The Therapeutic Revolution: Essays in the Social History of American Medicine*, ed. M. J. Vogel and C. E. Rosenberg (Philadelphia: Univ. of Pennsylvania Press, 1979), pp. 67–90; Howell, "Cardiac physiology and clinical medicine?"; R. C. Maulitz, "Physician versus bacteriologist: The ideology of science in clinical medicine," in *The Therapeutic Revolution*, ed. Vogel and Rosenberg, pp. 91–107; J. H. Warner, "The fall and rise of professional mystery: Epistemology, authority and the emergence of laboratory medicine in nineteenth-century America," in *The Laboratory Revolution in Medicine*, ed. A. Cunningham and P. Williams (Cambridge: Cambridge Univ. Press, 1992), pp. 110–141; H. Evans, "Losing touch: The controversy over the introduction of blood pressure instruments into medicine," *Technology and Culture* 34 (1993): 784–807; J. H. Warner, "Ideals of science and their discontents in late nineteenth-century American medicine," *Isis* 82 (1991): 454–478; and M. Borell, "Training the senses, training the mind," in *Medicine and the Five Senses*, ed. W. F. Bynum and R. Porter (New York: Cambridge Univ. Press, 1993), pp. 244–261. Several turn-of-the-century articles on technology in medicine are reprinted in *Technology and American Medical Practice 1880–1930: An Anthology of Sources*, ed. J. D. Howell (New York: Garland, 1988). See also J. D. Howell, *Technology in the Hospital: Transforming Patient Care in the Early Twentieth Century* (Baltimore: Johns Hopkins Univ. Press, 1995).

26. The definitive study is K. M. Ludmerer, *Learning to Heal: The Development of American Medical Education* (New York: Basic Books, 1985). See also W. G. Rothstein, *American Medical Schools and the Practice of Medicine, a History* (New York: Oxford Univ. Press, 1987), and S. C. Wheatley, *The Politics of Philanthropy: Abraham Flexner and Medical Education* (Madison: Univ. of Wisconsin Press, 1988).

27. Howell, "Cardiac physiology and clinical medicine?," quote pp. 279–280. An important study of how medical students began to use physiological instruments is M. Borell, "Instruments and an independent physiology: The Harvard physiological laboratory, 1871–1906," in *Physiology in the American Context*, ed. Geison, pp. 293–

321. See also W. G. MacCallum, "On the teaching of pathological physiology," *Johns Hopkins Hosp. Bull.* 17 (1906): 251–254.

28. A. D. Bevan, "Chairman's address," *AMA Bull.* 5 (1910): 241–252, quotes pp. 242–243. See N. Gevitz, ed., *Other Healers: Unorthodox Medicine in America* (Baltimore: Johns Hopkins Univ. Press, 1988); W. G. Rothstein, *American Physicians in the Nineteenth Century: From Sects to Science* (Baltimore: Johns Hopkins Univ. Press, 1972); and M. Kaufman, *Homeopathy in America: The Rise and Fall of a Medical Heresy* (Baltimore: Johns Hopkins Univ. Press, 1971). See also J. H. Warner, "Science in medicine," *Osiris*, n.s., 1 (1985): 37–58.

29. D. W. Cathell and W. T. Cathell, *Book on the Physician Himself and Things That Concern His Reputation and Success,* twentieth century ed. (Philadelphia: F. A. Davis, 1903), quote p. 9.

30. See R. C. Maulitz and P. B. Beeson, "The inner history of internal medicine," in *Grand Rounds,* ed. Maulitz and Long (Philadelphia: Univ. of Pennsylvania Press, 1988), pp. 15–54, and R. Stevens, "The curious career of internal medicine: Functional ambivalence, social success," ibid., pp. 339–364.

31. W. Osler, "Internal medicine as a vocation," *Med. News* 71 (1897): 660–663, quote p. 660.

32. Baltimore physician John Hemmeter wrote a 788-page book on stomach diseases in 1898. A trained physiologist, he embraced the ideology of pathological physiology. Hemmeter described procedures and laboratory techniques that reflected the diffusion of physiological instruments into clinical practice. Plate III is a photograph captioned "Patient with intragastric tube within stomach and pneumograph in place, both connected with the kymograph." Gastroenterology was a *specialty,* in Hemmeter's opinion. J. C. Hemmeter, *Diseases of the Stomach* (Philadelphia: P. Blakiston, Son & Co., 1898), quote p. vii.

33. Krehl, *Principles of Clinical Pathology.*

34. S. J. Meltzer, "Our aims," *Med. News* 85 (1 October 1904): 642–644. See also J. B. Kirsner, *The Development of American Gastroenterology* (New York: Raven Press, 1990).

35. See R. V. Bennett, *Hope in Heart Disease: The Story of Louis Faugères Bishop* (Philadelphia: Dorrance, 1948); L. F. Bishop [Jr.], *Myself When Young: Growing up in New York 1901–1925* (New York: K. S. Giniger, 1985); P. Reichert and L. F. Bishop Jr., "Sir James Mackenzie and his polygraph: The contribution of Louis Faugeres Bishop, Sr.," *Am. J. Cardiol.* 24 (1969): 401–403; and L. F. Bishop Jr., *The Birth of a Specialty: The Diary of an American Cardiologist, 1926–1972* (New York: Vantage Press, 1977). Frank Fulton of Providence, R.I., was a practitioner cardiologist whose career path was similar to Bishop's. F. T. Fulton, *The Story of the Heart Station at the Rhode Island Hospital* (Providence: [Frank T. Fulton], 1955).

36. C. E. Rosenberg, "Making it in urban medicine: A career in the age of scientific medicine," *Bull. Hist. Med.* 64 (1990): 163–186, quote p. 163.

37. For nineteenth-century medical practice and specialization, see Rothstein, *American Medical Schools,* esp. chapter 4, and B. E. Blustein, "New York neurologists and the specialization of American medicine," *Bull. Hist. Med.* 53 (1979): 170–183.

38. J. Shrady, ed., *The College of Physicians and Surgeons, New York, and Its Founders, Officers, Instructors, Benefactors and Alumni. A History,* 2 vols. (New York: Lewis Publishing Co., 1903), quote 1: 210. For the implications of outpatient and

hospital appointments in this era, see C. E. Rosenberg, "Inward vision and outward glance: The shaping of the American hospital, 1880–1914," *Bull. Hist. Med.* 53 (1979): 346–391.

39. A list of New York City's hospitals and staff appointments is in *The Medical Directory of the City of New York* (New York: Medical Society of the County of New York, 1898), pp. 196–216. The Colored Home and Hospital (founded in 1839 to care for freed slaves) became Lincoln Hospital shortly after Bishop joined the staff. See J. J. Walsh, *History of Medicine in New York: Three Centuries of Medical Progress*, 5 vols. (New York: National Americana Society, 1919), 3: 754–755. An important source for New York medicine at the turn of the century is D. Rosner, *A Once Charitable Enterprise: Hospitals and Health Care in Brooklyn and New York, 1885–1915* (New York: Cambridge Univ. Press, 1982). Compare this with M. J. Vogel, *The Invention of the Modern Hospital: Boston 1870–1930* (Chicago: Univ. of Chicago Press, 1980). See also G. Rosen, "Urbanization, occupation and disease in the United States, 1870–1920: The case of New York City," *J. Hist. Med. Allied Sci.* 43 (1988): 391–425.

40. Cathell and Cathell, *Book on the Physician Himself* (1903), quote p. 33.

41. Bennett, *Hope in Heart Disease*, quote p. 127. Bishop began focusing his practice and publications on cardiovascular disease between 1903 and 1907 (pp. 276–299). An 1899 directory of New York City specialists listed twelve physicians (including Bishop) who specialized in diseases of the chest (heart and lungs) in Manhattan and three in Brooklyn. See *New York Medical Practitioners Engaged in Special Branches* (New York: Eugene R. Trott, 1899).

42. Rosenberg, "Making it in urban medicine," quote p. 164.

43. L. F. Barker, "The development of the science of diagnosis," *J. S.C. Med. Assoc.* 13 (1917): 278–284.

44. V. C. Vaughan to R. W. Corwin, 24 April 1916, in Michigan University, Medical School, misc. corres. box 32, July 1916, A.-N. Bentley Library, University of Michigan, Ann Arbor.

45. J. H. Honan, *Honan's Handbook to Medical Europe* (Philadelphia: P. Blakiston's Son, 1912), quote p. v. Bonner estimates that more than fifteen thousand American medical students and physicians studied in Germany between 1870 and 1914. T. N. Bonner, *American Doctors and German Universities: A Chapter in International Intellectual Relations, 1870–1914* (Lincoln: Univ. of Nebraska Press, 1963), p. 23.

46. D. W. Cathell and W. T. Cathell, *Book on the Physician Himself and Things That Concern His Reputation and Success*, 12th ed. (Philadelphia: F. A. Davis, 1913), quote p. 66. See also S. J. Peitzman, "'Thoroughly practical': America's polyclinic medical schools," *Bull. Hist. Med.* 54 (1980): 166–187.

47. See A. Mair, *Sir James Mackenzie, M.D. 1853–1925, General Practitioner* (Edinburgh: Churchill Livingstone, 1973), esp. p. 233. Although Bishop spent just one day with Mackenzie, he found the experience stimulating. See Bennett, *Hope in Heart Disease*, p. 121. Mackenzie's reputation as the leading heart specialist (a label he resisted) in the English-speaking world was due mainly to his book on heart disease. J. Mackenzie, *Diseases of the Heart* (London: Oxford Univ. Press, 1908). For Bishop's opinion of Mackenzie, see L. F. Bishop and L. F. Bishop Jr., "Recent advances in cardiology," *Clin. Med. Surg.* 41 (1934): 15–17. See also W. B. R. Monteith, ed., *Bibliography with Synopsis of the Original Papers of the Writings of Sir James Mackenzie* (London: Oxford Univ. Press, 1930).

48. Bishop's office-based electrocardiograph is pictured in L. F. Bishop, *Heart Troubles: Their Prevention and Relief,* 2d ed. (New York: Funk & Wagnalls, 1921), facing p. 152. It cost about $14 hundred (approximately $20 thousand in 1994 dollars; U.S. Bureau of Labor Statistics).

49. L. F. Bishop, "A cardiologic and sociologic experiment in the treatment of heart disease," *International Clinics* 32 (1922): 15–23.

50. S. Neuhof, *Clinical Cardiology* (New York: Macmillan, 1917). His apparatus is pictured facing pp. 23, 110, and 111.

51. L. F. Bishop, "The Nauheim methods in the management of cardiac disease," *Med. Rec.* 79 (1911): 531–532. See also J. M. Swan, "A resume of the opinions upon the Nauheim treatment of chronic disease of the heart," *Trans. Am. Clin. Climatol. Assoc.* 27 (1911): 28–59; J. T. Groedel, *Bad-Nauheim: Its Springs and Their Uses with Useful Local Information and a Guide to the Environs,* 5th ed. (Friedberg: Carl Bindernagel, 1909); and C. A. Pierach, S. D. Wangensteen, and H. B. Burchell, "Spa therapy for heart disease, Bad Nauheim (circa 1900)," *Am. J. Cardiol.* 72 (1993): 336–342.

52. Neuhof, *Clinical Cardiology,* quote p. 226. For Mitchell, see M. Olfson, "The Weir Mitchell rest cure," *Pharos* 51 (1988): 30–32.

53. L. F. Bishop, "The prevention of arteriosclerosis and heart disease in otherwise healthy individuals past middle life," *JAMA* 60 (1913): 803–806, quote p. 803. By this time, Bishop was communicating with dozens of leading American internists on the subject. For a list of correspondents and excerpts from their letters, see L. F. Bishop, *Arteriosclerosis* (London: Oxford Univ. Press, 1914), pp. 204–260 and index.

54. Cathell and Cathell, *Book on the Physician Himself,* 12th ed., quotes pp. 35, 121, 124.

55. L. F. Bishop, "Some practical observations on the diagnosis and prognosis of cardiac disease," *Medical Examiner and General Practitioner* 12 (1902): 718–719. During the first half of the twentieth century, most doctors who functioned as practitioner cardiologists officially identified themselves as internists. The 1921 AMA directory listed 101 self-designated internists in Manhattan and the Bronx. Doctors fulfilling my criteria for various types of cardiologists included Ernst Boas, Lewis Conner, Hubert Guile, Robert Halsey, Stuart Hart, Selian Neuhof, Bernard Oppenheimer, and John Wyckoff. Bishop was the only one who listed anything (his Fordham appointment) that would indicate a special interest in cardiology. See *American Medical Directory: A Register of Legally Qualified Physicians of the United States,* 7th ed. (Chicago: AMA, 1921). Harlow Brooks exemplifies this phenomenon. A contemporary of Bishop's, he published several papers and books on cardiovascular topics and was one of the first doctors in New York City to own an electrocardiograph, but Brooks viewed himself as an internist-diagnostician, not a heart specialist. J. J. Moorhead, *Harlow W. Brooks: Man and Doctor* (New York: Harper & Bro., 1937).

56. There were no full-time clinical positions for cardiologists in this era. W. B. Fye, "The origin of the full-time faculty system: Implications for clinical research," *JAMA* 265 (1991): 1555–1562.

57. O. Paul, *Take Heart: The Life and Prescription for Living of Dr. Paul Dudley White* (Boston: Francis A. Countway Library of Medicine, 1986).

58. D. L. Edsall, "The clinician, the hospital and the medical school," *Boston Med. Surg. J.* 166 (1912): 315–323, and J. C. Aub and R. K. Hapgood, *Pioneer in Modern Medicine: David Linn Edsall of Harvard* (Boston: Harvard Medical Alumni Association, 1970).

59. P. D. White diary entry, 6 February 1913, in Paul, *Take Heart,* quote p. 30. See F. A. Washburn, *The Massachusetts General Hospital: Its Development, 1900–1935* (Boston: Houghton Mifflin, 1939), p. 376; and *Anniversary Volume: Scientific Contributions in Honor of Joseph Hersey Pratt on His Sixty-Fifth Birthday by His Friends* (Lancaster, Pa.: Lancaster Press, 1937), p. xxx; and J. H. Pratt, "Recollections and letters of Sir James Mackenzie," *N. Engl. J. Med.* 224 (1941): 1–10.

60. P. D. White to T. Lewis, 5 June 1913, file PP/LEW/A.1/177-861, Lewis Papers.

61. P. D. White to H. W. White, 9 November 1913, in Paul, *Take Heart,* p. 35.

62. Paul, *Take Heart,* p. 37. The cost in 1994 dollars is approximately $20 thousand (U.S. Bureau of Labor Statistics). No American firms manufactured electrocardiographs at the time, and the Cambridge firm was the sole British manufacturer of electrocardiographs. Between 1907 and 1914, they sold 134 machines. Burnett, "The origins of the electrocardiograph," pp. 75–76. The first electrocardiograph manufactured in the United States was built by the Charles F. Hindle Company and delivered in 1915. See A. E. Cohn and H. B. Williams, "Recollections concerning early electrocardiography in the United States," *Bull. Hist. Med.* 29 (1955): 469–474.

63. P. D. White to J. W. White, 29 July 1915, in Paul, *Take Heart,* p. 40. White was not ambivalent about the opportunity. Oglesby Paul (his biographer and former pupil) explained that White rejected the notion of being an internist with "a special interest" in heart disease. He "deliberately chose to proceed down the new path of specialization, limiting his professional work to diseases of the heart." Paul, *Take Heart,* quote p. 42.

64. P. D. White, "An outline of the tour of duty of Base Hospital No. 6 in the World War," in *The History of U.S. Army Base Hospital No. 6 and Its Part in the American Expeditionary Forces, 1917–1918* (Boston: Massachusetts General Hospital, 1924), pp. 1–21.

65. P. D. White to C. K. Drinker, 1925, in Paul, *Take Heart,* pp. 53–54. Paul thinks that White "came to value increasingly his teaching role and to give it a significant portion of his time." Paul, *Take Heart,* p. 54. For White's patient volume, see P. D. White, "Observations on functional disorders of the heart," *Am. Heart J.* 1 (1926): 527–539.

66. White's residents and students are listed in P. D. White and H. Donovan, *Hearts: Their Long Follow-Up* (Philadelphia: W. B. Saunders, 1967), pp. xxiii–xxv. Many of them paid tribute to him in S. Dack, ed., "A special volume honoring Paul D. White," *Am. J. Cardiol.* 15 (1965): 433–603. See also H. J. Levine, "Samuel A. Levine (1891–1966)," *Clin. Cardiol.* 15 (1992): 473–476; C. S. Wooley, *Academic Heritage: The Transmission of Excellence, Cardiology at the Ohio State University* (Mount Kisco, N.Y.: Futura, 1992); C. S. Roberts, *Life and Writings of Stewart R. Roberts, M.D., Georgia's First Heart Specialist* (Spartanburg, S.C.: Reprint Company Publishers, 1993); and J. B. Vander Veer, *Cardiology at the Pennsylvania Hospital (1920–1980)* (Philadelphia: Pennsylvania Hospital, 1986), esp. pp. 92–95.

67. An obituary confirms that some individuals were viewed as public health cardiologists. Marcus Rothschild was characterized as "one of the pioneers in the *field* of public health aspects of the diseases of the heart." [emphasis added] "Obituaries," *Bull. Am. Heart Assoc.* 11 (1936) [4]. See also J. J. Smith, "Lewis Atterbury Conner," *Cornell Univ. Med. Coll. Alumni Quart.* 38 (winter 1974–75): 12–14; C. F. Wooley, "Lewis A. Conner, M.D. (1867–1950), and lessons learned from examining four million young men in World War I," *Am. J. Cardiol.* 61 (1988): 900–903; A. E. Cohn, "John Wyckoff: 1881–1937," *Bull. Hist. Med.* 6 (1938): 834–857; J. Duffy, "Haven Emerson," in *Dictionary of American Biography,* ed. J. A. Garraty (New York: Charles Scribner's Sons, 1980), suppl. 6: 192–193; H. Emerson, *Selected Papers of Haven Emerson* (Battle Creek, Mich.: W. K. Kellogg Foundation, 1949); L. I. Dublin, *After Eighty Years: The Impact of Life Insurance on Public Health* (Gainesville: Univ. of Florida Press, 1966), esp. p. 110 where he notes Cohn's and Emerson's special interest in the public health aspects of heart disease; P. F. Cranefield, "Alfred Einstein Cohn," in *Dictionary of American Biography,* suppl 6: 117–118. Although Cohn was primarily a physiological cardiologist, Cranefield noted his interest in public health. Cohn "initiated" the "statistical approach to the study of rheumatic fever." M. G. Wilson, *Rheumatic Fever: Studies of the Epidemiology, Manifestations, Diagnosis, and Treatment of the Disease During the First Three Decades* (New York: Commonwealth Fund, 1940), quote p. 6. See also J. Duffy, *A History of Public Health in New York City, 1866–1966* (New York: Russell Sage Foundation, 1974).

68. Minutes, AHA AM, 6 February 1928, AHA Archives.

69. See M. E. Teller, *The Tuberculosis Movement: A Public Health Campaign in the Progressive Era* (New York: Greenwood Press, 1988); A. M. Brandt, *No Magic Bullet: A Social History of Venereal Disease in the United States since 1880* (New York: Oxford Univ. Press, 1985); R. A. Meckel, *Save the Babies: American Public Health Reform and the Prevention of Infant Mortality, 1850–1920* (Baltimore: Johns Hopkins Univ. Press, 1990); B. G. Rosenkrantz, *Public Health and the State: Changing Views in Massachusetts, 1842–1936* (Cambridge: Harvard Univ. Press, 1972); and J. H. Cassedy, *Charles V. Chapin and the Public Health Movement* (Cambridge: Harvard Univ. Press, 1962). R. H. Wiebe, *The Search for Order, 1877–1920* (New York: Hill & Wang, 1967) is an important study of the Progressive Era.

70. J. Duffy, *The Sanitarians: A History of American Public Health* (Urbana: Univ. of Chicago Press, 1990), quote p. 196.

71. W. S. Thayer, "The problems of internal medicine," *Am. Med.* 8 (1904): 915–919, quote p. 917. For bacteriology and virology, see P. F. Clark, *Pioneer Microbiologists of America* (Madison: Univ. of Wisconsin Press, 1961); H. A. Lechevalier and M. Solotorovsky, *Three Centuries of Microbiology* (New York: McGraw-Hill, 1965); and S. S. Hughes, *The Virus: A History of the Concept* (New York: Science History Publications, 1977).

72. C. E. Rosenberg, "Social class and medical care in nineteenth-century America: The rise and fall of the dispensary," *J. Hist. Med. Allied Sci.* 29 (1974): 32–54, quote p. 40.

73. R. C. Cabot, "Suggestions for the reorganization of hospital out-patient departments, with special reference to the improvement of treatment," *Md. Med. J.* 1 (1907): 81–91, quotes pp. 81, 83. See also C. E. Rosenberg, *The Care of Strangers: The Rise of America's Hospital System* (New York: Basic Books, 1987).

74. Cabot, "Suggestions." One historian notes that Cabot's therapeutics was "rooted in 'pathological physiology'." C. R. Burns, "Richard Clarke Cabot (1868–1939) and the reformation in American medical ethics," *Bull. Hist. Med.* 51 (1977): 353–368. See also J. H. Warner, *The Therapeutic Perspective: Medical Practice, Knowledge, and Identity in America, 1820–1885* (Cambridge: Harvard Univ. Press, 1986).

75. Cabot, "Suggestions," quotes pp. 84, 85, 86. See also D. Neuhauser, "Ernest Amory Codman, M.D., and end results of medical care," *Int. J. Technol. Assess. Health Care* 6 (1990): 307–325.

76. A detailed summary of hospital social work in general and the MGH program in particular is I. M. Cannon, *Social Work in Hospitals: A Contribution to Progressive Medicine* (New York: Survey Associates, 1913), esp. pp. 6–17.

77. R. C. Cabot, "Traditions, standards, and prospects of the Massachusetts General Hospital," *Boston Med. Surg. J.* 182 (1920): 287–295, quote p. 290. Studies on early efforts to enhance the efficiency of medical care that mention Cabot and the clinic movement are G. Rosen, "The efficiency criterion in medical care, 1900–1920," *Bull. Hist. Med.* 50 (1976): 28–44, and S. J. Kunitz, "Efficiency and reform in the financing and organization of American medicine in the Progressive Era," *Bull. Hist. Med.* 55 (1981): 497–515. See also R. E. Pumphrey, "Michael Davis and the transformation of the Boston dispensary, 1910–1920," *Bull. Hist. Med.* 49 (1975): 451–465.

78. Cabot, "Suggestions," quote p. 90.

79. J. Mackenzie to J. H. Pratt, 5 November 1907, in Pratt, "Recollections of Mackenzie," pp. 10–12. See also P. D. White and C. Thacher, "Massachusetts General Hospital cardiac department," in *Methods and Problems of Medical Education*, 8th ser. (New York: Rockefeller Foundation, 1927). By 1920, the MGH had specialty clinics for patients with diabetes, cardiac disease, polio, and asthma. See Washburn, *Massachusetts General Hospital*, pp. 375–381. For a detailed study of clinics, see M. M. Davis Jr. and A. R. Warner, *Dispensaries: Their Management and Development* (New York: Macmillan, 1918).

80. *Twenty Years of Social Service at Bellevue and Allied Hospitals, 1907–1926* ([New York: Bellevue and Allied Hospitals], 1927). For the Bellevue clinic, see D. Giles, *A Candle in Her Hand: A Story of the Nursing Schools of Bellevue Hospital* (New York: G.P. Putnam's Sons, 1949); M. E. Wadley to A. E. Cohn, 9 February 1938, in A. E. Cohn, "The first cardiac clinic," *JAMA* 121 (1943): 70; J. Wyckoff, "The organization of the cardiac clinic," *N.Y. State J. Med.* 25 (1925): 995–1001; and Cohn, "John Wyckoff."

81. L. A. Conner, "The value to the community of organized effort to control heart diseases," *Trans. Coll. Phys. Phila.*, 3d ser., 43 (1921): 53–63, quote p. 57.

82. M. J. Rosenau, *Preventive Medicine and Hygiene* (New York: D. Appleton, 1913). In the fifth edition, pubished three years after the incorporation of the AHA, Roseneau briefly mentions the prevention of heart disease. M. J. Roseneau, *Preventive Medicine and Hygiene*, 5th ed. (New York: D. Appleton, 1927), p. 496.

83. K. Tyng, "A survey of the Bellevue experiment in preventive work for 'cardiacs'," *Bellevue and Allied Hospitals Social Service Reports* (1914): 13–36, quote p. 15. This report describes the clinic's organization and summarizes ten typical cases.

84. Ibid.

85. Conner, "Organized effort to control heart diseases," quote p. 57.

86. Tyng, "Bellevue experiment," quotes pp. 17, 24. A contemporary perspective on the cost of illness is R. J. Behan, "Economics of health," *N.Y. Med. J.* 90 (1909): 798–801. The savings in 1994 dollars was approximately $6,250 (U.S. Bureau of Labor Statistics). Conner thought the Bellevue experience "formed the basis of all the cardiac clinics that have since been formed throughout the city." Conner, "Organized effort to control heart diseases," quote p. 58. Alfred Cohn, who witnessed the emergence of the cardiac clinics, thought they signaled "a new era" in the care of heart patients. Cohn, "The first cardiac clinic."

87. Conner, "Organized effort to control heart diseases," quote p. 58. See also J. Bryant, *Convalescence: Historical and Practical* (New York: Burke Foundation, 1927), and C. E. Obermann, *A History of Vocational Rehabilitation in America* (Minneapolis: T. S. Denison, 1965), esp. chapter 6.

88. Conner, "Organized effort to control heart diseases," quote p. 59. See also E. P. Maynard Jr., "Origin and development of the medical programs," in *The New York Heart Association: Origins and Development 1915–1965*, ed. C. de la Chapelle (New York: NYHA, 1966), pp. 14–27. See also E. P. Maynard, "The cardiac clinics of New York: Their origin, aims and accomplishment," *Am. Heart J.* 5 (1930): 660–666.

89. H. Emerson, "The founding of the New York Heart Association," in *The New York Heart Association*, ed. de la Chapelle, pp. 1–13. Another useful source, written by one of the founders, is R. H. Halsey, "History and Development of the American Heart Association." Attached to R. H. Halsey to H. M. Marvin, 7 February 1938, AHA Archives.

90. Statistics from W. Osler, "On the study of tuberculosis," *Phila. Med. J.* 6 (1900): 1029–1030.

91. B. Bates, *Bargaining for Life: A Social History of Tuberculosis, 1876–1938* (Philadelphia: Univ. of Pennsylvania Press, 1992), quote p. 317. See also Teller, *The Tuberculosis Movement;* C.-E. A. Winslow, *The Life of Hermann Biggs* (Philadelphia: Lea & Febiger, 1929); and S. A. Knopf, *A History of the National Tuberculosis Association: The Anti-Tuberculosis Movement in the United States* (New York: National Tuberculosis Association, 1922). A comprehensive summary of the medical profession's views about tuberculosis in this era is A. C. Klebs, ed., *Tuberculosis: A Treatise by American Authors* (New York: D. Appleton, 1909).

92. Conner, "Organized effort to control heart diseases," quote p. 59.

93. Emerson, "The founding of the New York Heart Association," quote p. 5.

94. C. Lynch, F. W. Weed, and L. McAfee, *The Surgeon General's Office. Volume 1 [of] The Medical Department of the United States Army in the World War* (Washington, D.C.: GPO, 1923) 1: 373. The war also shaped British cardiology. J. D. Howell, "'Soldier's heart': The redefinition of heart disease and speciality formation in early twentieth-century Great Britain," *Med. Hist.* suppl. 5 (1985): 34–52.

95. L. A. Conner, "Cardiovascular section," in Lynch, Weed, and McAfee, *The Surgeon General's Office*, 1: 377–381, quote p. 379. The Army established intensive three-week courses to train doctors to examine recruits for evidence of occult heart disease. They screened apparently healthy men and did not deliver care. See also A. E. Cohn to R. Cole, 6 March 1918, record group 450 C661-U, box 16, file 1, Cohn Papers, in which Cohn discusses using "cardio-vascular specialists" at the base hospitals.

96. T. C. Janeway to T. Lewis, 28 September 1917, file PP/LEW/C.1/4, Lewis Papers.

97. Conner, "Cardiovascular section," pp. 379–380.

98. By August 1918, twenty-five Americans were with Lewis. See H. Cushing, *The Life of Sir William Osler* (London: Oxford Univ. Press, 1925) 2: 613. Americans assigned to the Heart Hospital included Samuel Levine (Boston), Frank Wilson (then at St. Louis), Bernard Oppenheimer, Marcus Rothschild, and William St. Lawrence (New York). See S. A. Levine to H. C. Christian, October 1917, in C. F. Wooley and J. M. Stang, "Samuel A. Levine's First World War encounters with Mackenzie and Lewis," *Br. Heart J.*, 64 (1990): 166–170; J. Mackenzie to J. Parkinson, 13 January 1916, in Mair, *Sir James Mackenzie*, p. 264; and W. Osler to W. Francis, 12 April 1916, in Cushing, *Life of Osler*, 2: 524–525.

99. T. McMillan, "The standardization of the diagnosis and treatment of heart disease in cardiac clinics," *Trans. Coll. Phys. Phila.*, 3d ser., 46 (1924): 720–726. For Lewis on the organization of cardiology, see Howell, "Soldier's heart," p. 46.

100. Quote from Walsh, *History of Medicine in New York*, 2: 592. See also Bonner, *American Doctors and German Universities*, pp. 157–160, and R. G. Frank Jr., "American physiologists in German laboratories, 1865–1914," in *Physiology in the American Context*, ed. Geison, pp. 11–46.

101. Conner, "Organized effort to control heart diseases," quotes pp. 53–54. For organized efforts to prevent other noncommunicable diseases, see G. M. Kober and W. C. Hanson, eds., *Diseases of Occupation and Vocational Hygiene* (Philadelphia: P. Blakiston's Son, 1916), and W. S. Bainbridge, *The Cancer Problem* (New York: Macmillan, 1915). For a contemporary assessment of Conner's key role in the cardiac clinic movement, see J. Sailer, "The growth and work of the National Association for the Prevention and Relief of Heart Disease," *Trans. Coll. Phys. Phila.*, 3d ser., 46 (1924): 709–713. See also H. Emerson, "The prevention of heart disease—a new practical problem," *Boston Med. Surg. J.* 184 (1921): 587–607.

102. Conner, "Organized effort to control heart diseases," quote p. 56. See also Conner, "Cardiac diagnosis in the light of experiences with army physical examinations," *Am. J. Med. Sci.* 158 (1919): 773–782, and Wooley, "Lewis A. Conner, M.D." The systematic medical examination of schoolchildren was begun in some of America's largest cities at the turn of the century. A comprehensive 614-page guide for examiners published in 1913 made no mention of cardiac disease or of examining the heart. W. S. Cornell, *Health and Medical Inspection of School Children* (Philadelphia: F. A. Davis, 1913). Soon, the public health cardiologists would emphasize the importance of examining schoolchildren for evidence of cardiac disease. See also D. Dwork, "Childhood," chapter 45 in *Companion Encyclopedia of the History of Medicine*, 2 vols., ed. W. F. Bynum and R. Porter (New York: Routledge, 1993), 2:1072–1091, and C. R. King, *Children's Health in America* (New York: Twayne Publishers, 1993).

103. Conner, "Organized effort to control heart diseases," quotes pp. 56, 59.

104. Ibid., p. 59. See also T. G. Benedek, "Rheumatic fever and rheumatic heart disease," in *The Cambridge World History of Human Disease*, ed. K. F. Kiple (Cambridge: Cambridge Univ. Press, 1993), pp. 970–977; P. C. English, "Emergence of rheumatic fever in the nineteenth century," in *Framing Disease*, ed. Rosenberg and Golden, pp. 20–32; and A. L. Bloomfield, "Rheumatic fever," in *A Bibliography of Internal Medicine: Communicable Diseases* (Chicago: Univ. of Chicago Press, 1958),

pp. 133–163. A contemporary summary is C. F. Coombs, *Rheumatic Heart Disease* (Bristol: John Wright & Sons, 1924).

105. Conner, "Organized effort to control heart diseases," quote p. 61.

106. J. E. Talley, discussion following Conner, "Organized effort to control heart diseases," pp. 67–68. Conner characterized Sailer as "among the first to recognize the public health aspects of heart diseases." [L. Conner], "Joseph Sailer," *Am. Heart J.* 4 (1929): 367–368.

107. T. McCrae, discussion following Conner, "Organized effort to control heart diseases," pp. 68–69.

108. G. W. Norris, discussion following Conner, "Organized effort to control heart diseases," pp. 70–71. Norris pointed to the success of the Pennsylvania Society for the Prevention of Tuberculosis, which he thought could serve as a model for the public education campaign that Conner and other public health cardiologists thought was crucial. See E. R. Long, "Development of the voluntary health movement in America as illustrated in the pioneer National Tuberculosis Association," *Proc. Am. Phil. Soc.* 101 (1957): 142–148, and R. H. Shryock, *National Tuberculosis Association, 1904–1954: A Study of the Voluntary Health Movement in the United States* (New York: National Tuberculosis Association, 1957).

109. J. M. Anders, discussion following Conner, "Organized effort to control heart diseases," pp. 71–72.

110. Emerson, "The prevention of heart disease," quote p. 589. Emerson was a champion of the concept of preventive medicine. See Emerson, "A health program for New York City," *N.Y. Med. J.* 21 (1915): 393–396.

111. See Knopf, *A History of the National Tuberculosis Association,* and Davis and Warner, *Dispensaries,* esp. p. 13.

112. Krehl, "Diseases of the myocardium," quote p. 422.

113. R. C. Cabot, "The four common types of heart-disease," *JAMA* 63 (1914): 1461–1463. White thought this paper was a "landmark." P. D. White, "Richard Clarke Cabot," *N. Engl. J. Med.* 220 (1939): 1049–1052.

114. R. T. McKenzie, discussion following Conner, "Organized effort to control heart diseases," pp. 69–70. See also G. Gritzer and A. Arluke, *The Making of Rehabilitation: A Political Economy of Medical Specialization, 1890–1980* (Berkeley: Univ. of California Press, 1985); J. D. Howell, "Soldier's heart"; and C. F. Wooley, "From irritable heart to mitral valve prolapse: World War I—the U.S. experience and the origin of neurocirculatory asthenia," *Am. J. Cardiol.* 59 (1987): 1183–1186.

115. P. D. White and M. M. Myers, "The classification of cardiac diagnosis," *JAMA* 77 (1921): 1414–1415, quote p. 1414.

116. A. E. Cohn, "Clinical charts recommended by the Association for the Prevention and Relief of Heart Disease," *JAMA* 78 (1922): 1559–1562. But most clinics had inadequate clerical staff and had to "content themselves with less complete records." J. E. Talley, "The organization and results of the cardiac clinic," *Trans. Coll. Phys. Phila.* 46 (1924): 713–720, quote p. 717.

117. W. St. Lawrence, E. P. Maynard, H. E. B. Pardee, M. A. Rothschild, and J. Wyckoff, "Requirements for an ideal cardiac clinic and a system of nomenclature," *Boston Med. Surg. J.* 189 (1923): 762–768. St. Lawrence and Rothschild had worked

with Thomas Lewis during the war. See also Wyckoff, "The organization of the cardiac clinic."

CHAPTER 2 *Organizing the American Heart Association*

1. By 1921 there were cardiac clinics in Boston (eight), Chicago (four), Philadelphia (four), Minneapolis (two), St. Louis, Cleveland, Des Moines, Detroit, Iowa City, Long Branch, Calif., Milwaukee, and Rochester, N.Y. Most were modeled after the New York program. See H. Emerson, "The prevention of heart disease—a new practical problem," *Boston Med. Surg. J.* 184 (1921): 587–607.

2. O. Paul, *Take Heart: The Life and Prescription for Living of Dr. Paul Dudley White* (Boston: Francis A. Countway Library of Medicine, 1986), esp. pp. 116–119. Joseph Pratt, Samuel Levine, and William Robey Jr. helped White in these efforts.

3. Twenty clinics cared for 2,800 patients in Philadelphia by 1924. J. Talley, "The organization and results of the cardiac clinic," *Trans. Coll. Phys. Phila.*, 3d ser., 46 (1924): 713–720.

4. J. B. Herrick, *Memories of Eighty Years.* (Chicago: Univ. of Chicago Press, 1949). For tensions in Chicago's medical community, see T. N. Bonner, *Medicine in Chicago, 1850–1950* (Madison, Wis.: American History Research Center, 1957), esp. pp. 199–217. See also M. Fishbein, *History of the Chicago Heart Association* (Chicago: Chicago Heart Association, 1972).

5. H. Emerson, "Estimated needs for organized care of the sick [Boston 1930]," in *Selected Papers of Haven Emerson* (Battle Creek, Mich.: Kellogg Foundation, 1949), pp. 257–263, quote p. 260.

6. J. Wyckoff and C. Lingg, "Etiology in organic heart disease," *Am. Heart J.* 1 (1926): 446–470, quote p. 450.

7. F. Overton and W. J. Denno, *The Health Officer* (Philadelphia: W. B. Saunders, 1919), quote p. 25. A few years later, one doctor stated that "there has been a considerable amount of annoyance shown by the medical profession over the invasion, by public health services, of . . . the field of private practice." G. Fleming, "The medical aspects of national health insurance," *Ann. Intern. Med.* 8 (1934): 220–228.

8. Herrick, *Memories*, quote p. 203. Many doctors resisted attempts to organize medical care, fearing that each success would take them closer to socialized medicine. See R. L. Numbers, ed., *Compulsory Health Insurance: The Continuing American Debate* (Westport, Conn.: Greenwood Press, 1982), and R. Stevens, *American Medicine and the Public Interest* (New Haven: Yale Univ. Press, 1971). For practitioners' concerns about competition from dispensaries, see J. G. Burrow, *Organized Medicine in the Progressive Era: The Move Toward Monopoly* (Baltimore: Johns Hopkins Univ. Press, 1977), pp. 105–113.

9. J. B. Herrick, "Relation between the specialist and the practitioner," *JAMA* 76 (1921): 975–978, quote p. 795. See also Herrick, *Memories*, pp. 202–205.

10. A. E. Cohn, "Clinical charts recommended by the Association for the Prevention and Relief of Heart Disease," *JAMA* 78 (1922): 1559–1562, quote p. 1562.

11. The standard history of the AHA is W. M. Moore, *Fighting for Life: The Story of the American Heart Association* (Dallas: AHA, 1983). See also J. Sailer, "The growth

and work of the National Association for the Prevention and Relief of Heart Disease," *Trans. Coll. Phys. Phila.*, 3d ser., 46 (1924): 709–713; R. Halsey, "History and Development of the American Heart Association [1938]," with Halsey to H. M. Marvin, 7 February 1938, AHA Archives; and "A beginning and a future," *Bull. Am. Heart Assoc.* 1 (1925): 1. American doctors and scientists had formed dozens of specialty societies by 1920. G. Rosen, "Special medical societies in the United States after 1860," *Ciba Symp.* 9 (1947): 785–792. A list of them is in J. B. Kirsner, *The Development of American Gastroenterology* (New York: Raven Press, 1990), pp. 146–149.

12. A. E. Cohn, "Heart disease from the point of view of the public health," *Am. Heart J.* 2 (1927): 275–301, 386–407, quote p. 404. For similarities between the tuberculosis movement and the public health cardiologists' agenda, see J. D. Howell, "The changing face of twentieth-century American cardiology," *Ann. Intern. Med.* 105 (1986): 772–782. See also M. E. Teller, *The Tuberculosis Movement: A Public Health Campaign in the Progressive Era* (New York: Greenwood Press, 1988).

13. Emerson quoted in R. H. Halsey, "The founding of the American Heart Association," in *The New York Heart Association: Origins and Development, 1915–1965*, ed. C. E. de la Chapelle (New York: NYHA, 1966), pp. 8–13, quote p. 10.

14. Conner had chaired a committee to organize the AHA that also included Halsey (ex-officio), White, Herrick, Sailer, and Hugh McCullough (a Washington University pediatric heart specialist). The AHA founders are listed in Table A1.

15. Howell, "The changing face of twentieth-century American cardiology," quote p. 772. For the AHA's name, see Sailer, "The growth and work of the National Association."

16. Minutes, AHA AM, 7 February 1927, AHA Archives. Conner edited the *American Heart Journal* until 1938. See also *Archives des maladies du coeur, des vaisseaux et du sang* (Paris, 1908); *Zentralblatt für Herz- und Gefässkrankheiten* (Vienna, 1909); and *Heart: A Journal for the Study of the Circulation* (London, 1909). The annual AHA meeting was held in conjunction with the annual AMA meeting until 1955.

17. L. A. Conner, "The American Heart Journal," *Am. Heart J.* 1 (1925): 115–116.

18. The editorial board members were listed in each issue of the journal. The names of the AHA board members were published periodically in *Bull. Am. Heart Assoc.*

19. See "Society transactions. American Heart Association meeting of May 26, 1925," *Am. Heart J.* 1 (1925): 117–123, and "Atlantic City meeting," *Bull. Am. Heart Assoc.* 1, no. 2 (1925).

20. J. G. Carr, "The economic phases of cardiac disease," *Am. Heart J.* 1 (1925): 62–66. See also H. Emerson, "Economic aspects of heart disease," *Am. Heart J.* 4 (1929): 251–267, and A. Nugent, "Fit for work: The introduction of physical examinations in industry," *Bull. Hist. Med.* 57 (1983): 578–595.

21. See Howell, "The changing face of twentieth-century American cardiology" and "Similarity of tuberculosis and heart disease," *Bull. Am. Heart Assoc.* 2 (1927): 22.

22. R. H. Halsey, "Heart disease: The broad view," *N.Y. State J. Med.* 29 (1929): 1246–1248.

23. H. E. B. Pardee, J. H. Bainton, W. C. Munly, and R. L. Levy, *Criteria for the Classification and Diagnosis of Heart Disease* (New York: Paul B. Hoeber, 1928).

24. L. E. Holt Jr. to A. E. Cohn, 25 June 1928, record group 450 C661-U, box 17, file 32, Cohn Papers.

25. A. D. Hirschfelder, "Some applications of the laboratory viewpoint in clinical medicine," *Trans. Coll. Phys. Phila.*, 3d ser., 48 (1926): 16–35, quote p. 31. For the value of technology in cardiac diagnosis, see L. F. Bishop, "A cardiologic and sociologic experiment in the treatment of heart disease," *International Clinics* 32 (1922): 15–23, and W. D. Stroud, "The clinical importance of the myocardial reserve," *Trans. Coll. Phys. Phila.*, 3d ser., 47 (1925): 31–38.

26. J. B. Herrick, "In defense of the stethoscope," *Ann. Intern. Med.* 4 (1930): 113–116, quote p. 114.

27. "Jimmy was wizened," *Am. Heart J.* 9, no. 3 (1934): ads. p. 1.

28. One "truly portable" electrocardiograph was carried in two cases (40 and 49 pounds) and cost $1,290 in 1931. "Announcing the new Sanborn Portocardiograf," *Am. Heart J.* 6, no. 4 (1931): ads. p. 11. Another manufacturer offered machines for $780 to $2,650. "Amplifier type hellige electrocardiographs," *Am. Heart J.* 7, no. 2 (1931): ads p. 7. Average net incomes that year were: all practitioners $4,065; general practitioners $3,603; specialists $6,402. "Incomes of physicians," *JAMA* 111 (1938): 2311.

29. J. D. Howell, ed., *Technology and American Medical Practice 1880–1930: An Anthology of Sources* (New York: Garland, 1988), quote p. ix.

30. E. P. Maynard Jr., "The practice of medicine in 1921," *Bull. N.Y. Acad. Med.*, 2d ser., 48 (1972): 807–817.

31. S. C. Smith, *Heart Records: Their Interpretation and Preparation* (Philadelphia: F. A. Davis, 1923), quote p. 5.

32. F. A. Willius, *Clinical Electrocardiography* (Philadelphia: W. B. Saunders, 1922).

33. The University of Michigan did 1,600 electrocardiograms in 1930 and charged $3.50 per test. The charge is approximately $25 in 1994 dollars. (U.S. Bureau of Labor Statistics). For a description of the nation's best-equipped electrocardiographic department, see F. N. Wilson and P. S. Barker, "The heart station of the University of Michigan Hospital," in *Methods and Problems of Medical Education*, 18th ser. (New York: Rockefeller Foundation, 1930), pp. 89–93.

34. M. A. Rabinowitz, "Review of F. A. Willius, *Clinical Electrocardiography*," *N.Y. State J. Med.* 22 (1922): 340.

35. H. N. Segall, "Introduction of electrocardiography in Canada," *Can. J. Cardiol.* 3 (1987): 358–361.

36. Cambridge Instrument Co., Inc., *Am. Heart J.* 1, no. 3 (1925): ads. p. 1. The machines located in most hospitals and clinics were usually controlled by one or more practitioner cardiologists, because the academic cardiologists were limited to a few major teaching hospitals at this time.

37. "Over 300 Victor electrocardiographs now in use," *Am. Heart J.* 4, no. 5 (1929): ads p. 3. Advertisements in unbound issues of the *American Heart Journal* provide insight into the growth and marketing strategies of the electrocardiograph industry.

38. G. Lane, "Making your heart write," *Hygeia* (January 1930): 34–35.

39. AHA founder Robert Halsey reported that the incidence of heart disease increased steadily between 1917 and 1926. R. H. Halsey, "Observations on the mortality of heart disease in New York state," *Am. Heart J.* 4 (1928): 94–102. For a discussion of whether the incidence was actually increasing, see A. E. Cohn and C. Lingg, "Heart disease from the point of view of the public health—1933," *Am. Heart J.* 9 (1934): 283–297. Paul White thought that more accurate diagnostic techniques also contributed to the apparent increase in heart disease. P. D. White, *Heart Disease* (New York: Macmillan, 1931), pp. 296–298. For the decline of infectious diseases, see T. Smith, "The decline of infectious diseases in its relation to modern medicine," *Trans. Cong. Am. Phys. Surg.* 14 (1929): 1–18; B. Bates, *Bargaining for Life: A Social History of Tuberculosis, 1876–1938* (Philadelphia: Univ. of Pennsylvania Press, 1992), pp. 313–327; L. G. Wilson, "The historical decline of tuberculosis in Europe and America: Its causes and significance," *J. Hist. Med. Allied Sci.* 45 (1990): 366–396; and N. J. Tomes, "The white plague revisited," *Bull. Hist. Med.* 63 (1989): 467–480. The causes of the declining death rate from infectious diseases such as tuberculosis, diphtheria, scarlet fever, and typhoid fever were multifactorial: bacteriological techniques facilitated the identification of microorganisms; vaccines prevented a few diseases such as diphtheria; improved sanitation and quarantine programs reduced the transmission of some contagious diseases; and an improved standard of living and new laws meant that fewer Americans lived in overcrowded conditions. See J. Duffy, *The Sanitarians: A History of American Public Health* (Urbana, Ill.: Univ. of Chicago Press, 1990); W. W. Spink, *Infectious Diseases: Prevention and Treatment in the Nineteenth and Twentieth Centuries* (Minneapolis: Univ. of Minnesota Press, 1978); and G. Rosen, *A History of Public Health* (New York: MD Publications, 1958).

40. L. I. Dublin, "Statistical aspects of the problem of organic heart disease," *Am. Heart J.* 1 (1926): 359–367, quote p. 359.

41. Emerson, "The prevention of heart disease," quotes pp. 589, 607.

42. Ibid., p. 604. For conflicts resulting from the self-interest of medical practitioners and the aims of the public health movement, see J. Duffy, "The American medical profession and public health: From support to ambivalence," *Bull. Hist. Med.* 53 (1979): 1–22, and H. Emerson, "The relation of the medical profession to preventive medicine," *Boston Med. Surg. J.* 21 (1915): 603–606.

43. Emerson, "The prevention of heart disease," quote p. 606. See also Emerson, "Periodic medical examinations of apparently healthy persons," *JAMA* 80 (1923): 1376–1381, and M. H. Charap, "The periodic health examination: Genesis of a myth," *Ann. Intern. Med.* 95 (1981): 733–735.

44. C.-E. A. Winslow, *The Evolution and Significance of the Modern Public Health Campaign* (New Haven: Yale Univ. Press, 1923), quote pp. 60–61. See also G. Rosen, *Preventive Medicine in the United States, 1900–1975* (New York: Science History Publications, 1975).

45. J. A. Tobey, "Heart Disease," *American Mercury* 4 (1925): 462–465. See also A. B. Davis, "Life insurance and the physical examination: A chapter in the rise of American medical technology," *Bull. Hist. Med.* 55 (1981): 392–406.

46. "A beginning and a future," *Bull. Am. Heart Assoc.* 1 (1925): 1. In 1928 the AHA circulated a total of 26,000 copies of this publication. Minutes, AHA AM, 3 February 1930, AHA Archives.

47. Minutes, AHA AM, 6 February 1928, AHA Archives. See also W. L. Deadrick and L. Thompson, *The Endemic Diseases of the Southern States* (Philadelphia: W. B. Saunders, 1916). A popular 1500-page internal medicine textbook devoted just 14 pages to acute rheumatic fever (compared to 26 pages for typhoid fever) and only 19 pages to chronic valvular heart disease of all etiologies (compared to 21 pages for cardiac arrhythmias). See R. L. Cecil, ed., *A Text-Book of Medicine by American Authors* (Philadelphia: W. B. Saunders, 1929).

48. M. G. Wilson, *Rheumatic Fever* (New York: Commonwealth Fund, 1940), quote p. 6. In 1929 Paul White claimed that the "campaign now underway to prevent" heart disease was "more important than the discovery of surgical or other methods of treatment." P. D. White, "Chronic valvular disease," in *Text-Book of Medicine,* Cecil, ed., pp. 1031–1049, quote p. 1049.

49. These conclusions are drawn from a review of the "Heart" section in *Index-Catalogue of the Library of the Surgeon General's Office, United States Army,* 3d ser. (Washington, D.C.: GPO, 1926), 6: 489–603.

50. In 1929 the AHA summarized a study of "adult ward and private patients" in New York City that reported the etiology of heart disease as arteriosclerosis 40%; rheumatism 25%; syphilis 10%; various causes 15%; and unidentified 10%. See "The incidence of heart disease," *Bull. Am. Heart Assoc.* 1, no. 5 (1929): 1. Contemporary cardiology textbooks also support the conclusion that although rheumatic heart disease concerned contemporary practitioners, they did not place as much emphasis on it as did the public health cardiologists. See W. D. Reid, *The Heart in Modern Practice: Diagnosis and Treatment* (Philadelphia: J.B. Lippincott, 1923), and S. Neuhof, *Clinical Cardiology* (New York: Macmillan, 1917).

51. J. Wyckoff, "A consideration of the possibility of the prevention of arteriosclerotic heart disease," *Trans. Coll. Phys. Phila.,* 3d ser., 51 (1929): 95–110, quote p. 106. Although Louis Bishop had proposed that arteriosclerosis was preventable by "proper regulation of the chemistry of the body" as early as 1913, his formulation of the problem was unrelated to later concepts of prevention. See L. F. Bishop, "The prevention of arteriosclerosis and heart disease in otherwise healthy individuals past middle life," *JAMA* 60 (1913): 803–806, and Bishop, "The relation of diet to heart and blood-vessel disease," *Med. Rec.* 82 (1912): 559–561. Academic and practitioner cardiologists were slow to adopt the prevention ideology for coronary artery disease. See A. S. Hyman and A. E. Parsonnet, *The Failing Heart of Middle Life: The Myocardosis Syndrome, Coronary Thrombosis, and Angina Pectoris* (Philadelphia: F. A. Davis, 1932), and E. V. Cowdry, ed., *Arteriosclerosis: A Survey of the Problem* (New York: Macmillan, 1933).

52. Wyckoff and Lingg, "Etiology in organic heart disease." For background on the recognition of the clinical syndrome of acute myocardial infarction, see W. B. Fye, "The delayed diagnosis of acute myocardial infarction: It took half a century," *Circulation* 72 (1985): 262–271, and J. O. Leibowitz, *The History of Coronary Heart Disease* (London: Wellcome Institute of the History of Medicine, 1970). A provocative interpretation is C. Lawrence, "'Definite and material': Coronary thrombosis and cardiologists in the 1920s," in *Framing Disease,* ed. C. E. Rosenberg and J. Golden (New Brunswick, N.J.: Rutgers Univ. Press, 1992), pp. 50–82.

53. See Hyman and Parsonnet, *The Failing Heart,* esp. pp. 124–136. See also J. A. Myers, *Vital Capacity of the Lungs* (Baltimore: Williams & Wilkins, 1925).

54. A. M. Master, "The two-step test of myocardial function," *Am. Heart J.* 10 (1935): 495–510, and Master, "Reminiscences of fifty years in cardiology at Mount Sinai with special reference to the two-step test," *Mt. Sinai J. Med.* 39 (1972): 486–505.

55. L. M. Warfield, "How is your heart?" *Hygeia* 7 (1929): 127–128. See also H. C. Greene, *Listen in: Radio Health Talks* (Boston: American Red Cross, 1923).

56. A. S. Hyman, "Sudden heart failure as a public health menace," *Am. J. Public Health* 19 (1929): 1103–1110, quote p. 1103.

57. Hyman and Parsonnet, *The Failing Heart,* quote p. 3.

58. Ibid., p. 101.

59. This conclusion was reached after reviewing every issue of the *American Heart Journal* published between 1925 and 1950.

60. One academic internist's opinion: "In some respects it is unfortunate that diseases of the heart have become a highly specialized field of medicine." D. Riesman, "Preface," in Hyman and Parsonnet, *The Failing Heart,* p. v. Compare with F. W. Peabody, *Doctor and Patient* (New York: Macmillan, 1930), p. 17.

61. W. A. Pusey, *Medical Education and Medical Service* (Chicago: American Medical Association, 1925).

62. H. G. Weiskotten, "Present tendencies in medical practice," *Proc. Ann. Cong. Med. Educ.* (1928): 74–79, quote p. 79.

63. G. Shrady, "Specialism in general medicine," *Med. Rec.* 10 (1875): 255–256. The following year he stated, "Specialism, in the mind of the medical student, is always associated with pecuniary success." G. Shrady, "Specialism and general practice," *Med. Rec.* 11 (1876): 631–632. For factors stimulating specialization around 1930, see Peabody, *Doctor and Patient,* pp. 1–26, and W. G. Ricker, "The needs and opportunities of specialists," *N. Engl. J. Med.* 202 (1930): 22–28.

64. J. B. Herrick, "The clinician of the future," *JAMA* 86 (1926): 1–6. An academic internist noted that "professionally and socially the specialist is often looked up to as on a higher plane." Peabody, *Doctor and Patient,* quote p. 13. These statements support Sydney Halpern's conclusion that medical specialization historically has been "a status and market-driven phenomenon." S. A. Halpern, *American Pediatrics: The Social Dynamics of Professionalism, 1880–1980* (Berkeley: Univ. of California Press, 1988), quote p. 157.

65. H. H. Moore, *American Medicine and the People's Health* (New York: D. Appleton, 1927), quote p. 153.

66. H. Cabot, *The Doctor's Bill* (New York: Columbia Univ. Press, 1935), quote p. 116. Cabot's definition of "specialists" reflected the recognized specialties—mainly surgical. See Stevens, *American Medicine and the Public Interest,* p. 542.

67. J. B. Herrick, "The general practitioner," *Calif. West. Med.* 27 (1927): 179–185, quote p. 180. By this time, "people who could afford to, increasingly chose specialists . . . in many cases calling on the specialists directly," according to Rosemary Stevens. R. Stevens, *American Medicine and the Public Interest* (New Haven: Yale Univ. Press, 1971), quote p. 134.

68. Herrick, "The clinician of the future."

69. W. St. Lawrence, E. P. Maynard, H. E. B. Pardee, M. A. Rothschild, and J. Wyckoff, "Requirements for an ideal cardiac clinic and a system of nomenclature,"

Boston Med. Surg. J. 189 (1923): 762–768, quotes pp. 762, 764. See also J. Wyckoff, "The organization of the cardiac clinic," *N.Y. State J. Med.* 25 (1925): 995–1001.

70. J. A. Hartwell, "Presidential address," *Bull. N.Y. Acad. Med.* 7 (1931): 135–149, quote p. 136. Hartwell's comments reflected the opinion of many doctors that America was headed toward socialized medicine. See L. C. Taylor Jr., *The Medical Profession and Social Reform, 1885–1945* (New York: St. Martin's Press, 1974), and P. Starr, *The Social Transformation of American Medicine* (New York: Basic Books, 1982), esp. pp. 198–232. An academic internist observed that "any reorganization of the medical profession that threatens the personal bond between doctor and patient is to be viewed with suspicion." Peabody, *Doctor and Patient,* quote p. 3. For comments about "the spread of state medicine," see Hyman and Parsonnet, *The Failing Heart,* pp. 2–3.

71. D. M. Fox, *Health Policies, Health Politics: The British and American Experience, 1911–1965* (Princeton: Princeton Univ. Press, 1986), quote p. 49.

72. During the first two decades of the twentieth century, most of America's medical schools adopted the full-time faculty system for the scientific departments and encouraged those professors to perform research. This resulted in a dramatic increase in research output from the nation's medical schools. See W. B. Fye, *The Development of American Physiology: Scientific Medicine in the Nineteenth Century* (Baltimore: Johns Hopkins Univ. Press, 1987), esp. pp. 205–230, and Fye, "The origin of the full-time faculty system: Implications for clinical research," *JAMA* 265 (1991): 1555–1562. For town-gown tensions, see M. J. Lepore, *Death of the Clinician: Requiem or Reveille?* (Springfield, Ill.: Charles C. Thomas, 1982); K. M. Ludmerer, *Learning to Heal: The Development of American Medical Education* (New York: Basic Books, 1985), esp. pp. 213–218; and W. G. Rothstein, *American Medical Schools and the Practice of Medicine, a History* (New York: Oxford Univ. Press, 1987), esp. pp. 160–178.

73. "The future of medicine and the medical profession," *Cincinnati J. Med.* 3 (1922): 1–5, quote p. 2. See also J. H. Pratt, "Better training for academic careers in internal medicine," *JAMA* 91 (1928): 446–448, quote p. 447.

74. See note 14 for AHA board members. Boston internist James Means characterized the Association of American Physicians (of which he was a member) as "a self-appointed elite." Its members were academics whose shared interest was research. J. H. Means, *The Association of American Physicians: Its First Seventy-Five Years* (New York: McGraw-Hill, 1961), quote p. 29.

75. S. S. Goldwater to J. J. Golub, [c1928], record group 450 C661, box 11, file 8, Cohn Papers.

76. Minutes, AHA AM, 6 February 1928, AHA Archives.

77. "Activities of the AHA since February 1, 1927," with minutes, AHA AM, 6 February 1928, AHA Archives. See "Members of the A.H.A.," *Bull. Am. Heart Assoc.* 2, no. 2 (1927): 10–12.

78. H. M. Marvin to H. B. Sprague, 26 December 1934, Sprague Papers.

79. "The future of the hospital social service movement," *Hosp. Soc. Serv.* 5 (1922): 46. Quoted in R. Lobove, *The Professional Altruist: The Emergence of Social Work as a Career, 1880–1930* (Cambridge: Harvard Univ. Press, 1965), p. 29.

80. L. F. Bishop, "The practice of cardiology," *Ann. Intern. Med.* 2 (1928): 352–366, quotes p. 364.

81. Ibid.

82. L. F. Bishop, *Heart Troubles: Their Prevention and Relief,* 2d ed. (New York: Funk & Wagnalls, 1921), quote p. [vii].

83. Minutes, Sir James Mackenzie Cardiological Society, 22 October 1926, xerox copy in the author's possession. I thank Paul Kligfield and Arthur Hollman for recognizing the significance of these minutes and sharing them with me. Hollman obtained a copy of them from the estate of Mackenzie's relative, Lord Amulree. The persons present at the organizational meeting of the Sir James Mackenzie Cardiological Society are listed in Table A2.

84. Ibid. Bishop did not coin the word cardiology; it was first used in the nineteenth century.

85. Ibid.

86. L. F. Bishop, "History of cardiology," *N.Y. State J. Med.* 28 (1928): 140–141. Sailer's presence is noted in Minutes, Annual Meeting of the American Section of the International Association of Medical History, 3 May 1927, American Association for the History of Medicine Archives, Library of the College of Physicians of Philadelphia, Philadelphia, Pa. See also E. B. Krumbhaar, "Notes on the early days of the American Association of the History of Medicine," *Bull. Hist. Med.* 23 (1949): 577–582.

87. Minutes, Sir James Mackenzie Cardiological Society, 28 September 1928, xerox copy in the possession of the author. See note 83.

88. Ibid.

89. A. S. Hyman to J. Witkin, 19 January 1929, xerox copy in the possession of the author. See note 83.

90. The NYCS was formally incorporated in April 1935. Its stated purpose was "to conduct, assist and encourage investigations in the science of medicine and special problems relating to diseases of the heart and circulation, and to the study of the terminology, pathology, aetiology and symptomatology, directly or indirectly related to these diseases, and to make knowledge thereof available for the protection of the health of the public and the improved treatment of these diseases." *The New York Cardiological Society. Constitution and By-Laws As Amended* (New York: NYCS, 1941).

91. Minutes, NYCS, 30 April 1934, Reichert Papers, NYH Archives. The "charter members" present at the "[re]organizational" meeting of the NYCS are listed in Table A3.

92. Minutes, NYCS, 30 April 1934, Reichert Papers, NYH Archives.

93. Ibid.

94. In 1929 the president of the Rockefeller Foundation told members of the ACP, "You can't select the few from the many without leaving most of the many outside. . . . If you can't get into an existing elite, start one of your own." G. E. Vincent, "Address," *Ann. Intern. Med.* 3 (1929): 295–308.

95. The NYHA board (which included laypersons) was dominated during the 1920s and early 1930s by public health cardiologists John Wyckoff, Haven Emerson, Robert Halsey, William St. Lawrence, Alfred Cohn, and (until 1925) Lewis Conner. See *New York Heart Association, American Heart Association New York City Affiliate: A Quarter Century of Progress, 1966–1991* (New York: NYHA, 1991), pp. 106–116.

96. See M. Danzis, "Jewish hospitals and facilities for graduate training," *Medical Leaves* 3 (1940): 65–74.

97. These six individuals were listed in J. Cattell, ed., *American Men of Science: A Biographical Directory,* 5th ed. (New York: Science Press, 1933). Of the NYCS founders, only Bishop Sr. and Burton-Opitz were listed. But Burton-Opitz had been forced to resign from Columbia University's College of Physicians and Surgeons faculty for many reasons, including a complaint that he had made anti-Semitic remarks (which suggests that anti-Semitism was not the main reason for organizing the NYCS). See A. C. Laszlo, "Physiology of the future: Institutional styles at Columbia and Harvard," in *Physiology in the American Context, 1850–1940,* ed. G. L. Geison (Bethesda, Md.: American Physiological Society, 1987), pp. 67–96. See also *New York Heart Association,* pp. 106–116. Several sources for the history of anti-Semitism in the United States are listed in the bibliography.

98. "Remarks of Dr. Louis Faugeres Bishop, New York City, before the Organization Meeting of the American Cardiovascular Society [*sic*], 30 April 1934," Appendix A to Minutes, NYCS, 30 April 1934, Reichert Papers, NYH Archives. Bishop had made these points earlier; see Bishop, "History of cardiology," esp. p. 141. Bishop's son, a participant in the incorporation of the NYCS, recalls that his father sensed the need for an organization that emphasized "the continuing education of physicians" and would "help those in the active practice of cardiology by bringing together those physicians whose primary interest was the care of their patients." L. F. Bishop Jr., "Cardiology as a specialty," *N.Y. State J. Med.* 76 (1976): 1170–1174.

99. Minutes, NYCS, 30 April 1934, Reichert Papers, NYH Archives.

100. These conclusions are drawn from the minutes of the NYCS, Reichert Papers, NYH Archives. See also L. F. Bishop Jr., *The Birth of a Specialty: The Diary of an American Cardiologist, 1926–1972* (New York: Vantage Press, 1977), esp. pp. 26–28.

101. J. B. Herrick, "Comments on the treatment of heart disease," *Trans. Cong. Am. Phys. Surg.* 14 (1928): 76–90.

102. White, *Heart Disease,* esp. table 2 (pp. 302–303), pp. 498, 491, 400, and 424. For operations on heart valves, see E. C. Cutler and C. S. Beck, "The present status of the surgical procedures in chronic valvular disease of the heart," *Arch. Surg.* 18 (1929): 403–416.

103. P. D. White, "Therapeutic research," *JAMA* 85 (1925): 81–82.

104. For American physiology, see G. L. Geison, "International relations and domestic elites in American physiology, 1900–1940," in *Physiology in the American Context,* ed. Geison, pp. 115–154.

105. E. C. Andrus to A. E. Cohn, 30 September [1934], record group "processed," box 1, file 5, Cohn Papers. See also A. M. Harvey, "Cardiovascular research at Johns Hopkins," in *Adventures in Medical Research: A Century of Discovery at Johns Hopkins* (Baltimore: Johns Hopkins Univ. Press, 1976), pp. 261–287.

106. See Fye, "The origin of the full-time faculty system."

107. F. N. Wilson to A. E. Cohn, 20 February 1934, box 2, file 2, Cohn Papers. See also A. M. Harvey, *Science at the Bedside: Clinical Research in American Medicine, 1905–1945* (Baltimore: Johns Hopkins Univ. Press, 1981), esp. pp. 104–129.

108. W. O. Fenn, *History of the American Physiological Society: The Third Quarter Century, 1937–1962* (Washington, D.C.: American Physiological Society, 1963), quote p. 92.

109. L. N. Katz to Dear Doctor, 28 February 1933, record group 450 C661, box 17, file 1, Cohn Papers. The list of recipients suggests who belonged (or once belonged) to the category of physiological cardiologists: E. C. Andrus, R. Ashman, G. Bachmann, H. C. Bazett, C. S. Beck, H. L. Blumgart, D. W. Bronk, A. E. Cohn, O. M. Cope, P. M. Dawson, M. Dresbach, D. J. Edwards, J. Erlanger, J. A. E. Eyster, G. Fahr, W. E. Garrey, S. Goldschmidt, C. W. Greene, A. A. Grollman, C. M. Gruber, W. F. Hamilton, A. D. Hirschfelder, Y. Henderson, D. R. Hooker, F. P. Knowlton, P. D. Lamson, C. D. Leake, F. C. Mann, F. D. McCrea, D. A. McGinty, J. C. Meakins, W. J. Meeks, J. S. Robb, R. W. Scott, F. M. Smith, I. Starr, M. B. Visscher, J. T. Wearn, S. Weiss, P. D. White, C. J. Wiggers, and F. N. Wilson. Some of these individuals focused their efforts on cardiovascular pharmacology (like Leake and Hirschfelder). A few others had become more clinically oriented academic cardiologists (like Andrus and White). Louis Katz, Walter Meek, and Carl Wiggers were elected to the original steering committee. R. S. Alexander, "History of the cardiovascular section," *Physiologist* 27 (1984): 67–68.

110. Fenn, *History of the American Physiological Society,* quote p. 95.

111. Pardee's comments are in "Committee for the coordination of investigation," *Bull. Am. Heart Assoc.* 8, no. 1 (1933): 1–2. See also Minutes, AHA AM, 4 February 1929, AHA Archives, where research support is broken down into "statistical, social, and medical." The only "medical" research discussed was in the planning stages and dealt with the etiology, treatment, and prevention of rheumatic fever.

112. Moore, *Fighting for Life,* quote p. 36. See also "Program of the American Heart Association," *Bull. Am. Heart Assoc.* 7, no. 2 (1932): 1–3.

113. H. M. Marvin to H. B. Sprague, 26 December 1934, Sprague papers. See also A. J. Badger, *The New Deal: The Depression Years, 1933–1940* (New York: Noonday Press, 1989).

114. Comparison of income and expenses, American Heart Association, Inc. [1936], box 12, file 4, White Papers. See also Moore, *Fighting for Life,* p. 32.

115. "Program of the American Heart Association" (1932).

116. S. A. Levine, "Foreword," *Mod. Concepts Cardiovasc. Dis.* 1 (1932): 1.

117. The changes are summarized in "Twelfth annual meeting," *Bull. Am. Heart Assoc.* 11, no. 1 (1936): 1.

118. "Eighth annual meeting," *Bull. Am. Heart Assoc.* 7, no. 2 (1932): 5–6.

119. See H. M. Marvin to P. D. White, 8 February 1936, box 12, file 4, White Papers. See also "Miscellaneous," *Bull. Am. Heart Assoc.* 10, no. 1 (1935): [2]. The members of the enlarged board are listed in *Bull. Am. Heart Assoc.* 12, no. 1 (1937): [2]. The conclusion that most board members fit my definition of academic cardiologist was drawn after reviewing their institutional affiliations listed in standard biographical directories.

120. White purposely selected the title "Heart Disease" instead of "Cardiovascular Disease" or "Circulatory Disease." White, *Heart Disease,* quote p. viii.

121. Minutes, AHA AM, 4 February 1935, AHA Archives. See also R. L. Mueller, "Irving S. Wright: Innovator in cardiovascular medicine," *Clin. Cardiol.* 18 (1995): 181–183. Brown and Allen, each the author of several dozen papers on peripheral vascular disease, pushed the same agenda. See "The History of the

Medical Vascular Section of the Mayo Clinic." [c 1957]. Archives, Mayo Medical Library, Rochester, Minn.

122. I. H. Page, *Hypertension Research: A Memoir, 1920–1960* (New York: Pergamon Press, 1988), quote p. 6. Hypertension and atherosclerosis were not originally seen as preventable, even by the public health cardiologists.

123. Bishop, "The practice of cardiology," quote p. 364.

124. All but one of the twenty-four charter members had academic appointments at prominent medical schools, most of which encouraged clinical research. The names and institutional affiliations of the founders of the vascular section are in "New vascular section," *Bull. Am. Heart Assoc.* 10, no. 4 (1935): [2]. See also "Notes on Certain Significant Developments in the AHA, 1933–1950," in AHA General Histories, file 3, AHA Archives.

125. Irving S. Wright, interview by W. Bruce Fye, 14 August 1991, New York.

126. Minutes, AHA EC, 23 October 1935, AHA Archives.

127. [L. A. Conner], "Retrospect and prospect," *Am. Heart J.* 10 (1935): 830–831. See also "New vascular section." The most convenient summary of contemporary thought about arteriosclerosis is Cowdry, *Arteriosclerosis.*

128. *A History of the Scientific Councils of the American Heart Association* (New York: AHA, 1967).

129. "Section of the American Heart Association for the Study of the Peripheral Circulation," *Bull. Am. Heart Assoc.* 13, no. 3 (1938): 1.

130. In 1939 the AHA balance sheet revealed expenses of $13,327, income of $11,555, and deficit of $1,772. Minutes, AHA Board of Directors, 6 February 1939, box 12, file 6, White Papers.

131. H. B. Sprague to F. R. Taylor, 19 October, 1932, Sprague Papers. The AHA continued to emphasize the concept of periodic health examinations to detect asymptomatic heart disease. See "He and his father would have been great pals," *Bull. Am. Heart Assoc.* 10, no. 3 (1935): [5]. See also E. F. Bland, "Howard B. Sprague," *Clin. Cardiol.* 13 (1990): 888–889.

CHAPTER 3   *Declaring War on Heart Disease*

1. H. J. Morgan, "Memorandum from chairman of committee on postgraduate instruction," *Ann. Intern. Med.* 12 (1939): 1541–1546. See also note 27.

2. "Washington University School of Medicine," *Am. Heart J.* 1, no. 1 (1925): ad. p. 8. See also "Postgraduate courses in heart disease," *Bull. Am. Heart Assoc.* 5, no. 3 (1930): 2; "Postgraduate course in St. Louis," *Bull. Am. Heart Assoc.* 2, no. 3 (1927): 15; and "Postgraduate courses in heart disease," *Bull. Am. Heart Assoc.* 6, no. 3 (1931): 3; and "Postgraduate course on the heart," *Bull. Am. Heart Assoc.* 11, no. 2 (1936): [4].

3. P. D. White and H. Donovan, *Hearts: Their Long Follow-Up* (Philadelphia: W. B. Saunders, 1967), pp. xxiii–xxiv. See also J. B. Vander Veer, *Cardiology at the Pennsylvania Hospital (1920–1980)* (Philadelphia: Pennsylvania Hospital, 1986).

4. J. A. Hartwell, "The continued education of the doctor," *Bull. N.Y. Acad. Med.* 7 (1931): 446–463, quote p. 449.

5. W. C. Rappleye, "Further notes on present-day medical education," *South Med. J.* 23 (1930): 150–155.

6. G. M. Piersol, "Presidential address," *Ann. Intern. Med.* 8 (1934): 1–9, quote p. 1. See also "Incomes of physicians," *JAMA* 111 (1938): 2311.

7. "Current medical problems," *N. Engl. J. Med.* 203 (1930): 996. After survey-ing two thousand American physicians in 1937, the American Foundation con-cluded, "there are too many poor specialists, and there are not enough good ones." E. E. Lape, *American Medicine: Expert Testimony out of Court* (New York: American Foundation, 1937), quote 1: 459.

8. G. E. Follansbee, "The profession and the public," *Ann. Intern. Med.* 5 (1931): 224–230, quote p. 225. The survey is summarized in I. S. Falk, C. R. Rorem, and M. D. Ring, *The Costs of Medical Care: A Summary of Investigations on the Economic Aspects of the Prevention and Care of Illness* (Chicago: Univ. of Chicago Press, 1933), p. 205.

9. R. Stevens, *American Medicine and the Public Interest* (New Haven: Yale Univ. Press, 1971), quote p. 205. Stevens's perceptive account of the development of specialty boards supplements this necessarily brief overview. See also J. D. Howell, "The invention and development of American internal medicine," *J. Gen. Intern. Med.* 4 (1989): 127–133.

10. J. B. Herrick, "Report [of the committee of graduate instruction in internal medicine]," *AMA Bull.* 15 (1921): 18–21, quote p. 18. See also J. G. Burrow, *Organized Medicine in the Progressive Era: The Move Toward Monopoly* (Baltimore: Johns Hopkins Univ. Press, 1977).

11. R. Stevens, "The curious career of internal medicine: Functional ambiva-lence, social success," in *Grand Rounds: One Hundred Years of Internal Medicine*, ed. R. C. Maulitz and D. E. Long (Philadelphia: Univ. of Pennsylvania Press, 1988), pp. 339–364, quote p. 346. See also W. G. Morgan, *The American College of Physicians: Its First Quarter Century* (Philadelphia: ACP, 1940), esp. pp. 1–8; F. Smithies, "Presi-dential address," *Ann. Intern. Med.* 1 (1928): 861–874; and G. M. Piersol, *Gateway of Honor: The American College of Physicians 1915–1959* (Philadelphia: ACP, 1962). Louis Bishop (a prominent practitioner, but not a member of internal medicine's elite) was one of the original eleven members of the ACP.

12. [M. Pincoffs], "The certification of internists and the proposed examina-tions for fellowship in the college," *Ann. Intern. Med.* 8 (1935): 1162–1165. Several specialty societies were positioning themselves to participate in the creation of certifying boards in the face of attempts by the AMA and the newly created Advisory Board for Medical Specialties (ABMS) to gain control of the process. See Stevens, *American Medicine*, esp. table A1, p. 542, and Stevens, "The curious career of internal medicine," esp. pp. 348–350.

13. W. L. Bierring, "The American Board of Internal Medicine" in Morgan, *American College of Physicians*, pp. 87–102, quote p. 87.

14. F. M. Pottenger, "President's address," *Ann. Intern. Med.* 6 (1933): 1517–1534, quote p. 1522.

15. Minutes ACP BOG, 19 April 1937. *Ann. Intern. Med.* 11 (1937): 427.

16. "The American Board of Internal Medicine (Inc)," *JAMA* 107 (1936): 375–376.

17. T. R. Harrison to H. M. Marvin, 18 May 1943, box 12, file 39, White Papers. See also Bierring, "American Board of Internal Medicine." Sydney Halpern attri-

butes decisions like this to a desire on the part of leaders of established specialties (such as internal medicine) "to protect their markets by obstructing the further proliferation of specialty boards." S. A. Halpern, *American Pediatrics: The Social Dynamics of Professionalism, 1880–1980* (Berkeley: Univ. of California Press, 1988), quote p. 27. The American Board of Surgery unsuccessfully attempted to require trained surgical subspecialists to have completed a three-year general surgical residency and pass the general surgery examination before they could take their subspecialty board examination. See J. S. Rodman, *History of the American Board of Surgery, 1937–1952* (Philadelphia: J. B. Lippincott, 1956), esp. pp. 55–56. See also P. D. Olch, "Evarts A. Graham, the American College of Surgeons, and the American Board of Surgery," *J. Hist. Med. Allied Sci.* 27 (1972): 247–261.

18. L. F. Bishop and J. Neilson Jr., *History of Cardiology* (New York: Medical Life Press, 1927), quote p. 71.

19. Bierring, "American Board of Internal Medicine," esp. pp. 98–99.

20. H. M. Marvin to AHA EC, 18 December 1939, box 12, file 8, White Papers. See also Marvin to AHA EC, 9 October 1939, box 12, file 7, White Papers.

21. S. A. Levine, "Electrocardiography and the general practitioner," *Med. Clin. North Am.* 24 (September 1940): 1325–1345, quote p. 1340.

22. S. A. Levine, "Cardiology as a specialty," *Phi Delta Epsilon News Sci. J.* (October 1937): 138–140.

23. P. W. Morgan to H. B. Sprague, 27 May 1940, Sprague Papers.

24. H. B. Sprague to H. M. Marvin, 20 November 1940, Sprague Papers.

25. H. M. Marvin to W. S. Middleton, 8 May 1941, Sprague Papers. The decision had already been made to certify subspecialists when Irons became chair of the ABIM. See Bierring, "American Board of Internal Medicine," p. 100.

26. Minutes of the AHA BOD, 5 February 1940, AHA Archives.

27. H. M. Marvin to R. D. Friedlander, 21 August 1941, box 12, file 26, White Papers. After surveying "physicians, groups, medical societies, etc., throughout the country," the AHA leaders separated heart specialists into two groups: the "A" group included "the best men in the community," while the "B" group consisted of "the less competent ones." The AHA's final list of 205 men (and they were all men) was forwarded to the ABIM. See "Memorandum Concerning the Selection of the Founders' Group in Cardiovascular Disease," 8 November 1941, AHA History 1940s file, folder 2, AHA Archives. It is interesting to compare the AHA's final list with the ACP membership. The 1941 ACP directory included 4,654 persons, of whom 742 listed cardiology as a special interest (of these, 44 listed cardiology first, followed by internal medicine). *Directory, American College of Physicians* (Philadelphia: ACP, 1941). There were between 6,500 and 7,000 internists in America in 1940. See also Stevens, *American Medicine*, esp. pp. 162, 543. These statistics suggest that there were approximately one thousand American doctors who viewed themselves as heart specialists in 1941. See also "Specialties and sub-specialties among members of the American College of Physicians," *Ann. Intern. Med.* 17 (1942): 1042–1043.

28. Minutes, AHA BOD, 30 May 1941, Sprague Papers.

29. T. R. Harrison to H. M. Marvin, 18 May 1943, box 12, file 39, White Papers.

30. H. M. Marvin to P. D. White, 25 February 1942, box 12, file 29, White Papers. For a comparison of the ABIM and the American Board of Surgery, see

Howell, "Invention and development of American internal medicine." Some elite academic internists protested the entire certification movement. See J. H. Means, *The Association of American Physicians: Its First Seventy-Five Years* (New York: McGraw-Hill, 1961), pp. 193–194. Several important papers on professionalization are in A. Oleson and J. Voss, eds., *The Organization of Knowledge in Modern America, 1860–1920* (Baltimore: Johns Hopkins Univ. Press, 1979). See also L. Veysey, "Who's a professional? Who cares?" *Rev. Am. Hist.* 3 (1975): 419–423.

31. Between 1942 and 1951, the number of internists certified annually ranged from 9 in 1949 to 34 in 1950. H. R. Kimball [President, ABIM] to W. B. Fye, 26 October 1993, which includes a detailed listing of "diplomates certified by the American Board of Internal Medicine broken down by year."

32. Numbers and quotation from W. C. Rappleye, ed., *Graduate Medical Education: Report of the Commission on Graduate Medical Education* (Chicago: Univ. of Chicago Press, 1940), quote p. 15. Surgeons were expected to have completed an internship and a three-year hospital-based residency before they were eligible to take their boards. See Rodman, *History of the American Board of Surgery,* esp. pp. 6–7.

33. Bierring, "American Board of Internal Medicine," quotes pp. 96, 97.

34. "The American Board of Internal Medicine," *Ann. Intern. Med.* 10 (1936): 411–414.

35. Minutes, AHA BOD, 8 February 1943, box 12, file 37, White Papers.

36. See M. M. Wintrobe, *Hematology, the Blossoming of a Science: A Story of Inspiration and Effort* (Philadelphia: Lea & Febiger, 1985); C. J. Smyth, R. H. Freyberg, and C. McEwen, *History of Rheumatology* (Atlanta: Arthritis Foundation, 1985), esp. pp. 21–36; and C. S. Livingood, "History of the American Board of Dermatology, Inc. (1932–1982)," *J. Am. Acad. Dermatol.* 7 (1982): 821–850.

37. Stevens, *American Medicine,* quote pp. 234–235. Sydney Halpern agrees. Discussing these dynamics in a general sense, she notes, "Whether a segment is currently institutionalized as an autonomous specialty or as a subspecialty is determined largely by the timing of its development." Halpern, *American Pediatrics,* quote pp. 27–28.

38. O. H. P. Pepper, "What is an internist?" *Ann. Intern. Med.* 13 (1940): 1791–1798, quote p. 1796.

39. E. E. Irons to P. D. White, 3 July 1940, box 12, file 10, White Papers.

40. P. D. White to C. S. Burwell, 21 May 1941, Sprague Papers.

41. Sprague's committee included cardiologists from Los Angeles, Atlanta, Syracuse, N.Y., Emporia, Kan., and Toronto. Jack Marvin and William Stroud were ex-officio members. Minutes, AHA BOD, 7 June 1940, AHA Archives.

42. Minutes, AHA, Inc., "Preliminary Meeting of the Executive Secretaries of Local Heart Associations," 11 June 1940, AHA Archives.

43. Minutes, AHA BOD, 7 June 1940, AHA Archives.

44. "A General Program for the American Heart Association Prepared by the Committee on Activities," [cMarch 1941], Sprague Papers. See also "Report of the Committee on Activities," [1941], box 12, file 23, White Papers.

45. H. M. Marvin to AHA EC, 22 July 1942, AHA History 1940s, file 2, AHA Archives.

46. H. M. Marvin to H. E. Ungerleider, 6 January 1942, AHA History 1940s, file 2, AHA Archives.

47. J. R. Paul, *A History of Poliomyelitis* (New Haven: Yale Univ. Press, 1971), esp. pp. 308–323, quote p. 309. For the National Foundation for Infantile Paralysis, see N. Rogers, *Dirt and Disease: Polio before FDR* (New Brunswick, N.J.: Rutgers Univ. Press, 1992), esp. pp. 170–171. For financial information on the National Foundation and other voluntary health organizations, see S. M. Gunn and P. S. Platt, *Voluntary Health Agencies: An Interpretive Study* (New York: Ronald Press, 1945), esp. pp. 206–227.

48. H. M. Marvin to AHA EC, 22 July 1942.

49. "Proposal for a Public Relations and Fund Raising Program for the American Heart Association," 21 July 1942, AHA History 1940s, file 2, AHA Archives.

50. H. M. Marvin to AHA EC, 22 July 1942.

51. H. M. Marvin to P. D. White, 30 July 1942, box 12, file 34, White Papers. At this time the AHA had 2,364 members, 97 affiliated cardiac clinics, and 16 local (or regional) heart associations. See Marvin to Ungerleider, 6 January 1942.

52. P. D. White to H. M. Marvin, 5 August 1942, box 12, file 34, White Papers.

53. P. D. White to I. H. Page, 20 January 1943, box 12, file 37, White Papers.

54. H. M. Marvin to Dear Doctor, 6 August 1942, box 12, file 34, White Papers.

55. There AHA leaders debated whether their new research program should focus on rheumatic heart disease or arteriosclerosis and hypertension. See H. M. Marvin, Memorandum to the [AHA] BOD, 26 September 1945, box 12, file 51, White Papers.

56. Minutes, AHA BOD, 8 February 1943, box 12, file 37, White Papers. The AHA remained committed to its public health agenda. Marvin listed twenty-two projects (many related to public health and education) that the AHA hoped to undertake in 1942. See Marvin to Ungerleider, 6 January 1942.

57. Marvin, Memorandum to the [AHA] BOD, 26 September 1945. For the role of the war in delaying the AHA's reorganization, see L. N. Katz to H. M. Marvin, 18 May 1943, box 12, file 39, White Papers.

58. Gunn and Platt, *Voluntary Health Agencies,* quotes pp. 218–219. The March of Dimes was a great success, and the American Cancer Society had recently launched an effective fund-raising campaign. See W. S. Ross, *Crusade: The Official History of the American Cancer Society* (New York: Arbor House, 1987); J. T. Patterson, *The Dread Disease: Cancer and Modern American Culture* (Cambridge: Harvard Univ. Press, 1987); and V. A. Triolo and M. B. Shimkin, "The American Cancer Society and cancer research origins and organization: 1913–1943," *Cancer Res.* 29 (1969): 1615–1641.

59. Marvin, Memorandum to the [AHA] BOD, 26 September 1945.

60. Marvin to E. Stetson, 23 September 1946, AHA Archives.

61. P. D. White to H. M. Marvin, 17 January 1946, box 12, file 52, White Papers.

62. D. G. Price to officers and directors of the NYHA, December 1945, in Council for Heart Disease, 1946 file, AHA Archives. See also "Certificate of Incorpo-

ration of the Council for Heart Diseases, Inc.," 16 May 1946, in Council for Heart Disease, 1946 file, AHA Archives.

63. H. M. Marvin to E. P. Maynard Jr., 21 May 1946, in Council for Heart Diseases, 1946 file, AHA Archives.

64. H. B. Sprague to [R. Scott], cJune 1946, in "Conference on Organization of the American Heart Association," AHA Archives.

65. I. H. Page to H. M. Marvin, 28 January 1946, exhibit D of Minutes, AHA BOD, 5 February 1946, box 12, file 53, White Papers.

66. Ibid. Physiological cardiologist Frank Wilson also protested the AHA's emphasis on rheumatic heart disease. See "Relationship of the American and Local Heart Associations," 27 January 1948, AHA History 1940s, folder 2, AHA Archives. The AHA had formed a committee on rheumatic fever in 1939 that evolved into the American Council on Rheumatic Fever five years later. The council's executive committee included lay members, and its agenda included soliciting donations for rheumatic fever research. See Minutes, American Council on Rheumatic Fever, 8 May 1945, box 12, file 49, White Papers.

67. "Report on Steps Leading to Merger of American Foundation for High Blood Pressure with American Heart Association," 1949, Sprague Papers. See also I. H. Page to H. M. Marvin, 4 February 1946, exhibit D of Minutes, AHA BOD, 5 February 1946, box 12, file 53, White Papers.

68. H. Ungerleider in Minutes, AHA BOD, 28 June 1946, AHA Archives.

69. H. B. Sprague to [R. Scott], cJune 1946.

70. Ibid.

71. Ibid.

72. "The expanded program of the American Heart Association for 1947," *Am. Heart J.* 32 (1947): 679–680.

73. Win Nathanson and Associates, Inc., to Gentlemen, 19 September 1946, Sprague Papers. See also Minutes, AHA BOD, 20 September 1946, AHA Archives. This firm was selected by a committee consisting of Jack Marvin, Irving Wright, Brooklyn cardiologist Edwin Maynard, and New York cardiologist Clarence de la Chapelle. The AHA headquarters was in Manhattan, and three of the four members of the committee were from New York.

74. H. M. Marvin in Minutes, Chicago Heart Association Annual Meeting, 18 February 1947, Speeches file, AHA Archives.

75. 20th Anniversary Annual Dinner, American Heart Association, 24 November 1968, box 13, file 26, White Papers.

76. T. R. Harrison, Speech to the New England Heart Association, 7 February 1948, Speeches file, AHA Archives.

77. H. Chapman, *On Medical Education* (Philadelphia: Collins, 1876), quote pp. 12–13. I discuss the issue of research funding and full-time scientific careers in W. B. Fye, *The Development of American Physiology: Scientific Medicine in the Nineteenth Century* (Baltimore: Johns Hopkins Univ. Press, 1987).

78. E. V. Cowdry, ed., *Arteriosclerosis: A Survey of the Problem* (New York: Macmillan, 1933), quote p. ix.

384 *Notes to Pages 102–103*

79. R. B. Fosdick, *The Story of the Rockefeller Foundation* (New York: Harper & Bros., 1952). Foundations that supported cardiovascular research included the Josiah Macy Jr., Markle, and Commonwealth Foundations. See *The Josiah H. Macy, Jr. Foundation, 1930–1955: A Review of Activities* (New York: Josiah H. Macy, Jr., Foundation, 1955); T. G. Strickland and S. P. Strickland, *The Markle Scholars: A Brief History* (New York: Prodist, 1976); and A. M. Harvey and S. L. Abrams, *"For the Welfare of Mankind." The Commonwealth Fund and American Medicine* (Baltimore: Johns Hopkins Univ. Press, 1986). See also R. H. Shryock, *American Medical Research: Past and Present* (New York: Commonwealth Fund, 1947); R. L. Geiger, *To Advance Knowledge: The Growth of American Research Universities, 1900–1940* (New York: Oxford Univ. Press, 1986); and G. Jonas, *The Circuit Riders: Rockefeller Money and the Rise of Modern Science* (New York: W.W. Norton, 1989).

80. D. M. Fox, "The politics of NIH extramural program, 1937–1950," *J. Hist. Med. Allied Sci.* 42 (1987): 447–466, quote p. 466. See also V. A. Harden, *Inventing the NIH: Federal Biomedical Research Policy, 1887–1937* (Baltimore: Johns Hopkins Univ. Press, 1986); and S. P. Strickland, *The Story of the NIH Grants Program* (Lanham, Md.: Univ. Press of America, 1989).

81. For contemporary appraisals, see M. Fishbein, ed., *Doctors at War* (New York: E.P. Dutton, 1945), and P. H. Long, "Medical progress and medical education during the war," *JAMA* 130 (1946): 983–990.

82. It should be noted that there is debate about the role of World War II in stimulating the development of American science. I believe that its impact on medical science was significant, as discussed in the text. For an overview of the various interpretations of the development of what has been termed "big science," see J. H. Capshew and K. A. Rader, "Big science: Price to the present," *Osiris* 7 (1992): 3–25. See also R. L. Geiger, *Research and Relevant Knowledge: American Research Universities since World War II* (New York: Oxford Univ. Press, 1993).

83. V. Bush, *Science: The Endless Frontier* (Washington, D.C.: GPO, 1945). For Bush's perspective on Truman's response to the report, see V. Bush, *Pieces of the Action* (New York: William Morrow, 1970), esp. pp. 63–68. For the political dimensions of the debate over the government's postwar research programs, see D. J. Kevles, "The National Science Foundation and the debate over postwar research policy, 1942–1945," *Isis* 68 (1977): 5–26.

84. W. W. Palmer, "Appendix 2. Report of the medical advisory committee," in Bush, *Science: The Endless Frontier,* pp. 40–64, quote p. 43. See also F. A. Reister, ed., *Medical Statistics in World War II* (Washington, D.C.: GPO, 1975), esp. pp. 9–12.

85. Palmer, "Report of the medical advisory committee," quotes pp. 43, 44. See also S. P. Strickland, *Politics, Science, and Dread Disease: A Short History of United States Medical Research Policy* (Cambridge: Harvard Univ. Press, 1972).

86. V. E. Kinsey, "Fundamental research in the clinical specialties," *Science* 105 (1947): 373–378. See also C. J. Van Slyke, "New horizons in medical research," *Science* 104 (1946): 559–567; and E. M. Boyd, "Medical research in the university medical school," in *Medical Research: A Symposium,* ed. A. Smith (Philadelphia: J.B. Lippincott, 1946), pp. 80–109. For a discussion of the tensions (related to ideology and turf) between basic researchers, clinical investigators, and disease-oriented specialists in this era, see H. M. Marks, "Cortisone, 1949: A year in the political life of a drug," *Bull. Hist. Med.* 66 (1992): 419–439.

87. "Lasker Foundation for Medical Research," November 1934, record group 450 C661, box 16, file 6, Cohn Papers.

88. E. Boas, *The Unseen Plague of Chronic Disease* (New York: J.J. Augustin, 1940), quote p. 121.

89. D. M. Fox, "Health policy and changing epidemiology in the United States: Chronic disease in the twentieth century," in *Unnatural Causes: The Three Leading Killer Diseases in America,* ed. R. C. Maulitz (New Brunswick, N.J.: Rutgers Univ. Press, 1988), pp. 11–31. See also D. M. Fox, *Power and Illness: The Failure and Future of American Health Policy* (Berkeley: Univ. of California Press, 1993); A. E. Cohn and C. Lingg, "Heart disease from the point of view of the public health—1933," *Am. Heart J.* 9 (1934): 283–297; and A. E. Cohn and C. Lingg, *The Burden of Diseases in the United States* (New York: Oxford Univ. Press, 1950).

90. Patterson, *Dread Disease,* quotes pp. 172, 171.

91. Strickland, *Politics, Science, and Dread Disease,* quote pp. 32–33. For Lasker's support of the cause of arthritis, see Marks, "Cortisone," esp. pp. 434–435.

92. C. Pepper, Hearings on wartime health and education [1944], quoted in Strickland, *Politics, Science, and Dread Disease,* p. 39.

93. C. Pepper, Testimony, 1948 NHI Senate appropriation, History part 1, 1948–1967, pp. 6–8, NHLBI Archives.

94. "Stenographic Transcript of Hearings before the Committee on Interstate and Foreign Commerce, House of Representatives," 5 May 1948, Hearings, Diseases of the Heart, 1948 file, AHA Archives.

95. Ibid. For Scheele's ambivalence about the wholesale development of categorical research programs and institutes, see Marks, "Cortisone," esp. pp. 434–436.

96. Strickland, *Story of the NIH Grants Program.*

97. "Stenographic Transcript of Hearings," 5 May 1948.

98. Ibid.

99. *Public Law 655. 80th Cong. 2d sess. 1948. S. 2215. An Act to Amend the Public Health Service Act to Support Research and Training in Diseases of the Heart and Circulation* (Washington, D.C.: GPO, 1948).

100. Ibid., quote p. 4. See also Minutes, NAHC, 8 September 1948, NHLBI Archives.

101. L. N. Katz, "What Is Immediately Ahead," 5 June 1951, Speeches file, AHA Archives.

102. E. V. Allen to H. B. Sprague, 5 July 1950, Sprague Papers.

103. H. B. Sprague to E. V. Allen, 12 July 1950, Sprague Papers.

104. "American Heart Association," *N. Engl. J. Med.* 240 (1949): 239.

105. Original members included Tinsley Harrison, Howard Burchell, Myron Prinzmetal, Howard Sprague, Eugene Stead, Francis Wood, and Harry Goldblatt. See also W. M. Moore, *Fighting for Life: The Story of the American Heart Association 1911–1975* (Dallas: AHA, 1983), p. 173, and *Your Heart Program* (New York: AHA, 1950), which includes financial figures and a list of individuals and institutions that received AHA grants in 1949.

106. Marks, "Cortisone," quote p. 430. See also R. Bud, "Biotechnology in the twentieth century," *Soc. Stud. Sci.* 21 (1991): 415–457.

107. The *Time* article is quoted in Patterson, *Dread Disease*, pp. 145–146.

108. L. N. Katz to H. B. Sprague, 7 July 1949, Sprague Papers. For tensions regarding the role of the government in setting the agenda and controlling the resources for medical research, see Kevles, "National Science Foundation"; Strickland, *Politics, Science, and Dread Disease*; and Marks, "Cortisone." See also Palmer, "Report of the medical advisory committee."

109. C. A. R. Connor, "Research Policies of the Association," 2 September 1949, in AHA history 1940s, file 2, AHA Archives.

110. *Announcement of Clinical Investigator Program* (New York: NYHA, 1950). See also *Your Heart Program*.

111. Win Nathanson & Associates, "Recommendations for 1949 Campaign," June 1948, in AHA History 1940s, AHA Archives.

112. "Attacking the No. 1 Killer," *Business Week*, 12 July 1947, 21–22.

113. E. Sullivan, "Little Old New York," *[New York] Sunday News*, 11 January 1948, record group 450 C661-U, box 14, file 30, Cohn Papers.

114. "Why executives drop dead," *Fortune* 1 (1950): 88–91.

115. "Remarks," Minutes, AHA BOD, 7 December 1950, AHA Archives.

116. Gunn and Platt, *Voluntary Health Agencies*, quote p. 219.

117. "Remarks," Minutes, AHA BOD, 7 December 1950, AHA Archives.

118. Nathanson, "Recommendations for 1949 Campaign."

119. "Stenographic Transcript of Hearings," 5 May 1948.

120. P. D. White, *My Life and Medicine: An Autobiographical Memoir* (Boston: Gambit, 1971), quote p. 58.

121. I. S. Wright to M. Lasker, 26 May 1950, box 2, miscellaneous correspondence, 1950, Wright Papers.

122. Irving S. Wright, interview by W. Bruce Fye, 14 August 1991, New York.

123. I. H. Page, *Hypertension Research: A Memoir, 1920–1960* (New York: Pergamon Press, 1988), quote p. 36.

124. "National conference on cardiovascular diseases," *The American Heart* 1, no. 1 (1950): 5–6. See also *Proceedings First National Conference on Cardiovascular Diseases* (New York: AHA, 1950).

125. C. K. Friedberg, *Diseases of the Heart* (Philadelphia: W.B. Saunders, 1949), quote p. v.

126. J. P. Swazey and R. C. Fox, "The clinical moratorium: A case study of mitral valve surgery," in *Experimentation with Human Subjects*, ed. P. A. Freund (New York: George Brazillier, 1970), pp. 315–357. See also H. B. Shumacker Jr., *The Evolution of Cardiac Surgery* (Bloomington: Indiana Univ. Press, 1992).

127. W. Forssmann, "Catheterization of the right heart," in *Classics of Cardiology*, ed. J. A. Callahan, T. E. Keys, and J. D. Key (Malabar, Fla.: Robert E. Krieger, 1983), 3: 253–255. See also W. Forssmann, *Experiments on Myself: Memoirs of a Surgeon in Germany* (New York: Saint Martin's Press, 1974).

128. R. J. Bing, "The Johns Hopkins: The Blalock-Taussig Era," *Perspect. Biol. Med.* 32 (1988): 85–90. See also L. Dexter, "Early days of cardiac catheterization," *J. Appl. Cardiol.* 4 (1989): 343–344. Scientists had used cardiac catheterization to study

cardiac physiology since the mid-nineteenth century. See A. Cournand, "Cardiac catheterization: Development of the technique, its contributions to experimental medicine, and its initial applications in man," *Acta Med. Scand.* suppl. 579 (1975): 3–32. Before 1950, however, most physiological cardiologists concerned themselves with electrocardiography. In 1928 Carl Wiggers stated that the number of investigators working on hemodynamics "can be counted on the digits of two hands." C. J. Wiggers, *The Pressure Pulses in the Cardiovascular System* (London: Longmans, Green, 1928), quote p. vii.

129. For different perspectives on the innovation, see H. B. Taussig, *History of the Blalock-Taussig Operation and Some of the Long Term Results on Patients with a Tetralogy of Fallot* (Cooperstown, N.Y.: Mary Imogene Bassett Hospital, 1970), pp. 13–38; W. P. Longmire Jr., *Alfred Blalock: His Life and Times* ([Los Angeles]: William P. Longmire Jr., 1991), esp. pp. 88–89, 94–113; V. T. Thomas, *Pioneering Research in Surgical Shock and Cardiovascular Surgery: Vivien Thomas and His Work with Alfred Blalock* (Philadelphia: Univ. of Pennsylvania Press, 1985), esp. pp. 80–104; and Bing, "Johns Hopkins."

130. Denton A. Cooley, interview by W. Bruce Fye, 11 April 1992, Houston.

131. W. H. B[arker], "Brighter blood for blue babies," *Ann. Intern. Med.* 24 (1946): 285–288.

132. A. Cournand to A. Blalock, 4 October 1946, Blalock Papers.

133. Shumacker, *Evolution of Cardiac Surgery,* quote p. 66.

134. Longmire, *Alfred Blalock,* quote p. 109.

135. Richard J. Bing, interview by W. Bruce Fye, 11 February 1992, Pasadena. Denton Cooley believes that "surgery was the real stimulus to cardiologists to make exact and precise diagnoses." Cooley interview.

136. A. Cournand, R. J. Bing, L. Dexter, C. Dotter, L. N. Katz, J. V. Warren, et al., "Report of committee on cardiac catheterization and angiocardiography of the American Heart Association," *Circulation* 7 (1953): 769–773.

137. Lewis Dexter, interview by W. Bruce Fye, 15 November 1992, Boston.

138. Dwight E. Harken, interview by W. Bruce Fye, 14 April 1992, Dallas. T. Holmes Sellors, a British pioneer of heart surgery, emphasized the significance of Harken's experience: "The heart could not only be sutured: it could be safely opened and closed." T. H. Sellors, "Fifty years on—surgery of the heart and circulation," *Br. J. Tuberculosis Dis. Chest* 50 (1956): 72–76.

139. A. Blalock to C. Bailey, 1 December 1949, Bailey file, Blalock Papers.

140. J. H. Gibbon Jr. to A. Blalock, 25 March 1949, Blalock Papers.

141. See W. G. Bigelow, *Mysterious Heparin: The Key to Open Heart Surgery* (Toronto: McGraw-Hill Ryerson, 1990), and Shumacker, *Evolution of Cardiac Surgery.*

142. P. B. Beeson, "Infectious diseases in the decade 1940–50," *Year Book of Medicine* (1950): 9–17.

143. A. Fleming, *Chemotherapy: Yesterday, Today, and Tomorrow* (Cambridge: Cambridge Univ. Press, 1946), quote p. 36. See also J. Parascandola, ed., *The History of Antibiotics: A Symposium* (Madison, Wis.: American Institute of the History of Pharmacy, 1980).

144. A. Fleming, ed., *Penicillin: Its Practical Application* (London: Butterworth, 1946), quote p. v. For problems associated with the introduction and expanded use

of antibiotics, see J. C. Whorton, "'Antibiotic abandon': The resurgence of therapeutic rationalism," in *History of Antibiotics,* ed. Parascandola, pp. 125–136.

145. P. D. White, *Heart Disease* (New York: Macmillan, 1931), quote p. 347. Friedberg, *Diseases of the Heart,* quote p. v. See also B. F. Massell, C. G. Chute, A. M. Walker, and G. S. Kurland, "Penicillin and the marked decrease in morbidity and mortality from rheumatic fever in the United States," *N. Engl. J. Med.* 318 (1988): 280–286.

146. R. H. Meade, *A History of Thoracic Surgery* (Springfield, Ill.: Charles C. Thomas, 1961).

CHAPTER 4   *Doctors with a Different Vision: The American College of Cardiology*

1. H. B. Sprague to H. M. Marvin, 20 November 1940, Sprague Papers. A listing of the AHA officers, executive committee, and board or directors is in "American Heart Association, Inc." *Am. Heart J.* 20 (1940): 128.

2. "Report of the Committee on Activities," [1941], box 12, file 23, White Papers. AHA influential Irvine Page contends that the AHA was an "elitist" organization during the 1940s. See I. H. Page, *Hypertension Research: A Memoir, 1920–1960* (New York: Pergamon Press, 1988), quote p. 13.

3. L. N. Katz to H. M. Marvin, 18 May 1943, box 12, file 39, White Papers.

4. H. M. Marvin to P. D. White, 7 January 1942, box 12, file 28, White Papers.

5. H. V. Rice, "Medical research, its trends and portents," *Can. Med. Assoc. J.* 57 (1947): 95–101, quote p. 99. Regarding "academic snobbishness," see E. M. Boyd, "Medical research in the university medical school," in *Medical Research: A Symposium,* ed. A. Smith (Philadelphia: J. B. Lippincott, 1946), pp. 80–109, quote p. 107.

6. "Conference on Organization of the American Heart Association," 28 June 1946, in AHA History 1940s file, AHA Archives. Louis Katz was the most vocal supporter of research on this thirty-five-member committee (whose members are listed in this reference).

7. J. T. Patterson, *The Dread Disease: Cancer and Modern American Culture* (Cambridge: Harvard University Press, 1987), quote p. 173.

8. *A History of the Scientific Councils of the American Heart Association* (New York: American Heart Association, 1967). See also W. B. Fye, "A history of the American Heart Association's council on clinical cardiology," *Circulation* 87 (1993): 1057–1063.

9. "Report of Committee on Policies and Activities [of the AHA], 28 June 1946, AHA History 1940s file, AHA Archives.

10. "Members—Scientific Council of American Heart Association, Inc.," 31 July 1948, AHA History 1940s file, AHA Archives.

11. Certification numbers are from H. R. Kimball [President, ABIM] to W. B. Fye, 26 October 1993. Includes a listing of "diplomates certified by the American Board of Internal Medicine broken down by year." See also Minutes, AHA BOD, 5 February 1946, box 12, file 53, White Papers.

12. "A Planning Survey for the American Heart Association," June 1948, AHA Archives.

13. W. M. Moore, *Fighting for Life: The Story of the American Heart Association 1911–1975* (Dallas: American Heart Association, 1983), quote p. 129.

14. For Groedel's bibliography, see B. Kisch, ed., *Franz M. Groedel Anniversary Volume on the Occasion of His Seventieth Birthday* (New York: Brooklyn Medical Press, 1951), pp. 220–237.

15. See Ibid.; M. S. Schlepper and S. Dack, "Franz Groedel, Bruno Kisch and the founding of the American College of Cardiology," *Am. J. Cardiol.* 12 (1988): 577–580; M. Schlepper, "Franz Maximilian Groedel: Ein deutsches Schicksal von internationaler kardiologischer Bedeutung," *Z. Kardiol.* 77, suppl. 5 (1988): 155–177; and H. Mahr, "Franz M. Groedel: Kardiologe, Röntgen Spezialist, Balneologe und Weltmann," *CorVas* 3 (1987): 152–156.

16. W. B. Fye, "Carl Ludwig and the Leipzig Physiological Institute: A factory of new knowledge," *Circulation* 74 (1986): 920–928.

17. Arthur Dean Bevan quoted in T. N. Bonner, "Friedrich von Müller of Munich and the growth of clinical science in America, 1902–14," *J. Hist. Med. Allied Sci.* 45 (1990): 556–569, quote p. 556. See also A. M. Harvey, *Science at the Bedside: Clinical Research in American Medicine, 1905–1945* (Baltimore: Johns Hopkins Univ. Press, 1981), esp. pp. 28–30.

18. See F. M. Groedel, *Die Röntgendiagnostik der Herz- und Gefäberkrankungen* (Berlin: Hermann Meusser, 1912); Groedel, "Roentgen cinematography and its importance in medicine," *Br. Med. J.* 1 (1909): 1–3; and Groedel, "The present state of roentgen cinematography and its results as to the study of the movements of the inner organs of the human body," *Interstate Med. J.* 22 (1915): 281–290. This innovation was a precursor to later methods devised to record images of the moving cardiac chambers filled with x-ray contrast material (angiocardiography). British cardiologist Evan Bedford characterized Groedel as a "pioneer in cardiac radiology." *The Evan Bedford Library of Cardiology* (London: Royal College of Physicians, 1977), quote p. 119.

19. F. M. Groedel, *Das Extremitäten-, Thorax- und Partial-Elektrokardiogramm des Menschen* (Leipzig: Theodor Steinkopff, 1934), and Groedel, "The isolation of the left and right electrocardiogram," *South. Med. Surg. J.* 97 (1935): 353–355. See also F. N. Wilson, "[Review of Groedel] *Das Extremitäten-, Thorax- und Partial-Elektrokardiogramm des Menschen*," *Am. Heart J.* 10 (1935): 1127–1128; C. E. Kossmann, "Unipolar electrocardiography of Wilson: A half century later," *Am. Heart J.* 110 (1985): 901–904; and W. B. Fye, "A history of the origin, evolution, and impact of electrocardiography," *Am. J. Cardiol.* 73 (1994): 937–949.

20. F. M. Groedel, "Physiotherapeutics of diseases of the cardiovascular system," *Radiology* 11 (1928): 194–206. See also C. A. Pierach, S. D. Wangensteen, and H. B. Burchell, "Spa therapy for heart disease, Bad Nauheim (circa 1900)," *Am. J. Cardiol.* 72 (1993): 336–342, and T. W. Maretzki, "The Kur in West Germany as an interface between naturopathic and allopathic ideologies," *Soc. Sci. Med.* 24 (1987): 1061–1068.

21. W. Osler, *The Principles and Practice of Medicine*, 6th ed. (New York: D. Appleton, 1905), quote p. 829. See also W. B. Thorne, *The Schott Methods of the Treatment of Chronic Diseases of the Heart*, 5th ed. (London: J. & A. Churchill, 1906).

22. J. H. Pratt, "On the development of scientific hydrotherapy," *Boston Med. Surg. J.* 154 (1906): 85–91. See also Pratt, "The neglect of hydrotherapy in America," *Clifton Med. Bull.* 1 (1913): 21–27.

23. J. M. Groedel and T. Groedel, *Bad-Nauheim: Its Springs and Their Uses with Useful Local Information and a Guide to the Environs,* 5th ed. (Friedberg: Carl Bindernagel, 1909). See also J. M. Swan, "A resume of the opinions upon the Nauheim treatment of chronic disease of the heart," *Trans. Am. Clin. Climatol. Assoc.* 27 (1911): 28–59. For an overview of hydrotherapy in various countries, see A. T. Fripp, "A medical tour of some German spas," *Guy's Hosp. Gazette* 46 (1932): 410–417; E. H. L. Corwin, "Report on the spas of Europe," *Bull. N.Y. Acad. Med.* 6 (1930): 553–570; D. Cantor, "The contradictions of specialization: Rheumatism and the decline of the spa in inter-war Britain," *Med. Hist.* suppl. 10 (1990): 127–144; and H. B. Weiss and H. R. Kemble. *The Great American Water-Cure Craze: A History of Hydropathy in the United States* (Trenton, N.J.: Past Times Press, 1967).

24. P. S. Ward, "Simon Baruch: Rebel in the Ranks of Medicine, 1840–1921" (Ph.D. diss., University of Wisconsin-Madison, 1990), esp. pp. 392–424. See also S. Baruch, "The giving of Nauheim baths in this country," *Med. Rec.* 87 (1915): 972–975, and Baruch, "The Nauheim method," *Med. Rec.* 91 (1916): 1074–1081.

25. Corwin, "Report on the spas of Europe," p. 564. See also *Report of the Saratoga Springs Commission to the Legislature. Legislative Doc. 70* (Albany: State of New York, 1930), and G. M. Swanner, *Saratoga: Queen of Spas* (Utica, N.Y.: North Country Books, 1988).

26. Corwin, "Report on the spas of Europe," p. 566. See also "Saratoga Springs," *Bull. Am. Heart Assoc.* 7 (1932): 1–2. Correspondence between Groedel and Bernard Baruch regarding the Saratoga Springs Commission is in the Baruch Papers.

27. B. M. Baruch to F. D. Roosevelt, 8 December 1931, in Personal Papers as Governor, box 4, file Bart-Barv, Roosevelt Papers. Roosevelt (who had visited Nauheim with his father) supported the development of a spa at Saratoga Springs. He told Baruch that he recently had "a nice talk with Dr. Groedel whose father I knew very many years ago in Nauheim." F. D. Roosevelt to B. M. Baruch, 19 December 1931, in Personal Papers as Governor, box 4, file Bart-Barv, Roosevelt Papers. For a discussion of Roosevelt's interest in hydrotherapy, see N. Rogers, *Dirt and Disease: Polio before FDR* (New Brunswick, N.J.: Rutgers Univ. Press, 1992), esp. pp. 166–169.

28. P. T. O'Farrell, "Cardiological research at Bad-Nauheim," *Irish J. Med. Sci.,* ser. 6, 94 (1933): 579–586.

29. "New regulation of German medical practice," *JAMA* 100 (1933): 1550–1551.

30. D. Krasner, "Smith Ely Jelliffe and the immigration of European physicians to the United States in the 1930s," *Trans. Stud. Coll. Physicians Phila.,* ser. 5, 12, (1990): 49–67.

31. "Memorandum," 26 January 1942, record group 450 C661-U, box 19, file 27, Cohn Papers. Several printed primary and secondary sources dealing with anti-Semitism and the intellectual migration that resulted from the Nazi policies are listed in the bibliography.

32. L. Fermi, *Illustrious Immigrants: The Intellectual Migration from Europe, 1930–41* (Chicago: Univ. of Chicago Press, 1968), quote p. 303. See also D. L. Edsall, "The émigré physician in America, 1941," *JAMA* 117 (1941): 1881–1888.

33. G. Baehr, "Emergency committee in aid of displaced foreign physicians," *JAMA* 100 (1933): 1900.

34. D. Lewis, "The place of the clinic in medical practice," *JAMA* 100 (1933): 1905–1910. See also R. Kotelchuck, "The depression and the AMA," *Health PAC Bull.* 69 (March-April 1976): 13–18, and J. A. Johnson and W. J. Jones, *The American Medical Association and Organized Medicine: A Commentary and Annotated Bibliography* (New York: Garland Publishing, 1993).

35. W. L. Bierring, "Social dangers of an oversupply of physicians," *AMA Bull.* 29 (1934): 17–20.

36. A. E. Cohn to B. Warburg, 13 March 1934, record group 450 C661-U, box 1, file 26, Cohn Papers.

37. "Immigrant physicians," *JAMA* 104 (1935): 2357.

38. H. S. Leiper, "Those German refugees: Facts do not justify the propaganda about refugees displacing American jobholders," *Curr. Hist.* 50 (1939): 19–22, 63, quotes pp. 19, 20.

39. A. E. Cohn to F. Grünbaum, 16 May 1933, record group 450 C661, box 11, file 9, Cohn Papers.

40. J. H. Means to A. Gregg, 24 April 1933, record group 451 C661-U, box 1, file 27, Cohn Papers.

41. L. H. Kassel to A. E. Cohn, 11 March 1937, record group 450 C661, box 11, file 9, Cohn Papers.

42. A. E. Cohn to L. H. Kassel, 15 March 1937, record group 450 C661, box 11, file 9, Cohn Papers.

43. "Memorandum on the Problem of Refugee Physicians: Statement of Boston Committee on Medical Emigres," 1939, record group 450 C661-U, box 13, file 24, Cohn Papers.

44. A. E. Smith, "Can we make room for the refugees?" *New Outlook* (November 1933): 9–10.

45. H. Zinsser, *As I Remember Him: The Biography of R.S.* (Boston: Little, Brown, 1940), quote p. 42.

46. W. Coleman, "The physician in Nazi Germany," *Bull. Hist. Med.* 60 (1986): 234–240.

47. A. E. Cohn to N. A. Berwin & Co., 4 May 1934, record group 450 C661, box 11, file 9, Cohn Papers.

48. J. Wyckoff, "Address delivered at the laying of the cornerstone of the Simon Baruch Research Institute," *Publ. Saratoga Spa*, no. 3 (1935).

49. For Groedel's work in electrocardiography, see "[Review of Groedel] *Das Extremitäten-, Thorax- und Partial-Elektrokardiogramm des Menschen*," *JAMA* 104 (1935): 1932–1933, and "[Review of Groedel] *Direct Electrocardiography of the Human Heart and Intrathoracic Electrocardiography*," *JAMA* 139 (1949): 751.

50. "Presidential address," 3 May 1961, in Annual Reports of the ACC Secretary, 1952–1966, Reichert Papers, NYH Archives.

51. For Hyman on Groedel, see A. S. Hyman and A. E. Parsonnet, *The Failing Heart of Middle Life: The Myocardosis Syndrome, Coronary Thrombosis, and Angina Pectoris* (Philadelphia: F. A. Davis, 1932), pp. 424–425. For Beth David Hospital, see J. J. Walsh, *History of Medicine in New York: Three Centuries of Medical Progress* (New York:

National Americana Society, 1919) 3: 782–783, and R. Sheffield, "42nd Street Beth David Hospital," *New York Physician* 47 (1957): 18–20.

52. "German Physicians Placed in Hospitals," 30 May 1934, record group 450 C661-U, box 13, folder 31, Cohn Papers. The experience of one immigrant cardiologist provides insight into the dynamics of practicing medicine in Europe and America. Fritz Brunn, a Jewish doctor who emigrated to the United States from Austria in 1938, became a public health cardiologist in New York. See F. Brunn, *Memoirs of a Doctor of the Old and New Worlds* (New York: Crambruck Press, 1969).

53. H. M. Marvin to I. Page, 24 January 1943, box 12, file 37, White Papers.

54. B. Kisch, "Die Geschichte der Organisation der Kreislaufforschung in Deutschland," *Z. Kreislaufforschung* 44 (1955): 241–260.

55. F. M. Groedel to B. Wartenslaben, 20 April 1943, correspondence 1943–1947, Virchow Society Archives.

56. F. M. Groedel to J. S. Kenney, 12 October 1943, correspondence 1943–1947, Virchow Society Archives.

57. F. M. Groedel, "Address of the outgoing president," *Proc. Rudolf Virchow Med. Soc.* 4 (1945): 3–4. See also K. F. Hoffmann, "The history of the Rudolf Virchow Medical Society in the city of New York, 1860 to 1960," in *Rudolf Virchow Medical Society, Jubilee Volume, 100th Anniversary* (Basel: Karger, 1960), pp. 12–47.

58. C. H. Stember, "The recent history of public attitudes," in *Jews in the Mind of America*, ed. G. Salomon (New York: Basic Books, 1966), pp. 31–234, quotes pp. 53, 55.

59. P. D. White to F. Frankfurter, 27 September 1940, White Papers.

60. "Conference at Dr. Cohn's summer home, with Justice Felix Frankfurter and Dr. Alfred E. Cohn," 14 September 1940, box 34, file 6, White Papers. See also L. Dinnerstein, *Anti-Semitism in America* (New York: Oxford Univ. Press, 1994).

61. P. D. White to Bruno Kisch, 24 May 1955, box 1, file 28, White Papers. White expressed these same views in 1951. See P. D. White to J. C. Edwards, 15 October 1951, box 1, file 27, White Papers. In America in this era, promoting oneself as a specialist could engender hostility from other physicians. Historian George Rosen claimed, "At the present time the use of any form of publicity by specialists, even modest announcements, is roundly condemned." G. Rosen, *The Specialization of Medicine with Particular Reference to Ophthalmology* (New York: Froben Press, 1944), quote p. 66.

62. M. G. Synnott, "Anti-Semitism and American universities: Did quotas follow the Jews?" in *Anti-Semitism in American History*, ed. D. A. Gerber (Urbana: Univ. of Illinois Press, 1987), pp. 233–271, quote p. 238.

63. Minutes, NYCS, 30 October 1949, Reichert Papers, NYH Archives. Despite his exclusion from positions of influence in the AHA and NYHA, Groedel maintained his membership in these organizations. See *Who's Who in America*, vol. 25 (Chicago: A. N. Marquis, 1948).

64. For the challenges faced by immigrant physicians and medical scientists seeking authorship in American journals, see B. Kisch, *Wanderungen und Wandlungen: Die Geschichte eines Arztes im 20. Jahrhundert* (Cologne: Greven Verlag, 1966), esp. pp. 320–324, quote p. 323. A systematic review of the *American Heart Journal* from 1933 to 1949 reveals very few papers authored by immigrants. Elec-

trocardiographer David Scherf was one exception to the rule. Groedel's bibliography (see note 14) reveals the scope of his clinical research and shows that he continued to be a prolific author after arriving in the United States. His books on the venous pulse (1946) and direct electrocardiography (1948) received positive reviews in *JAMA*.

65. H. M. Marvin, "Foreword," *Circulation* 1 (1950): 1. See also Page, *Hypertension Research*, 27; Minutes, AHA EC, 29 September 1949, AHA Archives; and P. D. White to C. A. R. Connor, 24 October 1949, Sprague Papers.

66. Minutes, NYCS, 30 October 1949, Reichert Papers, NYH Archives. See also Minutes, NYCS, 13 October 1949, Reichert Papers, NYH Archives.

67. Minutes, NYCS, 30 October 1949. The concept of a new national society as an alternative to the AHA was first articulated in 1934 when the NYCS was reorganized by Albert Hyman and other New York City practitioners, as discussed in Chapter 2. That year Bensel made a motion that the NYCS "cooperate with other local cardiological societies in the formation of the American Cardiological Association." Minutes, NYCS, 30 April 1934, Reichert Papers, NYH Archives.

68. Minutes, NYCS, 30 October 1949.

69. Minutes, ACC (NYCS Group), 28 November 1949, Reichert Papers, NYH Archives. The founders of the American College of Cardiology are listed in Table A4.

70. P. Reichert, "A history of the development of cardiology as a medical specialty," *Clin. Cardiol.* 1 (1978): 5–15, quote p. 12. See also Minutes, ACC BOT, 23 December 1950, ACC Archives and Minutes NYCS, 25 April 1951, Reichert Papers, NYH Archives. Groedel held several meetings to plan the college with his physician colleagues and confidants Philip Reichert, Max Miller, and Bruno Kisch. See P. Reichert, "Heart House: The American College of Cardiology, Thirty Years," [1979], Reichert Papers, NYH Archives.

71. Minutes, [ACC] BOT, 2 December 1949, ACC Archives. Signatures on the original documents distinguish Groedel's lawyer Max Miller from his physician associate Max Miller (who collaborated with Groedel and Reichert in planning the ACC).

72. See E. Corday to W. D. Nelligan, 18 August 1965, Corday file, ACC Archives. The signers of the Delaware incorporation document included Samuel Blinder, Hannibal DeBellis, Seymour Fiske, Gabriel Greco, Albert Hyman, Samuel Korry, Alberto Robertiello, and Epaminonda Secondari. See "Certificate of Incorporation of American College of Cardiologists, Inc.," 6 December 1949, ACC Archives.

73. Minutes, ACC BOT, 5 February 1951, ACC Archives.

74. Minutes, ACC BOT, 2 December 1950, ACC Archives.

75. On 2 December 1950 the American College of Cardiology voted to increase the size of its board to thirteen members in order to absorb the trustees of the American College of Cardiologists, Inc. Two weeks later, the trustees of the American College of Cardiologists, Inc., approved a merger with the American College of Cardiology. Minutes, ACC BOT, 2 December 1950, ACC Archives. The "official" ACC founders were the men who signed the draft constitution on 28 November 1949, except for Bensel, who refused to participate. Epaminonda Secondari was added as a founder but was not an original signer. See Table A4.

76. J. L. Lochner, "Licensure evaluation of European medical graduates," *JAMA* 137 (1948): 16–17. For one immigrant's perspective, see B. Kisch, "The Jewish refugee and America," *Jewish Forum* (January-February 1942): 3–4, 27, 31

77. Minutes, ACC BOT, 23 December 1950, ACC Archives.

78. *Am. Coll. Cardiol. Bull.* (February 1951): 1–2.

79. "The American College of Cardiology, Its First Thirty Years," [1980], History file, ACC Archives. The practice of using society credentials to denote specialization was controversial. See C. Miller, "Should I designate my specialty?" *Med. Econ.* 27 (1949): 125–129.

80. T. D. Jones to F. M. Groedel, 31 January 1951, with Minutes, ACC BOT, 5 February 1951, ACC Archives. The American College of Chest Physicians was concerned about the impact the ACC might have on their organization. Groedel noted that they "became frightened also" and sent letters emphasizing that they "will do now more in the heart business." F. M. Groedel to M. van Adelsberg, 28 March 1951, in California chapter file, Reichert Papers, ACC Archives. See also J. A. Myers, *A History of the American College of Chest Physicians, 1935–1959* ([Chicago]: American College of Chest Physicians, 1959).

81. M. B. Visscher to R. A. Betts, 2 November 1950, Sprague Papers.

82. F. M. Groedel to T. D. Jones, 2 February 1951, with Minutes, ACC BOT, 1949–52, ACC Archives.

83. T. D. Jones to F. M. Groedel, 5 February 1951, with Minutes, ACC BOT, 1949–52, ACC Archives.

84. F. M. Groedel to T. D. Jones, 7 February 1951, with Minutes, ACC BOT, 1949–52, ACC Archives.

85. H. M. Marvin to AHA Scientific Council members, 31 January 1951, Sprague Papers.

86. F. M. Groedel to E. P. Maynard Jr., 6 February 1951, with Minutes, ACC BOT, 1949–52, ACC Archives.

87. H. B. Sprague to Dear Doctor, 23 February 1951, with Minutes, ACC BOT, 1949–52, ACC Archives.

88. *Rules and Regulations of the Scientific Council. Amended June 22, 1950* (New York: AHA, 1950).

89. H. B. Sprague to W. H. Lewis Jr., 23 March 1951, Sprague Papers.

90. H. B. Sprague to A. Graybiel, 9 July 1951, Sprague Papers. "L.M.D." stands for "local medical doctor," a term academicians and medical trainees sometimes apply to practitioners.

91. H. B. Sprague to M. A. Schnitker, 19 February 1951, Sprague Papers.

92. P. Reichert to L. F. Bishop Jr., 19 April 1960, in ACC correspondence 1960, Reichert Papers, NYH Archives. See Table A4 for a summary of the backgrounds of the ACC founders (all of whom were practitioner cardiologists).

93. H. B. Sprague to L. N. Katz, 5 July 1951, Sprague Papers.

94. H. B. Sprague to A. Graybiel, 9 July 1951, Sprague Papers.

95. A. Graybiel to H. B. Sprague, 17 July 1951, Sprague Papers.

96. H. B. Sprague to A. Graybiel, 21 July 1951, Sprague Papers.

97. I. S. Wright to H. M. Marvin, 7 November 1949, Wright Papers. See also L. N. Katz to H. B. Sprague, 29 June 1951, Sprague Papers.

98. L. F. Bishop Jr., *The Birth of a Specialty: The Diary of an American Cardiologist, 1926–1972* (New York: Vantage Press, 1977), quote pp. 120–121.

99. Irving S. Wright, interview by W. Bruce Fye, 14 August 1991, New York. For Wright's opinion of German medical education during the Nazi era, see I. S. Wright, "Medical education in Germany and Austria," *JAMA* 137 (1948): 5–8.

100. O. Hall, "The informal organization of the medical profession," *Can. J. Econ. Pol. Sci.* 12 (1946): 30–44, quotes pp. 36, 42–43. The ethnic heritage and national origins of the ACC founders are described in Table A4. One former AHA president thought that "if the New York Heart had been more broad minded and extended the hand to pull people aboard and make them feel wanted" the ACC might never have been formed. O. Paul, interview by W. B. Fye, 16 June 1992, Boston. Another former AHA president has the impression that the NYHA members at the time were "a very cliquey bunch" who "excluded the refugee physicians." R. S. Ross, interview by W. B. Fye, 11 June 1993, Baltimore. A member of the NYHA at the time recalled that the "antagonism" of members of that organization toward the NYCS "was very intense." C. S. Kossmann to W. B. Fye, April 1993.

101. L. N. Katz to H. B. Sprague, 20 June 1951, Sprague Papers.

102. See M. R. Walsh, *Doctors Wanted: No Women Need Apply* (New Haven: Yale Univ. Press, 1977), and D. C. Reitzes, *Negroes and Medicine* (Cambridge: Harvard Univ. Press, 1958).

103. "Founder's Group, Scientific Council, American Heart Association, Inc.," 7 April 1949, AHA History 1940s file, AHA Archives. This list does indicate that Jewish physicians and medical scientists were underrepresented in the Scientific Council, but they were underrepresented in American academic medicine at the time. Among the Jewish physicians and medical scientists invited to join the Scientific Council were Richard Bing, Herman Blumgart, Morris Fishbein, Arthur Fishberg, Harry Gold, Harry Goldblatt, Louis Katz, Richard Langendorf, Samuel Levine, Robert Levy, Arthur Master, Bernard Oppenheimer, Aaron Parsonnet, David Scherf, and Milton Winternitz. See also "Members—Scientific Council of American Heart Association, Inc.," 31 July 1948, AHA History file, AHA Archives; S. R. Kagan, *Jewish Contributions to Medicine in America from Colonial Times to the Present*, 2d ed. (Boston: Boston Medical Publishing Co., 1939); and N. Koren, *Jewish Physicians: A Biographical Index* (Jerusalem: Israel Universities Press, 1973).

104. H. F. K. Reichert to W. B. Fye, 15 July 1992. Simon Dack, an early influential in the ACC who knew all of the founders, agreed with Mrs. Reichert's assessment. Speaking of the founders, he explained, "They were nobodies as far as the Heart Association was concerned. They were nobodies." Simon Dack, interview by W. Bruce Fye, 21 October 1991, New York. Reflecting their lack of stature in New York's medical community, none of the ACC founders were included among the more than 150 individuals characterized as "friends, associates, and pupils" of Bernard S. Oppenheimer, a pioneering cardiologist and electrocardiographer at New York's Mt. Sinai Hospital. Reflecting the ethnic heritage of that institution, many of the persons listed were Jewish. Several prominent non-Jewish cardiologists (from around the country) were included: Arlie Barnes, Howard Burchell, Louis A. Conner, Tinsley Harrison, Edward Krumbhaar, Edwin Maynard, Irvine Page, Harold Pardee, Howard Sprague, Paul White, Frederick Willius, Frank Wilson, and Irving Wright. See

"Oppenheimer anniversary number," *J. Mt. Sinai Hosp.* 8 (January-February 1942), unpaginated.

105. Minutes, AHA EC, 28 April 1951, AHA Archives.

106. Minutes, AHA SC EC, 6 June 1951, AHA Archives.

107. Minutes, Committee for Reorganization of the Scientific Council, 26 September 1951, AHA Archives.

108. "Rules and regulations of the Section on Clinical Cardiology," 30 June 1952, with Minutes, AHA CCC EC, AHA Archives. See also Fye, "A history of the American Heart Association's council on clinical cardiology."

109. B. Kisch, "The American College of Cardiology," *Exp. Med. Surg.* 9 (1951): 206.

110. Minutes, ACC BOT, 24 March 1951, ACC Archives.

111. F. M. Groedel to M. van Adelsberg, 28 March 1951, California chapter file, Reichert Papers, ACC Archives.

112. J. P. Harvey to H. B. Sprague, 21 March 1951, Sprague Papers. See also Minutes, AHA EC, 28 April 1951, AHA Archives.

113. Harvey to Sprague, 21 March 1951.

114. H. B. Sprague, "What the Heart Association does for the practicing physician," *GP* 5 (1952): 91–95.

115. W. B. Bean to F. M. Groedel, 30 June 1951, ACC Minutes, 1949–1952, p. 82, ACC Archives. See also F. M. Groedel to W. B. Bean, 3 July 1951, ACC Minutes, p. 83, ACC Archives.

116. A. D. Dennison Jr. to F. M. Groedel, 1 May 1951, New Jersey chapter file, Reichert Papers, ACC Archives.

117. The original criteria for fellowship and other membership grades in the ACC are in *Am. Coll. Cardiol. Bull.* (March 1951): 1. Although only fellows were permitted to use the F.A.C.C. designation, associate fellows received a certificate (members did not). See also "F.A.C.S. or diplomate in surgery?" *J. Med. Soc. N.J.* 47 (1950): 292–294.

118. E. C. Andrus to P. D. White, 22 October 1954, box 1, file 27, White Papers.

119. Frank J. Gouze, interview by W. Bruce Fye, 27 May 1993, Marshfield, Wis.

120. M. C. Becker, "Review of *Cardiac Catheterization in Congenital Heart Disease* by André Cournand," *J. Med. Soc. N.J.* 46 (1949): 410.

121. "Report [on] ACC October 5 and 6, 1951," Sprague Papers. The ACC presentations were published in *Trans. Am. Coll. Cardiol.* 1 (1951): 24–138.

122. Kisch, *Wanderungen und Wandlungen,* esp. p. 337.

123. M. Miller to J. W. Bodlander, 1 November 1951, chapter file, Reichert Papers, ACC Archives.

124. Minutes, ACC Business Meeting, 6 June 1952, ACC BOT Minutes, ACC Archives.

125. "Approved internships and residencies 1952," *JAMA* 150 (1952): 301–363.

126. J. W. Bodlander to P. Reichert, 27 December 1951, chapter file, Reichert Papers, ACC Archives. See also "Constitution and by-laws," *Trans. Am. Coll. Cardiol.* 1 (1951): 11–22.

127. B. Kisch, "A year of activity," *Am. Coll. Cardiol. Bull.* (December 1951): 1–2.

128. J. W. Bodlander to F. M. Groedel, 24 July 1951, California file, Reichert Papers, ACC Archives.

129. Membership Session, October 1951, with ACC BOT Minutes, 1949–1952, pp. 228–245, ACC Archives.

130. F. M. Groedel to W. B. Parsons, 19 September 1951, ACC Minutes, 1949–1952, p. 207, ACC Archives. In 1947 fewer than 1 percent of the 378 persons certified in cardiovascular disease were women. In 1948, 2 percent of the AHA Scientific Council members were women, but some were medical scientists rather than physicians. Similarly, very few women joined the ACC in the 1950s. In 1952, 4 of 739 members were women (0.5 percent). In 1957, 9 of 1,444 members were women (0.6 percent). It must be recalled that only 5 percent of American physicians were women at this time. Sources: "Fellows, associate fellows and members," *Trans. Am. Coll. Cardiol.* 2 (1952): 6–27; "ACC membership roster," *Trans. Am. Coll. Cardiol.* 7 (1957): 294–333; "Candidates Certified in Cardiovascular Disease to September 8, 1947," in AHA History 1940s file, AHA Archives; and "Members, Scientific Council of American Heart Association, Inc.," 31 July 1948, in AHA History file, AHA Archives. See also C. Lopate, *Women in Medicine* (Baltimore: Johns Hopkins Univ. Press, 1968), and Walsh, *Doctors Wanted, No Women Need Apply,* esp. pp. 236–267. Three women (possibly spouses rather than physicians) and an African-American man were among the seventy-one people photographed at the banquet held during the ACC's first meeting in October 1951. At the time, approximately 2 percent of New York City physicians were African-Americans. See photograph published in *Cardiology* 13 (December 1984): [1], and Reitzes, *Negroes and Medicine,* table III-3, p. 386.

131. T. R. Harrison, "Progress in the cardiovascular field during the last decade," *Year Book Med.* (1950): 471–477.

132. Moore, *Fighting for Life,* appendix V, p. 270.

CHAPTER 5   *Cardiology and the Federal Funding of Academic Medicine*

1. E. Ginzberg, "The impact of World War II on U.S. medicine," *Am. J. Med. Sci.* 304 (1992): 268–271. See also J. Bordley III and A. M. Harvey, *Two Centuries of American Medicine, 1776–1976* (Philadelphia: W. B. Saunders, 1976), esp. pp. 353–361, and N. Reingold, "Science and government in the United States since 1945," *Hist. Sci.* 32 (1994): 361–385.

2. "Treatment of cardiovascular syphilis," *Cornell Conferences on Therapy* (New York: Macmillan), 4 (1951): 86–103, and G. H. Stollerman, "The use of antibiotics for the prevention of rheumatic fever," *Am. J. Med.* 17 (1954): 757–767.

3. L. A. Scheele, "A new era in medical research and practice," *Am. J. Med.* 9 (1950): 1–2. See also H. M. Marks, "Cortisone, 1949: A year in the political life of a drug," *Bull. Hist. Med.* 66 (1992): 419–439.

4. A. E. Cohn and C. Lingg, *The Burden of Diseases in the United States* (New York: Oxford Univ. Press, 1950).

5. D. M. Fox, *Power and Illness: The Failure and Future of American Health Policy* (Berkeley: Univ. of California Press, 1993), quotes pp. 42, 43. See also S. P. Strickland, *Politics, Science, and Dread Disease: A Short History of United States Medical Research Policy* (Cambridge: Harvard Univ. Press, 1972).

6. W. W. Palmer, "Appendix 2. Report of the medical advisory committee," in V. Bush, *Science: The Endless Frontier* (Washington, D.C.: GPO, 1945), pp. 40–64, quote p. 43. See also J. A. Shannon, "Federal support of biomedical sciences: Development and academic impact," *J. Med. Educ.* 51 (suppl.) (July 1976); L. A. Scheele and W. W. Sebrell, "Medical research and medical education," *Science* 114 (1951): 517–521; and E. C. Andrus, D. W. Bronk, G. A. Carden Jr., et al., eds., *Advances in Military Medicine Made by American Investigators Working under the Sponsorship of the Committee on Medical Research* (Boston: Little, Brown, 1948); and H. M. Marks, "Ideas as Reforms: Therapeutic Experiments and Medical Practice, 1900–1980" (Ph.D. diss., Massachusetts Institute of Technology, 1987), esp. chapters 3 and 4.

7. S. P. Strickland, *The Story of the NIH Grants Program* (Lanham, Md.: Univ. Press of America, 1989), quote p. 24.

8. See F. W. Reynolds and D. E. Price, "Federal support of medical research through the Public Health Service," *Am. Sci.* 37 (1949): 578–586, and D. C. Swain, "The rise of a research empire: NIH, 1930 to 1950," *Science* 138 (1962): 1233–1237. "Extramural" grants were disbursed to nongovernmental institutions and to individuals not employed directly by the NIH, in contrast to "intramural" grants given to NIH scientists.

9. E. Ginzberg and A. B. Dutka, *The Financing of Biomedical Research* (Baltimore: Johns Hopkins Univ. Press, 1989). See also J. H. Comroe Jr. and R. D. Dripps, *The Top Ten Clinical Advances in Cardiovascular-Pulmonary Medicine and Surgery 1945–1975* (Washington, D.C.: GPO, 1978).

10. M. M. Wintrobe, *Hematology, the Blossoming of a Science* (Philadelphia: Lea & Febiger, 1985), quote p. 179. See also E. E. Lape, ed., *Medical Research: A Midcentury Survey* (Boston: Little, Brown, 1955); and R. H. Shryock, *American Medical Research: Past and Present* (New York: Commonwealth Fund, 1947).

11. J. B. Kirsner, *The Development of American Gastroenterology* (New York: Raven Press, 1990).

12. For the cancer lobby, see J. T. Patterson, *The Dread Disease: Cancer and Modern American Culture* (Cambridge: Harvard Univ. Press, 1987).

13. Yeager quoted in Strickland, *NIH Grants Program*, p. 37. See also E. T. Lanahan, *A Salute to the Past: A History of the National Heart, Lung, and Blood Institute Based on Personal Recollections* (Bethesda, Md.: NHLBI, 1987), esp. pp. 29–30. The original structure and philosophy of the NHI is detailed in "The National Heart Institute: Information for Administrative Use on the Organization, Operations, Services, and Related Activities of the Public Health Service Heart Program," [Bethesda, MD]: Federal Security Agency, Public Health Service, National Institutes of Health, 1950. Typescript, 39 + iv pp. AHA Archives.

14. A detailed listing of institutions and the amounts requested is in C. J. Van Slyke to M. Lasker, 17 July 1951, Wright Papers. For a detailed list of grants awarded

through 13 September 1949, see "FSA-652, Federal Security Agency, Public Health Service, National Heart Institute, 13 September 1949." Typescript, 32 pp. Rutstein Papers.

15. By June 1951 the NAHC had distributed $6 million for 26 construction projects in 17 states. Minutes, NAHC, 25–27 June 1951, NHLBI Archives.

16. Minutes, NAHC, 23–25 February 1956, NHLBI Archives.

17. Cassius Van Slyke chaired the NAHC between 1948 and 1952. He was succeeded by James Watt (1952 to 1965). During the early years of the NHI, AHA leaders played a major role in the NAHC. See Lanahan, *Salute to the Past.* In 1949 Jack Marvin, Tinsley Harrison, Duckett Jones, and Paul White were on the council.

18. M. Lasker to I. S. Wright, 24 August 1954, Wright Papers. See also L. A. Scheele to I. S. Wright, 4 August 1954; I. S. Wright to L. Sheely [*sic*], 31 August 1954; and P. D. White to I. S. Wright, 6 September 1954. All in Wright Papers.

19. Minutes, NAHC, 10–11 December 1948, NHLBI Archives. See also Shannon, "Federal support of biomedical sciences," esp. p. 14. For the role of philanthropy in the emergence of a research tradition at Western Reserve, see D. H. Stapleton, "Abraham Flexner, Rockefeller philanthropy, and the Western Reserve School of Medicine," *Ohio Hist.* 101 (1992): 100–113.

20. C. J. Wiggers, *Reminiscences and Adventures in Circulation Research* (New York: Grune & Stratton, 1958), pp. 171, 384–387.

21. "Proposed Establishment of a Cardio-Vascular Institute or Division at Cornell University Medical College and New York Hospital," cJune 1948, box 2, misc. corres., 1950, Wright Papers.

22. J. F. Yeager to G. E. Burch, 3 September 1953, Burch Papers. Yeager had received 58 replies from a total of 86 program directors invited to participate. See J. F. Yeager to G. E. Burch, 14 August 1953, and "Names and addresses of program directors of undergraduate cardiovascular training grants," [1954], Burch Papers. An example of a cardiology curriculum developed for this program is A. A. Luisada, "Teaching cardiology to undergraduate students," *Dis. Chest* 25 (1954): 103–105.

23. Minutes, NAHC, 15–17 October 1951, NHLBI Archives.

24. R. H. Williams, "Departments of medicine in 1970," *Ann. Intern. Med.* 50 (1959): 1252–1276.

25. P. B. Beeson, "The changing role model, and the shift in power," *Daedalus* (Spring 1986): 83–97, quote p. 91.

26. See R. C. Maulitz and P. B. Beeson, "The inner history of internal medicine," in *Grand Rounds: One Hundred Years of Internal Medicine,* ed. R. C. Maulitz and D. E. Long (Philadelphia: Univ. of Pennsylvania Press, 1988), pp. 15–54, esp. p. 44.

27. Shannon, "Federal support of biomedical sciences," p. 7. Shannon's estimate includes government grants from all sources, not just the NIH. See also W. G. Rothstein, *American Medical Schools and the Practice of Medicine: A History* (New York: Oxford Univ. Press, 1987), table 12.1, p. 238.

28. H. M. Marvin, "Foreword," *Circulation* 1 (1950): 1.

29. "Foreword," *Circ. Res.* 1 (1953): 1–2.

30. See, for example, A. M. Harvey, V. A. McKusick, and J. D. Stobo, *Osler's Legacy: The Department of Medicine at Johns Hopkins, 1889–1989* (Baltimore: Johns Hopkins Univ. Press, 1990), p. 75.

31. *Public Law 655. 80th Cong. 2d sess. 1948. S. 2215. An Act to Amend the Public Health Service Act to Support Research and Training in Diseases of the Heart and Circulation* (Washington, D.C.: GPO, 1948), quote p. 2.

32. Minutes, NAHC, 10–11 December 1948, NHLBI Archives. See also "The National Heart Institute," 1950.

33. H. H. Hecht, "Training in cardiology," *Dis. Chest* 26 (1954): 239–241. See also W. B. Bean, "A department of internal medicine," *J. Med. Educ.* 29 (1954): 11–29.

34. Hecht, "Training in cardiology," p. 240. Tensions between academicians and practitioners increased in many institutions as the government endowed the full-time system and made research the centerpiece of the academic agenda. The issues are summarized in M. J. Lepore, *Death of the Clinician: Requiem or Reveille?* (Springfield, Ill.: Charles C. Thomas, 1982). See also J. Duffy, *The Tulane University Medical Center: One Hundred Fifty Years of Medical Education* (Baton Rouge: Louisiana State Univ. Press, 1984), pp. 175–177.

35. For a discussion of these and related themes, see H. H. Fudenberg and V. L. Melnick, eds., *Biomedical Scientists and Public Policy* (New York: Plenum Press, 1978); R. L. Geiger, *Research and Relevant Knowledge: American Research Universities since World War II* (New York: Oxford Univ. Press, 1993), esp. pp. 3–91; B. L. R. Smith, *American Science Policy since World War II* (Washington, D.C.: Brookings Institution, 1990); Strickland, *Politics, Science, and Dread Disease;* and Shannon, "Federal support of biomedical sciences."

36. C. A. Mills, "Distribution of American research funds," *Science* 107 (1948): 127–130. For conflicts over the ideology of science in America, see A. H. Dupree, *Science in the Federal Government: A History of Policies and Activities to 1940* (Cambridge: Harvard Univ. Press, 1957), and R. C. Tobey, *The American Ideology of National Science, 1919–1930* (Pittsburgh: Univ. of Pittsburgh Press, 1971).

37. S. L. Deignan and E. Miller, "The support of research in medical and allied fields for the period 1946 through 1951," *Science* 115 (1952): 321–343.

38. Shannon, "Federal support of biomedical sciences," quote p. 10.

39. See, for example, L. T. Coggeshall, "The influence of federal funds on medical education and research," *Am. J. Trop. Med.* 30 (1950): 351–356. See also J. D. Howell, "Lowell T. Coggeshall and American medical education: 1901–1987," *Acad. Med.* 67 (1992): 711–718.

40. Scheele and Sebrell, "Medical research and medical education," quotes pp. 517, 520. A decade later, University of Chicago anatomist Stanley Bennett, citing the "research revolution," claimed that "the primary responsibility of medical schools relates to knowledge rather than to students." H. S. Bennett, "Research and research training in medical schools in the United States," *J. Med. Educ.* 37 (1962): 581–587.

41. I examine this connection in W. B. Fye, "The origin of the full-time faculty system: Implications for clinical research," *JAMA* 265 (1991): 1555–1562. The architects of the clinical full-time system included medical scientists Lewellys Barker, Franklin Mall, and William Welch, and educational reformer Abraham

Flexner. For the intellectual origins of the full-time faculty system and the research ethic, see W. B. Fye, *The Development of American Physiology: Scientific Medicine in the Nineteenth Century* (Baltimore: Johns Hopkins Univ. Press, 1987). Many forces transformed American medical education during the early twentieth century. See K. M. Ludmerer, *Learning to Heal: The Development of American Medical Education* (New York: Basic Books, 1985); Rothstein, *American Medical Schools;* and S. C. Wheatley, *The Politics of Philanthropy: Abraham Flexner and Medical Education* (Madison: Univ. of Wisconsin Press, 1988).

42. Shannon, "Federal support of biomedical sciences," quote p. 18.

43. V. Johnson, "Implications of current trends toward specialization," in *Trends in Medical Education,* ed. M. Ashford (New York: Commonwealth Fund, 1949), pp. 173–178. For current statistics, see "Education update: 1995," *J. Am. Coll. Cardiol.* 26 (1995): 1092–1112.

44. "Approved internships and residencies 1952," *JAMA* 150 (1952): 301–363.

45. *Senate Committee on Appropriations. Labor-Federal Security Appropriations for 1951: Hearings Before the Subcommittee. 81st Cong., 2d sess.* (Washington, D.C.: GPO, 1950). Van Slyke's testimony is on pp. 492–500.

46. *House Committee on Appropriations. Hearings on the Department of Labor–Federal Security Agency Appropriations for 1953, 82nd Cong., 2d sess.* (Washington, D.C.: GPO, 1952), quote p. 748.

47. *House Committee on Appropriations. Hearings on Department of Labor–Federal Security Agency Appropriations for 1954, 83rd Cong., 1st sess.* (Washington, D.C.: GPO, 1953), quotes pp. 1048, 1051.

48. Ibid.

49. Minutes, NAHC, 14–16 February 1952, NHLBI Archives.

50. U.S. Dept. HEW, Public Health Service, *Design and Construction of General Hospitals* (New York: F. W. Dodge Corporation, 1953), pp. 1–3. See also D. M. Fox, *Health Policies, Health Politics: The British and American Experience, 1911–1965* (Princeton: Princeton Univ. Press, 1986), esp. pp. 115–131, 149–168. Another contemporary example of the principle is S. Proger, "Three eras in the developing relationship of medical education and care," in *Hospital Trends and Developments, 1940–1946,* ed. A. C. Bachmeyer and G. Hartman, (New York: Commonwealth Fund, 1948), pp. 223–232.

51. Fox points out in his discussion of regional hierarchies: "Medical knowledge apparently flowed down hierarchies serving particular geographic regions; patients should, in theory, be referred up the same hierarchies." Fox, *Health Policies,* p. 208.

52. T. R. Harrison to C. Connor, 14 February 1949, in AHA History 1940s, file 3, AHA Archives.

53. In fiscal year 1957 the NHI budget included $15 million for research grants, $5 million for intramural programs, $4.1 million for training grants, $2.25 million for grants to states, $1.7 million for research fellowships, and $0.5 million for technical assistance. Minutes, NAHC, 3–5 November 1955, NHLBI Archives. See also *National Heart, Lung, and Blood Institute Fact Book. Fiscal Year 1993* (Bethesda, Md.: NHLBI, 1994), esp. p. 63.

54. W. M. Moore, *Fighting for Life: The Story of the American Heart Association 1911–1975* (Dallas: AHA, 1983), esp. "Income history of the AHA," p. 270.

55. This pattern was well established by 1950, when academic internist Henry Christian complained, "The young man, keenly alert as to how to get along [in academic medicine] . . . seeks chiefly to investigate and publish, possibly even stressing the latter, since he thinks a bibliography of numerous titles will have much weight in the consideration of his promotional advancement." H. A. Christian, "Present day undesirable trends in the training of physicians and of teachers of internal medicine," *Ann. Intern. Med.* 33 (1950): 533–543, quote p. 535. See also W. B. Fye, "Medical authorship: Traditions, trends, and tribulations," *Ann. Intern. Med.* 113 (1990): 317–325. For an earlier discussion of the problems associated with linking academic advancement and publications, see H. Zinsser, "The next twenty years," *Science* 74 (1931): 397–404.

56. The status and prospects of American medicine at mid-century were considered by several authors in *Medicine Today* (New York: Columbia Univ. Press, 1947).

57. The list included morphine, digitalis, mecholyl (for paroxysmal atrial tachycardia), atropine, quinidine sulfate, mercurial diuretics, theophylline (for asthma and acute pulmonary edema), epinephrine (for shock), nitroglycerin, injectable penicillin, and an oral sulfonamide. W. H. Gordon, "The doctor's bag: What should be in it," *GP* 1 (1950): 51–54. Another doctor found that many physicians did not carry medicines to treat acute heart problems, however. See "The doctor's bag," in *Cornell Conferences on Therapy,* ed. H. Gold (New York: Macmillan, 1946) 1: 1–17. Compare these with a 1936 list of medications for the black bag published in W. M. Johnson, *The True Physician: The Modern "Doctor of the Old School"* (New York: Macmillan, 1936).

58. See J. P. Swann, *Academic Scientists and the Pharmaceutical Industry* (Baltimore: Johns Hopkins Univ. Press, 1988); M. Silverman and P. R. Lee, *Pills, Profits, and Politics* (Berkeley: Univ. of California Press, 1974); and J. S. Olson, ed., *The History of Cancer: An Annotated Bibliography* (New York: Greenwood Press, 1989), esp. pp. 327–342.

59. R. W. Gifford Jr., "Three decades of antihypertensive therapy," *Clin. Pharmacol. Ther.* 28 (1980): 1–5, quote p. 1.

60. For example, the vasodilator hydralazine (1951); the rauwolfia alkaloid reserpine (1952); the thiazide diuretics chlorothiazide and hydrochlorothiazide (1957); the postganglionic blocker guanethidine (1959); the potassium-sparing diuretics spironolactone and triamterine (1958–1964); and the central alpha$_2$-receptor agonist methyldopa (1964). See G. L. Bakris and E. D. Frohlich, "The evolution of antihypertensive therapy: An overview of four decades of experience," *J. Am. Coll. Cardiol.* 14 (1989): 1595–1608; and F. O. Simpson and J. V. Hodge, "The evolution of antihypertensive therapy," *N.Z. Med. J.* 67 (1968): 270–275.

61. J. Nolan, "A historical review of heart failure," *Scott. Med. J.* 38 (1993): 53–57.

62. Although effective, these and other cardiac drugs had definite side effects, and some of them could cause death.

63. An overview of the many diagnostic techniques in cardiology in this era is T. E. Lowe, H. B. Kay, and H. A. Luke, *The Practical Significance of Modern Cardiological Investigations* (Melbourne: Melbourne Univ. Press, 1951). Hospital privileges are

discussed in T. R. Ponton and M. T. MacEachern, *The Medical Staff in the Hospital,* 2d ed. (Chicago: Physicians' Record Company, 1953).

64. A. Blalock and T. R. Harrison, "The surgical treatment of certain types of heart disease," *J. Tenn. Med. Assoc.* 30 (1937): 292–297.

65. W. H. Witt, discussing ibid.

66. The years cited refer to the first published report of a successful case. See S. L. Johnson, *The History of Cardiac Surgery* (Baltimore: Johns Hopkins Univ. Press, 1970), and H. B. Shumacker Jr., *The Evolution of Cardiac Surgery* (Bloomington: Indiana Univ. Press, 1992).

67. In 1955 physiological cardiologist Herrman Blumgart cautioned that the value of operations for angina pectoris (including omentopexy, aortic-coronary sinus anastomosis, coronary sinus ligation, and myocardial implantation of internal mammary arteries) was unproven. H. L. Blumgart and M. H. Paul, "Surgical relief of myocardial ischemia," *Am. J. Med.* 18 (1955): 1–2.

68. The definitive study of the origins of physiological surgery in the United States is P. C. English, *Shock, Physiological Surgery, and George Washington Crile: Medical Innovation in the Progressive Era* (Westport, Conn.: Greenwood Press, 1980). It focuses on George Crile of Western Reserve University and (later) the Cleveland Clinic. Alexis Carrel was another pioneering physiological surgeon especially interested in the cardiovascular system. See W. S. Edwards and P. D. Edwards, *Alexis Carrel, Visionary Surgeon* (Springfield, Ill.: Charles C. Thomas, 1974). Physiological surgeons were performing human experiments when they first attempted new operations in people. For the early history of human experimentation, see S. E. Lederer, *Subjected to Science: Human Experimentation in America before the Second World War* (Baltimore: Johns Hopkins Univ. Press, 1995).

69. L. R. Dragstedt and J. S. Clarke, "The contributions of physiology to surgery, 1905–1955," in *Fifty Years of Surgical Progress, 1905–1955,* ed. L. Davis (Chicago: Franklin H. Martin Memorial Foundation, 1955), pp. 51–58, quote p. 52.

70. For example, Blalock's interest in research was stimulated by physiological cardiologist Tinsley Harrison, his roommate at Johns Hopkins and colleague on the Vanderbilt faculty. See W. P. Longmire Jr., *Alfred Blalock: His Life and Times* ([Los Angeles]: William P. Longmire Jr., 1991), esp. p. 31; V. T. Thomas, *Pioneering Research in Surgical Shock and Cardiovascular Surgery: Vivien Thomas and His Work with Alfred Blalock* (Philadelphia: Univ. of Pennsylvania Press, 1985), esp. pp. 30–33; and M. M. Ravitch, "Alfred Blalock, 1899–1964," in *The Papers of Alfred Blalock,* ed. M. M. Ravitch (Baltimore: Johns Hopkins Univ. Press, 1966), pp. xiii-lvii.

71. O. H. Wangensteen and S. D. Wangensteen, *The Rise of Surgery from Empiric Craft to Scientific Discipline* (Minneapolis: Univ. of Minnesota Press, 1978), quote p. 561.

72. See J. W. Kirklin, "Open-heart surgery at the Mayo Clinic: The 25th anniversary," *Mayo Clin. Proc.* 55 (1980): 339–341; and H. B. Burchell, "A cardiologist's view of modern cardiovascular surgery," *Dis. Chest* 55 (1969): 323–328.

73. A. Blalock to H. B. Taussig, 8 April 1946, Blalock Papers. An important source for the diffusion of medical knowledge to the public is J. C. Burnham, *How Superstition Won and Science Lost: Popularizing Science and Health in the United States* (New Brunswick, N.J.: Rutgers Univ. Press, 1987).

74. See H. B. Taussig to A. Blalock, 15 April [1946], and A. Blalock to H. B. Taussig, 16 April 1946, Blalock Papers. Taussig first approached Robert Gross with her concept of creating a shunt to treat patients with tetralogy of Fallot, but he was "not in the least interested in the idea." H. B. Taussig, *History of the Blalock-Taussig Operation and Some of the Long Term Results on Patients with a Tetralogy of Fallot* (Cooperstown, N.Y.: Mary Imogene Bassett Hospital, 1970), pp. 13–38, quote p. 17.

75. F. J. Lewis and M. Taufic, "Closure of atrial septal defects with the aid of hypothermia; experimental accomplishments and report of one successful case," *Surgery* 33 (1953): 52–59. An atrial septal defect is a birth defect in which an abnormal opening between the right atrium and left atrium can lead to heart failure. See also L. G. Wilson, *Medical Revolution in Minnesota: A History of the University of Minnesota Medical School* (St. Paul: Midewiwin Press, 1989), esp. pp. 481–528.

76. H. E. Warden, M. Cohen, R. C. Read, and C. W. Lillehei, "Controlled cross circulation for open intracardiac surgery. Physiologic studies and results of creation and closure of ventricular septal defects," *J. Thorac. Surg.* 28 (1954): 331–343, quote p. 331. Open-heart surgery refers to operations performed under direct vision using the heart-lung machine. Closed-heart surgery refers to operations (such as closed mitral commissurotomy) performed on the beating, blood-filled heart.

77. W. J. Rashkind, "Contributions of physiologic research to clinical cardiology," *Med. Clin. North Am.* (1954): 1565–1573, quote p. 1567. Americans heading efforts to develop heart-lung machines included John Gibbon Jr., Clarence Dennis, Charles Bailey, Forest Dodrill, Willem Kolff (originally from Holland), Richard Varco, and Richard DeWall, among others. See Shumacker, *Evolution of Cardiac Surgery,* pp. 242–279. P. M. Galletti and G. A. Brecher, *Heart-Lung Bypass* (New York: Grune & Stratton, 1962) is a valuable source for the early history and technology of heart-lung machines. See also P. M. Galletti, "Cardiopulmonary bypass: A historical survey," *Artif. Organs* 17 (1993): 675–686, and W. B. Fye, "H. Newell Martin and the isolated heart preparation: The link between the frog and open-heart surgery," *Circulation* 73 (1986): 857–864.

78. Warden et al., "Controlled cross circulation for open intracardiac surgery."

79. Kirklin, "Open-heart surgery at the Mayo Clinic."

80. D. E. Harken, "The surgical treatment of mitral insufficiency," in *Henry Ford Hospital International Symposium on Cardiovascular Surgery*, ed. C. R. Lam (Philadelphia: W.B. Saunders, 1955), pp. 212–269.

81. A. D. Crecca, J. J. McGuire, and N. A. Antonius, "Cardiovascular surgery at St. Michael's Hospital," *J. Med. Soc. N.J.* 50 (1953): 62–67.

82. C. P. Bailey, *Surgery of the Heart* (Philadelphia: Lea & Febiger, 1955), quote p. 483.

83. E. S. Hurwitt, "The organization of a cardiovascular surgical program: Preliminary observations on the surgical treatment of patients with mitral stenosis," *N.Y. State J. Med.* 53 (1953): 1209–1214, quote p. 1214.

84. J. L. Harrison, J. C. Davila, B. D. Iaia, and R. P. Glover, "An analysis of deaths following cardiac surgery," *J. Thorac. Cardiovasc. Surg.* 39 (1960): 91–108.

85. R. P. Glover, T. J. E. O'Neill, and O. H. Janton, "An analysis of fifty patients treated by mitral commissurotomy five or more years ago," *J. Thorac. Surg.* 30 (1955): 436–451.

86. F. C. Wood, "The Progress of Cardiac Surgery," [1953], Wood Papers. Emphasis in original.

87. Two textbooks illustrate how the scope of thoracic surgery expanded over a generation to include the heart. Compare H. Lilienthal, *Thoracic Surgery* (Philadelphia: W.B. Saunders, 1926) with G. E. Lindskog and A. A. Liebow, *Thoracic Surgery and Related Pathology* (New York: Appleton-Century-Crofts, 1953). See also R. H. Meade, *A History of Thoracic Surgery* (Springfield, Ill.: Charles C. Thomas, 1961). Regarding the training of thoracic surgeons just before the advent of heart surgery, see C. Eggers, "Special training for thoracic surgery," *J. Thorac. Surg.* 5, no. 6 (1936): 567–574. This shift is also described in D. C. McGoon, "Half a century of journal publication," *J. Thorac. Cardiovasc. Surg. Index to Vols. 1–84 (1931–1982)* (1983): v-xiv.

88. C. W. Lillehei, discussing J. W. Kirklin, F. H. Ellis, D. C. McGoon, J. W. DuShane, and H. J. C. Swan, "Surgical treatment for the tetralogy of Fallot by open intracardiac repair," *J. Thorac. Surg.* 37 (1959): 22–51.

89. The participants included Charles Bailey, Claude Beck, Wilfred Bigelow, Richard Bing, Russell Brock, Denton Cooley, Clarence Crafoord, Michael DeBakey, John Gibbon Jr., Dwight Harken, Charles Hufnagel, John Kirklin, Walton Lillihei, Andrew Morrow, William Mustard, Willis Potts, and Helen Taussig, among others. See Lam, *Cardiovascular Surgery,* v-xii.

90. R. Brock, "Foreword," in Lam, *Cardiovascular Surgery,* xv-xxiii, quotes pp. xvi, xxi.

91. Quoted in J. P. Swazey and R. C. Fox, "The clinical moratorium: A case study of mitral valve surgery," in *Experimentation with Human Subjects,* ed. P. A. Freund (New York: George Brazillier, 1970), pp. 315–357, quote p. 357.

92. Lillehei discussing Kirklin et al., "Surgical treatment for the tetralogy of Fallot."

93. P. D. White, *Personal Observations on the Evolution of Cardiovascular Surgery* (Leiden: Leiden Univ., 1957), quote p. 12.

94. Bailey, *Surgery of the Heart,* quotes p. 675.

95. B. Pearse, "Spare parts for defective hearts," *Saturday Evening Post* (30 August 1958): 18–19, 45–47. Hufnagel performed the first successful implantation of a prosthetic heart valve in 1952. See C. A. Hufnagel, "Surgical treatment of aortic insufficiency," in Lam, *Cardiovascular Surgery,* pp. 321–340, and C. A. Hufnagel, "Basic concepts in the development of cardiovascular prostheses," *Am. J. Surg.* 137 (1979): 285–300.

96. Catheterization provided "hemodynamic" information by measuring intracardiac pressures and flows through a tube inserted into the heart. Until 1950 the technique was limited to the right side of the heart; a catheter was advanced from a peripheral vein to the right atrium, right ventricle, and pulmonary artery. Angiocardiography (performed by injecting a radiopaque substance or "contrast agent" into the heart or aorta) made it possible to visualize the heart's cavities, identify leaking valves and intracardiac shunts, and characterize abnormalities of the aorta. See T. Doby, *Development of Angiography and Cardiovascular Catheterization* (Littleton, Mass.: Publishing Sciences Group, 1976); A. Cournand, "Cardiac catheterization: Development of the technique, its contributions to experimental medicine, and its initial applications in man," *Acta Med. Scand.* suppl. 579 (1975): 3–32. For contemporary assessments of these two procedures, see J. F. Goodwin, "The practical value of

cardiac catheterization," *Practitioner* 169 (1952): 40–48, and C. T. Dotter and I. Steinberg, "Clinical angiocardiography: A critical analysis of the indications and findings," *Ann. Intern. Med.* 30 (1949): 1104–1125.

97. Ibid., p. 1105.

98. In 1955 Charles Bailey concluded that combined right and left heart catheterization was "quite safe" and "should be employed more often." Bailey discussing D. L. Fisher, "The use of pressure recording obtained at transthoracic left heart catheterization in the diagnosis of valvular heart disease," *J. Thorac. Surg.* 30 (1955): 379–396, quote p. 395.

99. See, for example, R. B. Dickerson, "Performance of angiocardiography and cardiac catheterization as a combined procedure," *Am. Heart J.* 47 (1954): 252–269.

100. H. A. Zimmerman, R. W. Scott, and N. O. Becker, "Catheterization of the left side of the heart in man," *Circulation* 1 (1950): 357–359. See also A. A. Luisada and C. K. Liu, *Cardiac Pressure and Pulses: A Manual of Right and Left Heart Catheterization* (New York: Grune & Stratton, 1956).

101. Rashkind, "Contributions of physiologic research to clinical cardiology," quote p. 1573. An academic internist agreed: "Today's physician combines the clinician and the laboratory man." D. W. Atchley, "The changing physician," *Atlantic Monthly* 198 (1956): 29–31.

102. D. M. Green, A. D. Johnson, W. C. Bridges, J. H. Lehmann, J. Michel, F. Gray, et al., "Use of cardiac catheterization in medical practice," *Northwest Med.* 49 (1950): 27–29. Angiocardiography was thought to be very safe. Two pioneers of the field experienced no fatalities in an eleven-year experience with more than one thousand patients. See Dotter and Steinberg, "Clinical angiocardiography."

103. A. Cournand, R. J. Bing, L. Dexter, C. Dotter, L. N. Katz, J. V. Warren, et al., "Report of committee on cardiac catheterization and angiocardiography of the American Heart Association," *Circulation* 7 (1953): 769–773, quote p. 773. Academic and practitioner cardiologists who performed catheterization came to be called "invasive" cardiologists, reflecting the fact that their catheters entered the patient's arteries and veins.

104. K. L. White and M. A. Ibrahim, "The distribution of cardiovascular disease in the community," *Ann. Intern. Med.* 58 (1963): 627–636.

105. Statistics from: Rothstein, *American Medical Schools*, table 11.2, p. 225; "Directory of approved internships," *JAMA* 174 (1960): 637–662; "Directory of approved residencies. Thoracic surgery," *JAMA* 174 (1960): 803–806; "Directory of approved residencies. Cardiovascular disease," *JAMA* 174 (1960): 682–683; "Selected list of research training programs sponsored by the National Heart Institute," *Circulation* 21, part 2 (March 1960): 1–15; H. R. Kimball [President, ABIM] to W. B. Fye, 26 October 1993, which includes a list of "Diplomates certified by the American Board of Internal Medicine broken down by year." For personal health care expenditures (hospital care, professional services, drugs and medical sundries, and nursing home care) see *Source Book of Health Insurance Data, 1993* (Washington, D.C.: Health Insurance Association of America, 1994), table 4.4, p. 82. For health insurance statistics, see R. Stevens, *In Sickness and in Wealth: American Hospitals in the Twentieth Century* (New York: Basic Books, 1989), table 10.1, p. 259. For the diffusion of medical technology (including intensive care units, renal dialysis, and open-heart

surgery), see L. B. Russell, *Technology in Hospitals: Medical Advances and Their Diffusion* (Washington, D.C.: Brookings Institution, 1979).

106. A. F. Crocetti, "Cardiac diagnostic and surgical facilities in the United States," *Public Health Rep.* 80 (1965): 1035–1053.

107. W. B. Fye, "Coronary arteriography: It took a long time," *Circulation* 70 (1984): 781–787.

108. Selective coronary angiography is a technique in which a contrast agent [dye] is injected directly into a coronary artery through a catheter deliberately placed in the vessel. Sones was trained in internal medicine, pediatrics, and cardiac catheterization at the Henry Ford Hospital in Detroit. The Cleveland Clinic hired him in 1950 to establish a cardiac catheterization laboratory. See W. L. Proudfit, "F. Mason Sones, Jr., M.D. (1918–1985): The man and his work," *Cleve. Clin. Q.* 53 (1986): 121–124; and W. C. Sheldon, "F. Mason Sones, Jr.—Stormy petrel of cardiology," *Clin. Cardiol.* 17 (1994): 405–407.

109. *Program. Eighth Annual Convention. The American College of Cardiology. May 25–29, 1959* (New York: ACC, 1959). See also H. A. Baltaxe, K. Amplatz, and D. C. Levin, *Coronary Angiography* (Springfield, Ill.: Charles C. Thomas, 1975). Sones also presented a paper on the technique at the annual scientific sessions of the AHA later that year.

110. C. T. Dotter and L. H. Frische, "An approach to coronary arteriography," in *Angiography,* ed. H. L. Abrams (Boston: Little, Brown, 1961), 1: 259–273.

111. F. M. Sones Jr. and E. K. Shirey, "Cine coronary arteriography," *Mod. Concepts Cardiovasc. Dis.* 31 (1962): 735–738.

112. R. S. Kurtzman, "Coronary arteriography," *Med. Clin. North Am.* 46 (1962): 1583–1598, quote p. 1585. See also D. Littmann, "Coronary arteriography," *Am. J. Cardiol.* 9 (1962): 410–418; and H. J. Ricketts and H. L. Abrams, "Percutaneous selective coronary cine arteriography," *JAMA* 181 (1962): 620–624.

113. Russell, *Technology in Hospitals,* esp. pp. 41–70. Compare C. Butler and A. Erdman, *Hospital Planning* (New York: F.W. Dodge Corporation, 1946), which does not mention recovery rooms, with *Design and Construction of General Hospitals* (1953), which does.

114. N. A. Wilhelm, "Custom-built cardiovascular unit for research and treatment," *Hospitals* 27 (1953): 61–63. Eventually, Harken's cardiological colleague Samuel Levine began admitting nonsurgical heart patients to it. According to Harken, "Sam Levine always credited himself with having established the first CCU." Dwight E. Harken, interview by W. Bruce Fye, 14 April 1992, Dallas.

115. W. T. Mosenthal and D. D. Boyd, "Special unit saves lives, nurses and money," *Modern Hosp.* 89 (1957): 83–86.

116. P. F. Salisbury, "An *Intensive* treatment center meets special needs," *Hosp. Progress* 40 (1959): 92–94. See also A. R. Hunter, "Intensive care as a specialty," *Lancet* 1 (1967): 1151–1153. Experiences with respiratory care units during the early 1950s demonstrated the value of grouping nonsurgical patients who required specialized technologies and care. See J. Cule, "An historical view of intensive care," *Intensive Therapy and Clinical Monitoring* 10 (1989): 288–293, and R. R. Cadmus, "Intensive care reaches silver anniversary," *Hospitals* 54 (1980): 98–102.

117. W. B. Fye, "Ventricular fibrillation and defibrillation: Historical perspectives," *Circulation* 71 (1985): 858–865; and D. C. Schechter, *Exploring the Origins of*

Electrical Cardiac Stimulation: Selected Works of David Charles Schechter, M.D., F.A.C.S., on the History of Electrotherapy (Minneapolis: Medtronic, 1983).

118. C. S. Beck, "Reminiscences of cardiac resuscitation," *Rev. Surg.* 27 (1970): 77–86. For contemporary drug treatment of cardiac arrest, see A. M. Master, M. Moser, and H. L. Jaffe, *Cardiac Emergencies and Heart Failure: Prevention and Treatment* (Philadelphia: Lea & Febiger, 1952), esp. pp. 119–121.

119. H. D. Levine, *Cardiac Emergencies and Related Disorders* (New York: Landsberger Medical Books, 1960), quote p. 337. See also H. E. Stephenson Jr., *Cardiac Arrest and Resuscitation* (St. Louis: C. V. Mosby, 1958).

120. See C. S. Beck, E. C. Weckesser, and F. M. Barry, "Fatal heart attack and successful defibrillation: New concepts in coronary artery disease," *JAMA* 161 (1955): 434–436, and L. B. Reagan, K. R. Young, and J. W. Nicholson, "Ventricular defibrillation in a patient with probable acute coronary occlusion," *Surgery* 39 (1956): 482–486.

121. P. M. Zoll, A. J. Linenthal, W. Gibson, M. H. Paul, and L. R. Norman, "Termination of ventricular fibrillation in man by externally applied electric countershock," *N. Engl. J. Med.* 254 (1956): 727–732. See also W. B. Kouwenhoven, "The development of the defibrillator," *Ann. Intern. Med.* 71 (1969): 449–458.

122. P. M. Zoll, A. J. Linenthal, L. R. Norman, M. H. Paul, and W. Gibson, "External electric stimulation of the heart in cardiac arrest," *Arch. Intern. Med.* 96 (1955): 639–653.

123. Levine, *Cardiac Emergencies*, quote pp. 348–349.

124. W. B. Kouwenhoven, J. R. Jude, and G. G. Knickerbocker, "Closed-chest cardiac massage," *JAMA* 173 (1960): 94–97. See also Kouwenhoven, Jude, and Knickerbocker, "Heart activation in cardiac arrest," *Mod. Concepts Cardiovasc. Dis.* 30 (1961): 639–643, and Kouwenhoven and O. R. Langworthy, "Cardiopulmonary resuscitation: An account of forty-five years," *Johns Hopkins Med. J.* 132 (1973): 186–193. A detailed and well-illustrated description of the method is Jude and J. O. Elam, *Fundamentals of Cardiopulmonary Resuscitation* (Philadelphia: F.A. Davis, 1965). Alfred Blalock had been a longtime supporter of Kouwenhoven's resuscitation research. See A. P. Blalock to C. P. Crane, 20 February 1951, Blalock Papers.

125. "Ghastly ritual" is from Levine, *Cardiac Emergencies*, quote p. 348.

126. A. S. Hyman, "Resuscitation of the stopped heart by intercardial therapy. II. Experimental use of an artificial pacemaker," *Arch. Intern. Med.* 50 (1932): 283–305. See also Schechter, *Exploring the Origins of Electrical Cardiac Stimulation*, pp. 105–107.

127. P. M. Zoll, "Resuscitation of the heart in ventricular standstill by external electric stimulation," *N. Engl. J. Med.* 247 (1952): 768–771.

128. By the mid-1960s several effective intravenous antiarrhythmic drugs were available. See A. J. Moss and R. D. Patton, *Antiarrhythmic Agents* (Springfield, Ill.: Charles C. Thomas, 1973).

129. See D. G. Julian, "The history of coronary care units," *Br. Heart J.* 57 (1987): 497–502; and H. W. Day, "History of coronary care units," *Am. J. Cardiol.* 30 (1972): 405–407. Julian and Day were unaware of each other's work. D. G. Julian to W. B. Fye, 22 March 1994.

130. Another incentive for centralizing vulnerable patients was that the original defibrillators were large, and critical time was lost moving the machine to a patient who had suffered a cardiac arrest in a standard hospital room.

131. D. G. Julian, "Treatment of cardiac arrest in acute myocardial ischaemia and infarction," *Lancet* 2 (1961): 840–844.

132. H. W. Day, "A cardiac resuscitation program," *Journal-Lancet* 82 (1962): 153–156.

133. H. W. Day, "Preliminary studies of an acute coronary care area," *Journal-Lancet* 83 (1963): 53–55.

134. H. A. Day to C. S. Beck, 12 September 1969, in Beck, "Reminiscences of cardiac resuscitation," p. 86.

135. Thomas Killip, interview by W. Bruce Fye, 13 November 1994, Dallas. See also K. W. G. Brown, R. L. MacMillan, N. Forbath, F. Mel'Grano, and J. W. Scott, "Coronary unit: An intensive-care centre for acute myocardial infarction," *Lancet* 2 (1963): 349–352; L. E. Meltzer, "The concept and system for intensive coronary care," *Acad. Med. N.J. Bull.* 10 (1964): 304–311; and B. Lown, A. M. Fakhro, W. B. Hood, and G. W. Thorn, "The coronary care unit," *JAMA* 199 (1967): 188–198, which includes a detailed description of the coronary care unit at Boston's Peter Bent Brigham Hospital.

CHAPTER 6   *Continuing Medical Education: A Link between Academics and Practitioners*

1. W. C. Rappleye, ed., *Graduate Medical Education: Report of the Commission on Graduate Medical Education* (Chicago: Univ. of Chicago Press, 1940), quote p. 167.

2. O. W. Holmes, "Dedicatory address at the opening of the new building and hall of the Boston Medical Library Association," *Boston Med. Surg. J.* 99 (1878): 743–758, quote p. 748.

3. W. Osler, "The importance of post-graduate study," *Lancet* 2 (1900): 73–75, quote p. 73.

4. W. M. Johnson, *The True Physician: The Modern "Doctor of the Old School"* (New York: Macmillan, 1936), quotes pp. 59, 61.

5. See Rappleye, *Graduate Medical Education*, esp. pp. 167–223. An important summary (with a historical section) is R. K. Richards, *Continuing Medical Education: Perspectives, Problems, Prognosis* (New Haven: Yale Univ. Press, 1978). See also G. R. Shepherd, "History of continuation medical education in the United States since 1930," *J. Med. Educ.* 35 (1960): 740–758.

6. Rappleye, *Graduate Medical Education*, quote pp. 169–170.

7. D. D. Vollan, *Postgraduate Medical Education in the United States* (Chicago: AMA, 1955).

8. Ibid., quote p. [9].

9. R. C. Buerki, "Discussion of foregoing papers," in *Trends in Medical Education*, ed. M. Ashford (New York: Commonwealth Fund, 1949), pp. 239–241.

10. Vollan, *Postgraduate Medical Education*, fig. 33, p. 117.

11. Ibid., p. 35.

12. E. V. Allen, "The George E. Brown memorial lecture: Fifteen years of progress in cardiovascular disease," *Circulation* 11 (1950): 726–735, quote p. 735.

13. The AMA's annual scientific sessions were discontinued in 1978 because specialty societies offered many continuing medical education alternatives and the association chose to focus on socioeconomic issues. See W. Sodeman in Minutes, ACC BOT, 5 March 1978, ACC Archives.

14. These conclusions are drawn from reviewing AHA and ACC programs published between 1951 and 1969.

15. See L. B. Ellis, "Reflections on postgraduate medical education for practicing physicians," *N. Engl. J. Med.* 250 (1954): 243–245.

16. T. R. Harrison, "Progress in the cardiovascular field during the last decade," *Year Book of Medicine* (1950): 471–477, quote p. 477.

17. B. Kisch, "A year of activity," *Am. Coll. Cardiol. Bull.* (December 1951): [1–2].

18. F. M. Groedel, "Specialization in cardiology, its necessity, demarcation line and requirements," *Am. Coll. Cardiol. Bull.* (June 1951): [2–3].

19. B. Kisch, "Historical survey of graphic registration in cardiology," *Trans. Am. Coll. Cardiol.* 1 (1951): 161–167. Speakers discussed electrocardiography, vectorcardiography, ballistocardiography, electrokymography, phonocardiography, and microplethysmography. Their papers were published in *Trans. Am. Coll. Cardiol.* 2 (1952): 157–252. For the techniques that became obsolete, see B. R. Boone, G. F. Ellinger, and F. G. Gillick, "Electrokymography of the heart and great vessels: Principles and application," *Ann. Intern. Med.* 31 (1949): 1030–1056, and J. D. Howell, "The Rise and Fall of the Ballistocardiogram," unpublished essay kindly provided by Joel D. Howell, M.D., Ph.D.

20. H. B. Sprague to G. E. Burch, 10 November 1951, Sprague Papers.

21. "Rules and regulations of the Section on Clinical Cardiology," 30 June 1952, in Minutes, AHA CCC EC, AHA Archives.

22. Minutes, AHA CCC EC, 11 April 1953, AHA Archives.

23. "AHA scientific sessions," *Circulation* 5 (1952): 636–639.

24. Minutes, AHA CCC EC, 13 March 1954, AHA Archives.

25. *A History of the Scientific Councils of the American Heart Association* (New York: AHA, 1967).

26. Minutes, AHA CCC EC, 13 March 1954, AHA Archives.

27. Cardiovascular surgeons who participated in ACC meetings during the 1950s included Charles Bailey, Claude Beck, Michael DeBakey, Dewey Dodrill, Donald Effler, Robert Glover, Charles Hufnagel, Earle Kay, John Kirklin, Andrew Morrow, and Willis Potts.

28. W. S. Priest, "Message from the President," *Am. Coll. Cardiol. Bull.* (July-August 1955): 1–2, 7.

29. These conclusions are drawn from a review of the official ACC programs. In 1958 attendees had a choice of nineteen films, most showing surgeons performing operations they had devised or refined to treat various congenital and acquired cardiovascular lesions.

30. "Successful symposium," *Am. Coll. Cardiol. Bull.* (March-April 1957): 7.

31. D. D. Eisenhower, in Minutes, ACC BOT, 15 May 1957, ACC Archives.

32. Minutes, ACC BOT, 21 October 1960, ACC Archives. For comparison, the ACP earned a profit of $45 thousand from the exhibits at their 1956 meeting, which 6,380 physicians attended. E. C. Rosenow Jr., *History of the American College of Physicians: Executive Perspectives 1959–1977* (Philadelphia: ACP, 1984), p. 11.

33. P. Reichert to H. L. Conn Jr., 26 July 1963, in Bethesda workshop, September 1962 file, ACC Archives.

34. P. Reichert, "How medical advertising saves lives," *Printers' Ink* (14 December 1951): 37, and Helen F. Reichert, interview by W. Bruce Fye, 13 August 1991, New York.

35. "1963 annual convention American College of Cardiology," *Am. J. Cardiol.* 9 (1962): 620.

36. By 1993 the AHA and ACC annual meetings were the largest trade shows of any clinical specialty. *Trade Show 200: The 200 Largest Shows,* 19th ed. (np: Trade Show Week, 1993): 57–60.

37. Minutes, ACC BOT, 24 May 1960, ACC Archives.

38. C. D. May, "Selling drugs by 'educating' physicians," *J. Med. Educ.* 36 (1961): 1–23.

39. See, for example, J. T. Bennett and T. J. DiLorenzo, *Unhealthy Charities: Hazardous to Your Health and Wealth* (New York: Basic Books, 1994), esp. pp. 137–140; J. D. Coulter, *Guidelines for Faculty Involvement in Commercially Supported Continuing Medical Education* (Washington, D.C.: Association of American Medical Colleges, 1992); C. R. Conti, "The relation of cardiovascular specialists to industry, institutions and organizations," *J. Am. Coll. Cardiol.* 16 (1990): 30–33; and D. A. Kessler, "Drug promotion and scientific exchange: The role of the clinical investigator," *N. Engl. J. Med.* 325 (1991): 201–203.

40. "Constitution and by-laws," *Trans. Am. Coll. Cardiol.* 1 (1952): 11–22.

41. P. Reichert to D. E. Harken, 3 October 1962, in workshops, general documents, 1962–1965, Reichert Papers, ACC Archives.

42. Minutes, ACC BOT, 25 May 1959, ACC Archives.

43. Eugene Braunwald, interview by W. Bruce Fye, 13 November 1991, Anaheim, Calif.

44. Minutes, ACC BOT, 25 May 1959, ACC Archives.

45. Ibid.

46. Minutes, ACC BOT, 29 May 1962, ACC Archives. The exhibitors (and their products) are listed in the official programs for the annual meetings. ACC Archives.

47. A. G. W. Whitfield, "Postgraduate medical education in the United States," *Lancet* 2 (1963): 514–518, quote p. 517.

48. These conclusions are drawn from the official programs of the annual ACC meetings. ACC Archives.

49. J. S. Billings, "A century of American medicine. 1776–1876. Literature and institutions," *Am. J. Med. Sci.*, n.s., 72 (1876): 439–480. See also W. B. Fye, "The literature of American internal medicine: A historical view," *Ann. Intern. Med.* 106 (1987): 450–461, and D. de Solla Price, "The development and structure of the biomedical literature," in *Coping with the Biomedical Literature: A Primer for the Scientist*

and the Clinician, ed. K. S. Warren (New York: Praeger Special Studies, 1981), pp. 3–16.

50. Howard B. Burchell, interview by W. Bruce Fye, 13 January 1991, Minneapolis. Burchell edited *Circulation* from 1965 to 1970.

51. Minutes, NYCS, 27 July 1949, Reichert Papers, NYH Archives, and Minutes, NYCS, 7 September 1949, Reichert Papers, NYH Archives.

52. P. D. White to C. A. R. Connor, 24 October 1949, Sprague Papers. For Meakins and Canadian cardiology, see H. N. Segall, *Pioneers of Cardiology in Canada 1820–1970. The Genesis of Canadian Cardiology* (Willowdale, Ontario: Hounslow Press, 1988), esp. pp. 77–78.

53. R. C. Meakins, "Editorial," *Am. Heart J.* 29 (1950): 1.

54. B. Snow to H. B. Sprague, 25 September 1951, Sprague Papers.

55. Ibid.

56. H. B. Sprague to G. E. Burch, 10 November 1951, Sprague Papers.

57. Minutes, NYCS, 30 October 1949, Reichert Papers, NYH Archives.

58. "Constitution and by-laws," *Trans. Am. Coll. Cardiol.* 1 (1952): 11–22.

59. Minutes, ACC BOG, 6 June 1952, Reichert Papers, NYH Archives.

60. Minutes, ACC BOT, 11 November 1955, ACC Archives.

61. "Introducing the American Journal of Cardiology," *Am. Coll. Cardiol. Bull.* (January-February 1957): [1]

62. S. Dack, "Looking ahead," *Am. J. Cardiol.* 1 (1958): 1–2.

63. F. Tirella to S. Dack, 17 February 1957, in Journal 1956–57 file, Reichert Papers, ACC Archives.

64. "The American Journal of Cardiology, A New Approach. Advertising Rate Circular," [New York c1957], in Journal 1956–57 file, Reichert Papers, ACC Archives.

65. Minutes, *American Heart Journal* editorial board, 1 May 1960, box 13, file 47, White Papers.

66. P. Reichert to P. Porter, 14 December 1964, ACC corres. 1964, Reichert Papers, NYH Archives.

67. P. Reichert to C. S. Mill, 15 July 1965, in Journal 1961–65 file, Reichert Papers, ACC Archives.

68. Minutes, ACC BOT, 7 December 1953, ACC Archives.

69. A. A. Luisada, "Why an encyclopedia of cardiology?" *Am. J. Cardiol.* 4 (1959): 708–710.

70. S. Dack, "Book review of *Cardiology: An Encyclopedia of the Cardiovascular System,*" *Am. J. Cardiol.* 7 (1961): 466–467.

71. "Postgraduate courses for members of the college," *Ann. Intern. Med.* 11 (1938): 1354–1355.

72. W. S. Priest, "Message from the President."

73. J. B. Wolffe to P. D. White, 11 October 1955, White Papers.

74. E. C. Andrus to E. F. Bland, 31 October 1955, White Papers. White wrote on Wolffe's 11 October 1955 letter that he would respond "after consulting Ed Bland

and Coke Andrus." See also E. C. Andrus to P. D. White, 1 November 1955, White Papers.

75. P. D. White to William D. Stroud, 25 July 1956, box 1, file 28, White Papers.

76. The workshop programs are described in various issues of *Am. Coll. Cardiol. Bull.*, 1956–57.

77. "American College of Cardiology Workshop Program," *Am. J. Cardiol.* 8 (1961): 920. The speakers included Lewis Dexter, Lawrence Ellis, Richard Gorlin, Samuel Levine, Francis Moore, and Leroy Vandam.

78. W. D. Nelligan, "Report of the executive director American College of Cardiology," *Am. J. Cardiol.* 20 (1967): 887–890.

79. Minutes, AHA CCC EC, 11 May 1962, AHA Archives.

80. W. B. Fye, "A history of the American Heart Association's council on clinical cardiology," *Circulation* 87 (1993): 1057–1063.

81. E. G. Dimond, "The work shops," *Am. J. Cardiol.* 8 (1961): 606.

82. Eugene Braunwald, interview by W. Bruce Fye, 13 November 1991, Anaheim, Calif. Former ACC president Eliot Corday agrees: "We could maneuver, we could do things. They were a ponderous organization." He explained, "We didn't have too much red tape. Somebody had a good idea. . . . [if] we liked the idea, we moved." Eliot Corday, interview by W. Bruce Fye, 13 November 1991, Anaheim, Calif.

83. Eugene Braunwald, interview by W. Bruce Fye, 13 November 1991, Anaheim, Calif. Former AHA president Willis Hurst (an academic cardiologist trained by Paul White) agrees that the AHA "was not deeply involved in postgraduate courses" in the 1950s and 1960s. He believes the college "stimulated the American Heart to do more" in this area. J. Willis Hurst, interview by W. Bruce Fye, 11 November 1991, Anaheim, Calif.

84. S. Z. Levine, "Some impressions of teaching medical missions of the World Health Organization," *N. Engl. J. Med.* 251 (1954): 813–816.

85. E. G. Dimond, *Take Wing! Interesting Things That Happened on My Way to School* (Kansas City, Mo.: Lowell Press, 1991), quote p. 109. See also pp. 174–180. See also M. M. Alimurung, "Strokes of a painter's brush," *Am. J. Cardiol.* 15 (1965): 438–441, which includes a photograph of White's associates and trainees in 1948.

86. M. M. Alimurung to P. Reichert, 3 April 1960, in Reichert Papers, general correspondence, 1960–61, ACC Archives.

87. P. Reichert to M. M. Alimurung, 13 April 1960, in Reichert Papers, general correspondence 1960–61, ACC Archives.

88. E. Corday to A. O. Abbott, 5 April 1960, in circuit courses, 1961–65 file, ACC Archives.

89. E. Grey Dimond, interview by W. Bruce Fye, 28–29 January 1993, Kansas City, Mo.

90. P. N. Mayuga to the [ACC] President, 16 June 1961, in circuit courses, 1961–65 file, ACC Archives.

91. E. Valencia to the [ACC] President, 5 May 1961, in circuit courses, 1961–65 file, ACC Archives.

92. Report to Committee Members of the Postgraduate Program Overseas, 5 July 1961, in circuit courses, 1961–65 file, ACC Archives.

93. E. G. Dimond to E. Corday, 20 June 1961, in circuit courses, 1961–65 file, ACC Archives.

94. P. D. White to E. G. Dimond, 6 July 1961, box 1, file 31, White Papers.

95. H. M. Schmeck Jr. "Heart unit maps own Peace Corps," *New York Times,* 3 October 1961. See also E. G. Dimond and E. Corday, "Report on first international circuit course," *Am. J. Cardiol.* 9 (1962): 220–221, and E. G. Dimond, "Medicine, a universal language: The international circuit courses of the American College of Cardiology," *Medical Times* 95 (1967): 1058–1071.

96. E. Corday to E. G. Dimond, 22 May 1962, in circuit courses, 1961–65 file, ACC Archives.

97. D. Rusk to D. E. Harken, 17 February 1964, in circuit courses, 1964 file, ACC Archives. Participants were reimbursed for their expenses.

98. H. H. Humphrey to F. H. Adams, 24 January 1966, in circuit courses, 1963–73 file, ACC Archives.

99. E. Corday to J. H. Moyer, 12 November 1966, in circuit courses, 1963–73 file, ACC Archives.

100. By 1992, seventy-five circuit courses had been completed, and college teams had visited more than sixty countries. *Thirty Years of Sharing Cardiovascular Knowledge around the World* (Bethesda, Md.: ACC, 1992). See also "International Circuit Courses [1961–1992]," [Bethesda, Md.: ACC, 1993], 6 pp. typescript listing courses, countries visited, and speakers. ACC Archives.

101. Minutes, ACC BOT, 21 November 1968, ACC Archives.

102. Dennis M. Krikler, interview by W. Bruce Fye, 8 November 1993, Atlanta.

103. W. D. Nelligan, "Report of the executive director," *Am. J. Cardiol.* 20 (1967): 887–890.

104. F. M. Groedel to C. A. R. Connor, 24 February 1951, Minutes ACC BOT, 1949–52, ACC Archives.

105. Minutes of the special committee appointed by the president to confer with the committee of the AHA, 8 October 1952, Minutes ACC BOT, 1949–52, ACC Archives.

106. Otakar Pollak, interview by W. Bruce Fye, 21 September 1992, Wilmington, Del. See also T. B. Clarkson, G. C. McMillan, and H. C. McGill Jr., "The origin of the Council on Arteriosclerosis," *Arterioscler. Thromb.* 12 (1992): 543–547.

107. R. P. Glover to R. L. King, 22 July 1952, Sprague Papers.

108. H. B. Sprague to R. L. King, 8 August 1952, Sprague Papers.

109. Minutes, AHA EC, 19 February 1953, AHA Archives.

110. Minutes, ACC BOT, 16 May 1956, ACC Archives. Simon Dack acknowledges that several early ACC presidents (citing specifically Walter Priest, Robert Glover, George Meneely, and Osler Abbott) were promised the ACC presidency if they joined. The goal was to "give the college an academic cloak." Simon Dack, interview by W. Bruce Fye, 21 October 1991, New York.

111. Minutes, ACC BOT, 16 May 1956, ACC Archives. Although he was an influential advocate of the ACC, Prinzmetal did not become president.

112. Simon Dack, interview by W. Bruce Fye, 21 October 1991, New York. See also B. Kisch, *Wanderungen und Wandlungen: Die Geschichte eines Arztes im 20. Jahrhundert* (Cologne: Greven Verlag, 1966), p. 336.

113. "Circular Letter to the Board of Governors," 31 January 1957, Minutes, ACC BOG, 1955–58, ACC Archives.

114. A. Graybiel, "Report from the president," *Am. Coll. Cardiol. Bull.* (November–December 1954): 1–2.

115. Minutes, ACC AM, 16 May 1957, ACC Archives. The amendment was drafted by Osler Abbott, Irving Brotman, Elwyn Evans, Robert Glover, George Meneely, and Walter Priest.

116. Arthur Bernstein, interview by W. Bruce Fye, 19 May 1992, Newark, N.J.

117. Minutes, ACC BOT, 7 December 1957, ACC Archives.

118. Minutes, ACC BOT, 29 May 1962, ACC Archives.

119. A. Graybiel, "Inaugural address of the new president," *Trans. Am. Coll. Cardiol.* 4 (1954): 184–186. In May 1958 ACC trustees discontinued financial support for Bruno Kisch's electron microscope research institute at the New York City Hospital on Welfare Island, the sole research project they had funded. The origins and activities of the institute (created when the college purchased the microscope in 1952) are discussed in various issues of *Am. Coll. Cardiol. Bull.* between 1952 and 1957. See esp. A. Graybiel, "The electron microscope institute," *Am. Coll. Cardiol. Bull.* (March–April 1955): [8]. See also B. Kisch and J. M. Bardet, *Electron Microscopic Histology of the Heart* (New York: Brooklyn Medical Press, 1951); B. Kisch, "Electron microscopy of the atrium of the heart," *Exp. Med. Surg.* 14 (1956): 99–112; and ACC BOT, 20 May 1958, ACC Archives.

120. W. M. Moore, *Fighting for Life: The Story of the American Heart Association 1911–1975* (Dallas: AHA, 1983), appendix v, p. 270.

121. "Report of September 10, 1958, New York meeting of conference committees of the AHA and ACC," 15 September 1958, in Annual reports of the secretary, 1952–1966, Reichert Papers, NYH Archives. To compare the two associations' views on continuing medical education, see S. G. Wolf, "The physician's continuing education," *Circulation* 24 (1961): 543–548, and G. Griffith, "The role of the American College of Cardiology in the continuing lifetime education of the cardiovascular specialist," *Am. J. Cardiol.* 15 (1965): 879–881.

122. O. Abbott to A. Blalock, 27 April 1959, Blalock Papers.

123. Minutes, ACC AM, 27 May 1959, ACC Archives.

124. E. G. Dimond to P. D. White, 27 October 1959, box 1, file 29, White Papers.

125. E. G. Dimond to P. D. White, 23 June 1961, box 1, file 30, White Papers.

126. P. D. White to E. G. Dimond, 5 November 1959, box 1, file 29, White Papers.

127. P. D. White to W. D. Stroud, 25 July 1956, box 1, file 28, White Papers.

128. F. Smithies, "Presidential address," *Ann. Intern. Med.* 1 (1928): 861–874, quote p. 862.

129. P. D. White to G. Wakerlin, 17 March 1960, box 1, file 30, White Papers.

130. H. B. Taussig to D. E. Harken, 11 November 1959, convocations, 1953–63 file, ACC Archives.

131. P. D. White to O. Paul, 28 March 1960, box 1, file 30, White Papers.

132. Minutes, ACC BOT, 26 June 1965, ACC Archives. A "Basic Science Symposium" was added to the annual meeting in 1965.

133. ACC Archives.

134. Minutes, ACC BOG, 24 May 1960, ACC Archives.

135. P. Reichert to J. R. Setnor, 4 August 1960, in ACC-Bethesda correspondence file, ACC Archives.

136. O. A. Abbott, "Admission requirements of the American College of Cardiology," *Am. J. Cardiol.* 7 (1961): 159–160.

137. Minutes, ACC BOT, 24 May 1960, ACC Archives.

138. P. R. Reichert to [program directors], c1960, miscellaneous circulars, 1955–62 file, ACC Archives.

139. Minutes, ACC BOT, 22 October 1960, ACC Archives.

140. Minutes, ACC BOT, 21 October 1960, ACC Archives.

141. P. R. Reichert to E. G. Dimond, 31 October 1960, in Young Investigator Award, 1960–64 file, ACC Archives.

142. Thirty-two-year-old Jere Mitchell, a research fellow at NIH, won the competition. "The Young Investigator's Award for 1961," *Am. J. Cardiol.* 8 (1961): 308.

143. P. R. Manning, "George C. Griffith," *Clin. Cardiol.* 11 (1988): 59–60.

144. Dwight E. Harken, interview by W. Bruce Fye, 14 April 1992, Dallas.

145. California cardiologist David Carmichael recalls Griffith discouraging him from joining the college in the early 1950s: "Stick with the ACP and belong to the AHA, that's what you should do." David B. Carmichael, interview by W. Bruce Fye, 19 September 1991, Bethesda, Md.

146. G. C. Griffith to P. D. White, 27 June 1962, box 1, file 32, White Papers.

147. Minutes, ACC BOT, 6 October 1962, ACC Archives. See also G. C. Griffith to P. D. White, 17 July 1962, box 1, file 32, White Papers. Harken said White resisted giving the lecture until the name was changed. Dwight E. Harken, interview by W. Bruce Fye, 14 April 1992, Dallas.

148. P. D. White to E. G. Dimond, 14 August 1962, box 1, file 32, White Papers. White's lecture was published. P. D. White, "Reflections of a pioneer in cardiology," *Am. J. Cardiol.* 11 (1963): 697–703.

149. D. E. Harken to P. D. White, 24 January 1963, box 1, file 33, White Papers.

150. P. D. White to D. E. Harken, 29 January 1963, box 1, file 33, White Papers.

151. Oglesby Paul, interview by W. Bruce Fye, 16 June 1992, Boston.

152. Simon Dack, interview by W. Bruce Fye, 21 October 1991, New York.

153. G. E. Wakerlin to P. D. White, 15 March 1963, box 1, file 33, White Papers.

154. E. G. Dimond to B. L. Martz, 9 December 1968, box 1, file 47, White Papers.

155. Minutes, ACC BOT, 20 June 1965, ACC Archives. Grey Dimond characterized Harken as "a hell of a recruiter . . . he'd go to people and say, 'I want you,

and you've got to do it for me, do it for me.' And he got 'em." E. Grey Dimond, interview by W. Bruce Fye, 28–29 January 1993, Kansas City, Mo.

156. Minutes, AHA CCC EC, 12 January 1961, AHA Archives.

157. Ibid.

158. "Report of the Medical Director to the Assembly," 29 October 1962, AHA Archives.

159. O. Paul to P. D. White, 6 April 1961, box 1, file 31, White Papers.

160. L. E. January to D. Rutstein, 25 January 1963, Rutstein Papers.

161. Minutes, AHA CCC EC, 2 December 1964, AHA Archives.

162. "Summary notes, meeting of representatives of AHA and ACC," 7 January 1966, AHA 1965–67 file, ACC Archives.

163. "President's report" to the BOT, 28 January 1966, with unbound minutes, ACC BOT, 2 February 1966, ACC Archives.

164. *The President's Commission on Heart Disease, Cancer and Stroke. Report to the President. Volume 1* (Washington, D.C.: GPO, 1964), quote p. 44.

165. Richards, *Continuing Medical Education,* esp. pp. 67–95. See also J. C. Verner Nakamoto, *Continuing Education in the Health Professions: A Review of the Literature 1960–1970* (Syracuse, N.Y.: ERIC Clearinghouse on Adult Education, 1973).

166. Minutes, ACC BOT, 27 February 1968, ACC Archives.

167. S. G. Wolf, ed., *The Physician's Continuing Education* (New York: AHA, 1961), quote p. 21.

168. Minutes, ACC BOT, 21 November 1968, ACC Archives.

169. B. L. Martz to W. B. Fye, March 1993.

170. ACCESS, vol. 1, no. 1, 1969 [Bethesda, Md.: ACC].

171. "Report on ACCESS activity," 3 November 1969, Minutes ACC BOT, ACC Archives. See also Minutes, ACC BOT EC, 11 November 1970, ACC Archives.

172. Minutes, ACC BOT, 10 February 1974, ACC Archives.

173. Minutes, ACC BOT, 22 February 1976, ACC Archives. Dimond reported in 1977 that the market for the videotape series was small. Minutes, ACC BOT, 6 March 1977, ACC Archives.

CHAPTER 7   *Washington, Medicine, and the American College of Cardiology*

1. *Health in America: 1776–1976* (Washington, D.C.: DHEW, 1976), esp. pp. 195–211.

2. See, for example, "3 out of 5 heart specialists say Ike could serve a second term," *U.S. News & World Report* 40, no. 2 (1956): 19–29. For a perspective on how earlier American presidents concealed their health status from the public, see B. E. Park, *The Impact of Illness on World Leaders* (Philadelphia: Univ. of Pennsylvania Press, 1986).

3. P. D. White, *My Life and Medicine: An Autobiographical Memoir* (Boston: Gambit, 1971), quote p. 58. See also S. P. Strickland, *Politics, Science, and Dread Disease: A Short History of United States Medical Research Policy* (Cambridge: Harvard Univ. Press,

1972), p. 142. For Johnson's heart attack, see J. W. Hurst and J. C. Cain, *LBJ: To Know Him Better,* ed. R. L. Hardesty and T. Gittinger (np: LBJ Foundation, 1995).

4. "Moving force in medical research: Catalyst for action, Mary Lasker has sparked support for increased scientific efforts," *Med. World News* (20 November 1964): 83–89. See also E. B. Drew, "The health syndicate: Washington's noble conspirators," *Atlantic Monthly* (December 1967): 75–82, and Strickland, *Politics, Science, and Dread Disease,* which includes many examples of Lasker's role in lobbying Congress on behalf of research.

5. The NIH budget figures are from J. A. Shannon, "Federal support of biomedical sciences: Development and academic impact," *J. Med. Educ.* 51 (suppl. to July 1976, no. 2), table 6, p. 87. The NHI budget increased from $16.7 million in 1955 to $35.9 million in 1958. *National Heart, Lung, and Blood Institute Fact Book. Fiscal Year 1993* (Bethesda, Md.: NHLBI, 1994), p. 63. Hereafter, *NHLBI Fact Book 1993.*

6. S. Bayne-Jones, *The Advancement of Medical Research and Education Through the Department of Health, Education and Welfare* (Washington, D.C.: DHEW, 1958), table 5, p. 24. The remaining research funds came from philanthropy (21 percent), endowment (12 percent), and direct grants from industry (1 percent). For a summary of the nation's medical schools in the 1950s, see F. Bane, *Physicians for a Growing America* (Washington, D.C.: GPO, 1959), and J. E. Deitrick and R. C. Berson, *Medical Schools in the United States at Mid-Century* (New York: McGraw-Hill, 1953).

7. Bayne-Jones, *Medical Research,* quotes pp. 31, 1.

8. J. Fogarty, *Report to Accompany H.R. 6769. 86th Cong., 1st sess., 28 April 1959. Report No. 309* (Washington, D.C.: GPO, 1959). See also J. P. Crowley, "Health for peace: John E. Fogarty's vision of American leadership in health care and international biomedical research," *Rhode Island Medicine* 75 (1992): 561–582.

9. J. Fogarty, *Report to Accompany H.R. 7035. 87th Cong., 1st sess., 15 May 1961. Report No. 392* (Washington, D.C.: GPO, 1961).

10. B. Jones, *Federal Support of Medical Research* (Washington, D.C.: GPO, 1960), quote p. xiii.

11. Ibid., quotes pp. 107, 23. For the committee's history and a list of its members, see pp. 119–123. See also Strickland, *Politics, Science, and Dread Disease,* esp. pp. 160–162, quote p.160.

12. "Background: The President's Conference on Heart Disease and Cancer," 21 April 1961, Wright Papers. This typescript includes a list of the participants. The NIH budget figures are from Shannon, "Federal support of biomedical sciences."

13. "Background: The President's Conference," quote p. [1]. For the cancer lobby, see J. T. Patterson, *The Dread Disease: Cancer and Modern American Culture* (Cambridge: Harvard Univ. Press, 1987). See also Strickland, *Politics, Science, and Dread Disease,* and D. M. Fox, *Power and Illness: The Failure and Future of American Health Policy* (Berkeley: Univ. of California Press, 1993), esp. pp. 56–83.

14. "Background: The President's Conference," quotes p. 25. Emphasis in original.

15. Shannon's testimony in *House Subcommittee of the Committee on Government Operations. Hearings on Health Research and Training. 87th Cong., 1st sess.* (Washington, D.C.: GPO, 1961), quote p. 67.

16. Strickland, *Politics, Science, and Dread Disease,* quote p. 204.

17. *The President's Commission on Heart Disease, Cancer and Stroke. Report to the President.* vol. 1 (Washington, D.C.: GPO, 1964), quotes p. xi. For statistics on cardiovascular diseases in this era, see I. M. Moriyama, D. E. Krueger, and J. Stamler, *Cardiovascular Diseases in the United States* (Cambridge: Harvard Univ. Press, 1971), esp. pp. 49–118. For a detailed analysis of the lag between discovery and application of new knowledge, see J. H. Comroe Jr. and R. D. Dripps, *The Top Ten Clinical Advances in Cardiovascular-Pulmonary Medicine and Surgery 1945–1975* (Washington, D.C.: GPO, 1978).

18. Michael E. DeBakey, interview by W. Bruce Fye, 10 April 1992, Houston.

19. *The President's Commission on Heart Disease, Cancer and Stroke. Report to the President.* vol. 2 (Washington, D.C.: GPO, 1965), quotes pp. 1–3.

20. Ibid., quote p. 90.

21. *The President's Commission on Heart Disease, Cancer and Stroke. Report to the President.* vol. 1, quote p. 59.

22. Minutes, ACC BOT, 20 June 1965, ACC Archives.

23. M. E. DeBakey, "Report of President's Commission on Heart Disease, Cancer, and Stroke," *Circulation* 32 (1965): 686. In a sense, the program reflected a health care delivery policy historian Daniel Fox terms hierarchical regionalism because it linked patients to academic medical centers through a network of local facilities and practitioners. See Fox, *Power and Illness.*

24. *Senate Subcommittee on Health. Hearings on Combating Heart Disease, Cancer, Stroke, and Other Major Diseases. (S.596). 89th Cong., 1st sess.* (Washington, D.C.: GPO, 1965), pp. 127–128, 179–180.

25. *House Committee on Interstate and Foreign Commerce. Hearings on Regional Medical Complexes for Heart Disease, Cancer, Stroke, and Other Diseases. (H.R. 3140). 89th Cong., 1st sess.* (Washington, D.C.: GPO, 1965), esp. pp. 122–124.

26. Ibid., p. 139.

27. Minutes, ACC BOT, 20 June 1965, ACC Archives.

28. S. P. Strickland, "A History of Regional Medical Programs," 21 March 1994. Draft kindly provided by the author. See also T. S. Bodenhamer, "Regional medical programs: No road to regionalization," *Med. Care Rev.* 26 (1969): 1125–1166.

29. I. H. Page, *Hypertension Research: A Memoir, 1920–1960* (New York: Pergamon Press, 1988), quote p. 37.

30. E. T. Lanahan, *A Salute to the Past: A History of the National Heart, Lung, and Blood Institute Based on Personal Recollections* (Bethesda, Md.: NHLBI, 1987).

31. Appendix 2 [attached to summary minutes], Inter-Society Commission for Heart Disease Resources, first Advisory Committee meeting, 16 January 1969, Burch papers.

32. M. R. Laird, "Remarks," in *Proceedings: Conference Workshop on Regional Medical Programs.* 2 vols., ed. R. Q. Marston (Washington, D.C.: GPO, 1968), 1: 123. Vol. 1, appendix 6 (pp. 161–175) is a detailed list of Regional Medical Programs. Vol. 2 is a summary of sixty Regional Medical Programs.

33. T. R. Harrison, "The challenge of the regional medical program," *Ann. Intern. Med.* 68 (1968): 245–247.

34. Strickland, "A History of Regional Medical Programs," quote p. [v].

35. R. Stevens and R. A. Stevens, *Welfare Medicine in America: A Case Study of Medicaid* (New York: Free Press, 1974), quote p. 48. See also E. Witkin, *The Impact of Medicare* (Springfield, Ill.: Charles C. Thomas, 1971).

36. See R. L. Numbers, ed., *Compulsory Health Insurance: The Continuing American Debate* (Westport, Conn.: Greenwood Press, 1982); R. Munts, *Bargaining for Health: Labor Unions, Health Insurance, and Medical Care* (Madison: Univ. of Wisconsin Press, 1967); and H. M. Somers and A. R. Somers, *Medicare and the Hospitals: Issues and Prospects* (Washington, D.C.: Brookings Institution, 1967).

37. M. M. Poen, *Harry S. Truman versus the Medical Lobby: The Genesis of Medicare* (Columbia: Univ. of Missouri Press, 1979), p. ix. For the AMA perspective, see F. D. Campion, *The AMA and U.S. Health Policy Since 1940* (Chicago: Chicago Review Press, 1984).

38. A perceptive summary of how a major piece of health legislation was developed and signed into law is E. Redman, *The Dance of Legislation* (New York: Simon & Schuster, 1973). See also W. G. Magnuson and E. A. Segal, *How Much for Health?* (Washington, D.C.: Robert B. Luce, 1974); M. V. Pauly and W. L. Kissick, eds., *Lessons from the First Twenty Years of Medicare* (Philadelphia: Univ. of Pennsylvania Press, 1988); and J. M. Feder, *Medicare: The Politics of Federal Hospital Insurance* (Lexington, Mass.: Lexington Books, 1977).

39. Social Security Amendments of 1965, Public Law 89–97, 30 July 1965, 79 Stat.

40. R. J. Myers, *Medicare* (Bryn Mawr, Pa.: McCahn Foundation, 1970).

41. T. R. Marmor, "Reflections on Medicare," *J. Med. Philo.* 13 (1988): 5–29. For health laws passed during the 1960s, see *Health in America*, pp. 203–207. For the politics behind the focus on chronic disease, see D. M. Fox, "Health policy and changing epidemiology in the United States: Chronic disease in the twentieth century," in *Unnatural Causes: The Three Leading Killer Diseases in America*, ed. R. C. Maulitz (New Brunswick, N.J.: Rutgers Univ. Press, 1988), pp. 11–31, and Fox, *Power and Illness*, esp. pp. 70–78. See also R. A. Meckel, *Save the Babies: American Public Health Reform and the Prevention of Infant Mortality, 1850–1929* (Baltimore: Johns Hopkins Univ. Press, 1990), esp. pp. 178–236.

42. Charles Fisch, interview by W. Bruce Fye, 16 November 1992, New Orleans.

43. Lewis Dexter, interview by W. Bruce Fye, 15 November 1992, Boston.

44. For background on health care financing in America, see H. M. Somers and A. R. Somers, *Doctors, Patients, and Health Insurance: The Organization and Financing of Medical Care* (Washington, D.C.: Brookings Institution, 1961); R. Stevens, *American Medicine and the Public Interest* (New Haven: Yale Univ. Press, 1971), esp. pp. 426–495; S. E. Harris, *The Economics of American Medicine* (New York: Macmillan, 1964), esp. pp. 301–431; and O. W. Anderson, *Health Services in the United States: A Growth Enterprise since 1875* (Ann Arbor, Mich.: Health Administration Press, 1985).

45. *Cardiovascular Specialists and the Economics of Medicine* (Bethesda, Md.: ACC, 1994), figures 9.1 and 9.3, p. 65.

46. W. Mills interview c1980 quoted in L. E. Weeks and H. J. Berman, *Shapers of American Health Care Policy: An Oral History* (Ann Arbor, Mich.: Health Administration Press, 1985), p. 93.

47. Anderson, *Health Services in the United States*, quote p. 173. For the implications of Medicare for hospitals, see R. Stevens, *In Sickness and in Wealth: American Hospitals in the Twentieth Century* (New York: Basic Books, 1989), esp. pp. 256–283. Congress had acknowledged the increasing role of hospitals in health care delivery two decades earlier when it passed the "Hospital Survey and Construction Act" (PL 79-725), popularly known as the Hill-Burton Act, which gave grants to states to design and build hospital facilities.

48. H. Cabot, *The Doctor's Bill* (New York: Columbia Univ. Press, 1935), esp. pp. 266–271.

49. E. F. Butler discussing E. N. Packard, "The training of the thoracic surgeon from the standpoint of the phthisiologist," *J. Thorac. Surg.* 5 (1936): 583–589, quote p. 587. See also I. S. Falk, C. R. Rorem, and M. D. Ring, *The Costs of Medical Care: A Summary of Investigations on the Economic Aspects of the Prevention and Care of Illness* (Chicago: Univ. of Chicago Press, 1933), and N. Sinai, O. W. Anderson, and M. L. Dollar, *Health Insurance in the United States* (New York: Commonwealth Fund, 1946).

50. B. Bates, *Bargaining for Life: A Social History of Tuberculosis, 1876–1938* (Philadelphia: Univ. of Pennsylvania Press, 1992). See also R. Dubos and J. Dubos, *The White Plague: Tuberculosis, Man and Society* (Boston: Little, Brown, 1952).

51. B. B. Roe, "The UCR boondoggle: A death knell for private practice?" *N. Engl. J. Med.* 305 (1981): 41–45. The 1990 figure is from *Cardiovascular Specialists and the Economics of Medicine*, figure 9.1, p. 65.

52. G. E. Burch, "Changing concepts in cardiovascular therapy: A quarter century perspective," *Am. Heart J.* 93 (1977): 413–418, quote p. 417.

53. Ibid.

54. Earl Bakken, interview by W. Bruce Fye, 12 November 1991, Anaheim, Calif. See also J. D. Bronzino, V. H. Smith, and M. L. Wade, *Medical Technology and Society: An Interdisciplinary Perspective* (Cambridge: MIT Press, 1990), esp. pp. 38–77; M. Eden, "The engineering-industrial accord: Inventing the technology of health care," in *The Machine at the Bedside*, ed. S. J. Reiser and M. Anbar (Cambridge: Cambridge Univ. Press, 1984), pp. 49–64; and H. D. Banta, "Embracing or rejecting innovations: Clinical diffusion of health care technology," Ibid., pp. 65–92, esp. pp. 79–80.

55. S. J. Peitzman, "Nephrology in America from Thomas Addis to the artificial kidney," in *Grand Rounds: One Hundred Years of Internal Medicine*, ed. R. C. Maulitz and D. E. Long (Philadelphia: Univ. of Pennsylvania Press, 1988), pp. 211–241, quotes p. 226. The ESRD program is discussed extensively in A. L. Plough, *Borrowed Time: Artificial Organs and the Politics of Extending Lives* (Philadelphia: Temple Univ. Press, 1986). See also L. B. Russell, *Technology in Hospitals: Medical Advances and Their Diffusion* (Washington, D.C.: The Brookings Institution, 1979), esp. pp. 110–115, and E. G. Lowrie and C. L. Hampers, "The success of Medicare's end-stage renal-disease program," *N. Engl. J. Med.* 305 (1981): 434–438.

56. Minutes, ACC AM, 22 May 1958, ACC Archives.

57. Ibid.

58. M. V. Crafts, "American College of Cardiology, Inc." 15 March 1953–31 July 1965, with M. V. Crafts to W. B. Fye, 9 November 1991.

59. Minutes, ACC BOT, 19 October 1961, ACC Archives.

60. E. G. Dimond, *Take Wing! Interesting Things That Happened on My Way to School* (Kansas City, Mo.: Lowell Press, 1991), quote p. 180.

61. E. Grey Dimond, interview by W. Bruce Fye, 28–29 January 1993, Kansas City, Mo.

62. P. Reichert to J. Bodlander, 28 April 1960, ACC correspondence, 1960, Reichert Papers, NYH Archives.

63. Minutes, ACC EC, 26 February 1963, ACC Archives.

64. George Fry & Associates, General Survey, ACC, 1 May 1963, with BOT reports, 1959–1963, ACC Archives. They interviewed Louis Bishop Jr., Eliot Corday, Grey Dimond, Simon Dack, George Griffith, John LaDue, Philip Reichert, and Henry Russek. The college had 2,137 members at the time; their geographical distribution in 1960 is depicted in the figure on p. 61.

65. Fry & Associates, General Survey.

66. William D. Nelligan, interview by W. Bruce Fye, 28 December 1993, Bethesda, Md.

67. Dimond interview.

68. E. G. Dimond to G. E. Burch, 6 April 1965, correspondence Dim-Dis, Burch Papers. Nelligan was born in Halstead, Kansas.

69. E. Corday to W. D. Nelligan, cApril 1965, in Corday correspondence, ACC Archives.

70. W. D. Nelligan to E. Corday, 29 April 1965, in Corday file, ACC Archives.

71. There has been one exception to the ACC's one-year presidential term limit. Academic cardiologist Charles Fisch served two terms (1975–1977) when the college's executive committee asked president-elect Warren Taylor (a cardiothoracic surgeon who was a protégé of Dwight Harken) not to assume the presidency after the *Boston Globe* published an article reporting excessive mortality in the heart surgery program he ran at a suburban Boston hospital. Warren J. Taylor, interview by W. Bruce Fye, 15 June 1992, Boston.

72. "Office relocation committee," *Am. J. Cardiol.* 16 (1965): 311. Corday denied that discussions regarding the move to Washington included a consideration of the college's becoming politically active. Minutes, ACC BOT, 26 June 1965, ACC Archives.

73. L. T. Coggeshall, *Planning for Medical Progress through Education* (Washington, D.C.: Association of American Medical Colleges, 1965), quote p. 89.

74. G. Calver to S. Dack, 5 May 1965, papers and documents of prominent college members, file 1, ACC Archives.

75. I. Brotman to E. Corday, 7 June 1965, permanent headquarters site file, ACC Archives.

76. "Report," 11 June 1965, permanent headquarters site file, ACC Archives. See Minutes, ACC BOT, 20 June 1965, ACC Archives.

77. E. G. Dimond to P. D. White, 13 July 1965, box 41, file 32, White Papers.

78. "President's report" to the BOT, 28 January 1966, with unbound minutes, ACC BOT, 2 February 1966, ACC Archives. For the National Library of Medicine, see W. D. Miles, *A History of the National Library of Medicine* (Bethesda, Md.: National Library of Medicine, 1982).

79. Samuel M. Fox, interview by W. Bruce Fye, 17 March 1993, Anaheim, Calif.

80. W. D. Nelligan to E. Corday, 17 May 1965, in permanent headquarters site file, ACC Archives. Emphasis in original.

81. E. Corday to G. E. Burch, 6 May 1965, Burch Papers.

82. G. E. Burch to E. Corday, 11 May 1965, Burch Papers.

83. Dimond interview. Although he did not support the effort, Dimond feels that Corday was very effective in his dealings with legislators. Nelligan agrees: "Corday proved to be the most effective voice the college had on Capitol Hill." W. D. Nelligan to W. B. Fye, August 1994.

84. *Senate Subcommittee on Health. Hearings on Combating Heart Disease, Cancer, Stroke, and Other Major Diseases. (S.596). 89th Cong., 1st sess.* (Washington, D.C.: GPO, 1965), quote p. 251.

85. "Bethesda Conferences," *Am. J. Cardiol.* 17 (1966): 294–295. Between 1961 and 1967, Democratic Congressman Lawrence Fountain's Subcommittee on Intergovernmental Relations held a series of hearings on NIH policies and practices that raised questions of mismanagement and inefficiency. They are summarized in *The Administration of Research Grants in the Public Health Service, Ninth Report by the Committee on Government Operations. 90th Cong., 1st sess.* (Washington, D.C.: GPO, 1967), pp. 9–12.

86. Eliot Corday, interview by W. Bruce Fye, 13 November 1991, Anaheim, Calif.

87. "Training technics for the coronary care unit," *Am. J. Cardiol.* 17 (1966): 736–747. See also B. Lown, A. M. Fakhro, W. B. Hood, and G. W. Thorn, "The coronary care unit," *JAMA* 199 (1967): 188–198.

88. "Report on the Bethesda conference committee," Minutes ACC BOT, 26 June 1966. Also Corday interview.

89. L. Hill to E. Corday, 26 June 1966, Corday correspondence file, ACC Archives. Corday also encouraged Rhode Island Congressman John Fogarty to support government funding to help build and staff coronary care units in America's larger hospitals. E. Corday to J. Fogarty, 12 July 1966, Bethesda Conference 1965–66 file, ACC Archives.

90. Minutes, ACC BOT, 26 June 1966, ACC Archives. See also S. Sperling, *Animal Liberators: Research and Morality* (Berkeley: Univ. of California Press, 1988).

91. E. Freidson, "Foreword," in *The Making of Rehabilitation: A Political Economy of Medical Specialization, 1890–1980*, G. Gritzer and A. Arluke (Berkeley: Univ. of California Press, 1985), pp. xi–xxii, quote pp. xviii–xix.

92. J. Helwig Jr. to W. D. Nelligan, 25 May 1966, Nelligan general correspondence 1966 file, ACC Archives.

93. G. Griffith to W. D. Nelligan, [cJune 1966], written on W.D. Nelligan to J. Helwig Jr., 31 May 1966, ACC Archives.

94. W. D. Nelligan to J. Helwig Jr., 11 July 1966, Nelligan general correspondence 1966 file, ACC Archives.

95. W. C. Felch and C. C. Greene Jr., *Aspiration and Achievement: The Story of the American Society of Internal Medicine, 1956–1981* (Washington, D.C.: ASIM, 1981). See

also E. C. Rosenow Jr., *History of the American College of Physicians: Executive Perspectives 1959–1977* (Philadelphia: ACP, 1984), esp. pp. 15–16, 62.

96. NHI budget data from *NHLBI Fact Book 1993*, p. 63. See also Strickland, *Politics, Science, and Dread Disease,* esp. pp. 158–209.

97. Extracts from Congressional Record, 23 June 1967, quoted in E. Corday, "Report of the special committee for liaison with congress, the Surgeon General, and the National Institutes of Health," September 1967, Minutes, ACC BOT, 1965–1969, ACC Archives.

98. F. Arkus, "Roles, Shoals and Goals," 1967, speeches file, AHA Archives.

99. W. M. Moore, *Fighting for Life: The Story of the American Heart Association 1911–1975* (Dallas: AHA, 1983), p. 270, and *NHLBI Fact Book 1993*, p. 63.

100. Extracts from Congressional Record, 23 June 1967.

101. W. Likoff, "Appropriations for cardiovascular research," *Am. J. Cardiol.* 20 (1967): 289–291.

102. Nelligan interview.

103. DeBakey interview.

104. Minutes, ACC BOT, 19 October 1967, ACC Archives.

105. Ibid.

106. Ibid.

107. Nelligan interview.

108. W. Likoff, "A master plan for postgraduate education," *Am. J. Cardiol.* 19 (1967): 474–475.

109. H. M. Pollard, "The 'territorial imperative' of medicine," *Ann. Intern. Med.* 71 (1969): 407–413, quotes pp. 412–413.

110. E. G. Dimond to E. Corday, 4 September 1969, Burch Papers.

111. A. M. Katz to E. G. Dimond, 16 September 1969, Burch Papers.

112. Minutes, ACC BOT, 12 November 1970, ACC Archives.

113. *Health in America: 1776–1976,* pp. 205–210.

114. Minutes, ACC BOT, 17 November 1972, ACC Archives.

115. Minutes, ACC BOT, 14 February 1973, ACC Archives.

116. Ibid.

117. Minutes, ACC BOT, 10 February 1974, ACC Archives.

118. Moore, *Fighting for Life;* see esp. pp. 120–121.

119. DeBakey interview.

120. W. G. Austen, "Presidential address," *Circulation* 59 (1979): 614A-616A, quote p. 615A.

121. Minutes, ACC BOT, 12 November 1970, ACC Archives.

122. Minutes, ACC BOT, 19 October 1967, ACC Archives. See also E. G. Dimond to W. Likoff, 13 July 1967, Heart House Committee 1965–75 file, ACC Archives.

123. D. E. Harken, S. Dack, and G. C. Griffith to ACC governors, 20 April 1970, in Heart House committee 1970 file, ACC Archives.

124. Minutes, ACC BOT, 27 February 1968, ACC Archives. See also "Interim report: Budget, finance, resource and endowments committee," 21 November 1968, ACC Archives.

125. D. E. Harken to J. E. Doherty, 20 April 1970, Heart House Committee 1970 file, ACC Archives.

126. R. W. Gifford Jr. to D. E. Harken, 5 July 1970, Heart House Committee 1970 file, ACC Archives.

127. R. N. Class to D. E. Harken, 23 June 1970, Heart House Committee 1970 file, ACC Archives.

128. *Senate Subcommittee on Health. Hearings on Combating Heart Disease, Cancer, Stroke, and Other Major Diseases (S.596). 89th Cong., 1st sess.* (Washington, D.C.: GPO, 1965).

129. E. Corday to B. L. Martz, 12 August 1971, Heart House Committee 1971 file, ACC Archives.

130. T. G. Kummer to R. L. Herting, 10 September 1973, Heart House Committee 1973 file, ACC Archives.

131. Untitled Heart House fund raising pamphlet (4 pp.), Bethesda, Md., ACC, 1973, in Heart House Committee file, ACC Archives.

132. W. D. Nelligan to D. B. Carmichael, 27 November 1974, in Heart House Committee 1974 file, ACC Archives.

133. "The ASCP educational center: No other medical group has anything like it," *Lab. Med.* 2 (1971): 11–18, 21–28. Also B. L. Martz to W. B. Fye, March 1993.

134. T. Cooper to D. E. Harken, 24 October 1976, Heart House Committee 1976 file, ACC Archives.

CHAPTER 8   *Fueling the Growth of Cardiology: Patients, Procedures, and Profits*

1. I. M. Moriyama, D. E. Krueger, and J. Stamler, *Cardiovascular Diseases in the United States* (Cambridge: Harvard Univ. Press, 1971), esp. pp. 91–101. See also E. Braunwald, "The golden age of cardiology," in *An Era in Cardiovascular Medicine*, eds. S. B. Knoebel and S. Dack (New York: Elsevier Science Publishing, 1991), pp. 1–4.

2. R. D. Pruitt, "Coronary care units: A partisan view," *Cardiovascular Research Center Bulletin* 4 (1966): 67–68.

3. E. Corday, "The coronary care area: A tiger by the tail," *Am. J. Cardiol.* 16 (1965): 466–468, quote p. 466. See also Moriyama et al., *Cardiovascular Diseases in the United States*, esp. pp. 85–101.

4. Corday, "Coronary care area," quote p. 466.

5. Ibid.

6. *Proceedings of the National Conference on Coronary Care Units* (Washington, D.C.: GPO, 1968).

7. T. Killip and J. T. Kimball, "A survey of the coronary care unit: Concept and results," *Prog. Cardiovasc. Dis.* 11 (1968): 45–52, quote p. 50.

8. B. S. Bloom and O. L. Peterson, "Patient needs and medical-care planning: The coronary-care unit as a model," *N. Engl. J. Med.* 290 (1974): 1171–1177, quotes

pp. 1173, 1172. See also B. S. Bloom and O. L. Peterson, "End results, cost and productivity of coronary-care units," *N. Engl. J. Med.* 288 (1973): 72–78.

9. G. D. Curfman, "Shorter hospital stay for myocardial infarction," *N. Engl. J. Med.* 318 (1988): 1123–1125.

10. L. E. Meltzer and J. R. Kitchell, "The development and current status of coronary care," in *Textbook of Coronary Care* ed. L. E. Meltzer (Philadelphia: Charles Press Publishers, 1972), pp. 3–25. See also W. B. Fye, "Acute myocardial infarction: A historical summary," in *Acute Myocardial Infarction,* ed. B. J. Gersh and S. H. Rahimtoola (New York: Elsevier, 1991), pp. 3–13.

11. E. Braunwald, "Efforts to limit myocardial infarct size: Historical considerations," *Eur. Heart J.* 6 (1985): E1–E4.

12. H. J. C. Swan, W. Ganz, and J. S. Forrester, "Catheterization of the heart in man with the use of a flow-directed balloon-tipped catheter," *N. Engl. J. Med.* 283 (1970): 447–451. A comprehensive summary of all aspects of building, equipping, staffing, and operating a coronary care unit (illustrated with many photographs) is C. W. Clipson and J. J. Wehrer, *Planning for Cardiac Care* (Ann Arbor, Mich.: Health Administration Press, 1972).

13. A. F. Crocetti, "Cardiac diagnostic and surgical facilities in the United States," *Public Health Rep.* 80 (1965): 1035–1053. A summary of these 1961 data is presented in Chapter 5.

14. F. M. Sones Jr. and E. K. Shirey, "Cine coronary arteriography," *Mod. Concepts Cardiovasc. Dis.* 31 (1962): 735–738. See also W. B. Fye, "Coronary arteriography: It took a long time," *Circulation* 70 (1984): 781–787.

15. *Program. ACC 11th Annual Convention, 1962* (New York: ACC, 1962). The conference was moderated by William Likoff and J. Stauffer Lehman.

16. W. H. Sewell, "Coronary arteriography by the Sones technique: Technical considerations," *Am. J. Roentgenol.* 95 (1965): 673–683.

17. W. Heberden, "Some account of a disorder of the breast," *Medical Transactions, College of Physicians of London* 2 (1772): 59–67.

18. R. G. Favaloro, "Saphenous vein autograft replacement of severe segmental coronary artery occlusion: Operative technique," *Ann. Thorac. Surg.* 5 (1968): 334–339. See also R. G. Favaloro, *The Challenging Dream of Heart Surgery: From the Pampas to Cleveland* (Boston: Little, Brown, 1994).

19. D. B. Effler, L. K. Groves, F. M. Sones Jr., and E. K. Shirey, "Increased myocardial perfusion by internal mammary artery implant: Vineberg's operation," *Ann. Surg.* 158 (1963): 526–536.

20. H. A. Zimmerman, "The dilemma of surgery in the treatment of coronary artery disease," *Am. Heart J.* 77 (1969): 577–578. He listed most of the operations that had been invented to treat angina, including Vineberg's mammary implant procedure, omental grafts, endarterectomy, venous patching, splenic artery implantation, gastric epiploic implantation, the Senn procedure, gas endarterectomy, Dacron prosthesis, and poudrage. Other cardiologists shared Zimmerman's skepticism. Paul White thanked him for writing an "excellent editorial on the dilemma of surgery in the treatment of coronary artery disease." P. D. White to H. A. Zimmerman, 23 June 1969, Burch Papers. See also A. Selzer and W. J. Kerth, "Surgical treatment of coronary artery disease: Too fast, too soon?" *Am. J. Cardiol.* 28 (1971): 490–492.

21. D. B. Effler to H. A. Zimmerman, 16 May 1969, Burch Papers.

22. R. G. Favaloro, D. B. Effler, L. K. Groves, F. M. Sones Jr., and D. J. G. Fergusson, "Myocardial revascularization by internal mammary artery implant procedures," *J. Thorac. Cardiovasc. Surg.* 54 (1967): 359–368.

23. Minutes National Heart and Lung Advisory Council, 17–18 June 1971, NHLBI Archives.

24. Coronary artery by-pass surgery: Recommendations for a program of research, the ad-hoc policy advisory board on coronary artery surgery of the NHLI, 31 August 1972, Office of the Assistant Director, NHLBI. The author thanks Peter Frommer, M.D., for this reference.

25. Report to accompany HR 15417, 21 June 1972, 92nd Cong., 2d sess., calendar no. 854, report no. 92–894. Prevalence data from Moriyama et al., *Cardiovascular Diseases in the United States*, table 4.12, p. 87.

26. W. Murrell, "Nitro-glycerine as a remedy for angina pectoris," *Lancet* 1 (1879): 80–81, 113–115, 151—152, 225–227. See also W. B. Fye, "Vasodilator therapy for angina pectoris: The intersection of homeopathy and scientific medicine," *J. Hist. Med. Allied Sci.* 45 (1990): 317–340.

27. C. K. Friedberg, "Caution and coronary artery surgery: Timeo chirurgos et dona ferentes," *Circulation* 45 (1972): 727–730.

28. R. S. Ross, "Surgery for coronary artery disease placed in perspective," *Bull. N.Y. Acad. Med.* 48 (1972): 1163–1178, quote p. 1170.

29. E. Braunwald, "Coronary-artery surgery at the crossroads," *N. Engl. J. Med.* 297 (1977): 661–663. For a discussion of CASS, the Veterans Administration Cooperative Trial, and other controlled trials of surgical procedures for angina, see T. J. Moore, *Heart Failure* (New York: Random House, 1989), pp. 106–125.

30. In 1991 approximately 65 percent of America's 15,998 self-designated cardiologists performed cardiac catheterization. Source: *ACC Fact Sheet*, spring 1992 (Bethesda, Md.: ACC). This does not include the Swan-Ganz catheter, used by many practitioners.

31. J. A. Veiga-Pires and R. G. Grainger, eds., *Pioneers in Angiography: The Portuguese School of Angiography* (Lancaster, U.K.: MTP Press, 1982).

32. See T. Doby, *Development of Angiography and Cardiovascular Catheterization* (Littleton, Mass.: Publishing Sciences Group, 1976); A. Cournand, "Cardiac catheterization: Development of the technique, its contributions to experimental medicine, and its initial applications in man," *Acta Med. Scand.* suppl. 579 (1975): 3–32; and J. F. Goodwin, "The practical value of cardiac catheterization," *Practitioner* 169 (1952): 40–48. In some centers surgeons performed catheterizations and angiography, but that practice had virtually ceased by the 1960s.

33. D. S. Lukas, "The relation of cardiac catheterization to cardiovascular surgery," *Bull. N.Y. Acad. Med.* 29 (1953): 668–676, quote p. 671. See also R. B. Dickerson, "Performance of angiocardiography and cardiac catheterization as a combined procedure," *Am. Heart J.* 47 (1954): 252–269.

34. C. T. Dotter and I. Steinberg, *Angiocardiography* (New York: Paul B. Hoeber, 1951), quote p. 176.

35. For radiologists' perspective on why they lost coronary angiography, see J. M. Taveras, "Subspecialization in radiology: Response to a need," *Am. J.*

Roentgenol. 148 (1987): 465–469, and L. F. Rogers and O. W. Linton, "Turf and technology: Responsibilities and realities," *Radiology* 176 (1990): 319–320.

36. H. L. Stein, "An emergency angiocardiography service," *Radiology* 84 (1965): 115–116.

37. H. M. Marks, "Medical technologies: Social contexts and consequences," in *Companion Encyclopedia of the History of Medicine,* ed. W. F. Bynum and R. Porter (New York: Routledge, 1993), 2: 1592–1618, quote pp. 1596–1597. See also R. Brecher and E. Brecher, *The Rays: A History of Radiology in the United States and Canada* (Baltimore: Williams and Wilkins, 1959).

38. R. S. Ross, "Clinical applications of coronary arteriography," *Circulation* 27 (1963): 107–112, quote p. 111.

39. H. L. Abrams and D. F. Adams, "The coronary arteriogram: Structural and functional aspects," *N. Engl. J. Med.* 281 (1969): 1276–1285, 1336–1342.

40. S. Paulin, "Coronary arteriography: Radiologic aspects," *Adv. Cardiol.* 4 (1970): 258–266, quote p. 260. See also R. S. Kurtzman, "Coronary arteriography," *Med. Clin. North Am.* 46 (1962): 1583–1598, and K. Amplatz, "Technics of coronary arteriography," *Circulation* 27 (1963): 101–106.

41. W. W. L. Glenn, "Some account of the early years of cardiac surgery," *Conn. Med.* 44 (1980): 338–344.

42. "Coronary angiography," *Lancet* 1 (1966): 1084–1085.

43. H. A. Baltaxe, "The current uses of coronary angiography," *Radiol. Clin. North Am.* 9 (1971): 597–607, quotes pp. 597, 607. See also R. I. White, A. E. James, and M. W. Donner, "Cardiovascular radiology: Current status," *Am. J. Roentgenol.* 119 (1973): 636–638.

44. M. P. Judkins and M. P. Gander, "Prevention of complications of coronary arteriography," *Circulation* 49 (1974): 599–602.

45. C. E. Hansing, K. Hammermeister, K. Prindle, R. Twiss, R. R. Schwindt, B. Gowing, et al., "Cardiac catheterization experience in hospitals without cardiovascular surgery programs," *Cathet. Cardiovasc. Diagn.* 3 (1977): 207–214.

46. F. M. Sones Jr., "The Society for Cardiac Angiography," *Cathet. Cardiovasc. Diagn.* 4 (1978): 233–234. See also W. C. Sheldon, "A short history of the Society for Cardiac Angiography: The first decade," *Cathet. Cardiovasc. Diagn.* 17 (1989): 1–4. Reflecting the active involvement of radiologists in the field of cardiac imaging, the Society of Cardiovascular Radiology had been formed in 1974 during a meeting of the Radiological Society of North America. A. B. Crummy, "Chronological history of the Society of Cardiovascular and Interventional Radiology from 1973 to 1989," *Radiology* 174 (1990): 932–936.

47. "Standards for training in cardiac catheterization and angiography," *Cathet. Cardiovasc. Diagn.* 6 (1980): 345–348.

48. J. D. Howell, "Diagnostic technologies: X-rays, electrocardiograms, and CAT scans," *S. Calif. Law Rev.* 65 (1991): 529–564.

49. In 1993 only sixteen fellows were enrolled in the nation's nineteen cardiovascular radiology fellowship programs, and they were being trained to perform noncardiac vascular procedures. D. C. Levin and T. Matteucci, "'Turf battles' over imaging and interventional procedures in community hospitals: Survey results,"

Radiology 176 (1990): 321–324. See also R. D. White, L. M. Boxt, and L. Wexler, "Cardiac radiology: A survey of its current status," *Invest. Radiol.* 28 (1993): 545–549.

50. The diversity of early workers in diagnostic ultrasound is reflected in the participants in a 1965 conference; see C. C. Grossman, J. H. Holmes, C. J. Joyner, and E. W. Purnell, eds., *Diagnostic Ultrasound: Proceedings of the First International Conference, University of Pittsburgh, 1965* (New York: Plenum Press, 1966), pp. vii–xiii.

51. I. Edler to W. B. Fye, 10 May 1993.

52. I. Edler, "Cardiac studies by ultrasounds [*sic*]," in *Cardiology: An Encyclopedia of the Cardiovascular System,* ed. A. Luisada (New York: McGraw-Hill, 1962): suppl. 1, chapter 17, pp. 79–92, and L. J. Kotler, "The History of Echocardiography" (B.A. thesis, University of Pennsylvania, 1986). See also C. H. Hertz, "The interaction of physicians, physicists and industry in the development of echocardiography," *Ultrasound Med. Biol.* 1 (1973): 3–11. See also S. Effert, D. Bleifeld, F. J. Deupmann, and J. Karitsiotis, "Diagnostic value of ultrasonic cardiography," *Br. J. Radiol.* 37 (1964): 920–927.

53. The term "noninvasive" is used to differentiate echocardiography and nuclear cardiology techniques from invasive procedures in which a catheter is inserted into the vascular system.

54. H. Feigenbaum, J. A. Waldhausen, and L. P. Hyde, "Ultrasound diagnosis of pericardial effusion," *JAMA* 191 (1965): 107–110. See also H. Feigenbaum, *Echocardiography* (Philadelphia: Lea & Febiger, 1972), quote p. 3, and S. Chang and J. K. Chang, "A historical review of echocardiographic detection of pericardial effusion," *Jpn. Heart J.* 22 (1981): 789–800.

55. *Program, American College of Cardiology, Fifteenth Annual Convention, 1966, New York.* ACC Archives.

56. "History of the American Society of Echocardiography" (Raleigh, N.C.: American Society of Echocardiography, 1983). This society for specialists with an interest in this single-organ-specific technology was open to echocardiography technicians as well as physicians. It had 1,035 members by 1976, the year it was incorporated. The society's official journal, the *Journal of the American Society of Echocardiography,* appeared in 1988, and its first national scientific meeting was held two years later.

57. Harvey Feigenbaum, interview by W. Bruce Fye, 8 November 1993, Atlanta, Ga. See also J. H. Holmes, "Ultrasonic diagnostic techniques applied to the cardiovascular system," *National Conference on Cardiovascular Disease* 2 (1964): 279–281.

58. P. R. Manning and T. A. Denson, "How cardiologists learn about echocardiography: A reminder for medical educators and legislators," *Ann. Intern. Med.* (1979): 469–471.

59. B. Surawicz, "How to cope with the new technology? The knowledge and the prudence," *Am. J. Cardiol.* 43 (1979): 1249–1250.

60. H. J. C. Swan to R. Gorlin, 30 August 1973, general correspondence 1974 file, ACC Archives.

61. "ACC Long Range Planning Committee Report," with Minutes ACC BOT, 13 September 1975, ACC Archives.

62. C. V. Cimmino, "Let us not lose echocardiography," *Radiology* 130 (1979): 813–814.

63. See R. G. Evens, "Whose turf is imaging? Professional responsibility for imaging procedures in hospital practice," *Am. J. Roentgenol.* 151 (1988): 261–262.

64. H. N. Wagner Jr., "The development of cardiovascular nuclear medicine," in *Cardiovascular Nuclear Medicine*, eds. H. W. Strauss, B. Pitt, and A. E. James (St. Louis: C.V. Mosby, 1974), pp. 1–5.

65. S. C. Bushong, *The Development of Radiation Protection in Diagnostic Radiology* (Cleveland: CRC Press, 1973). See also J. S. Walker, "The Atomic Energy Commission and the politics of radiation protection, 1967–1971," *Isis* 85 (1994): 57–78.

66. Minutes, ACC BOT, 28 September 1975, ACC Archives.

67. "Nuclear cardiology," *Cardiology* 11, no. 2 (1982): 4. See also "NRC clarifies training requirements," *ACC Washington Update* (February 1992): 6.

68. W. M. Chardack, A. A. Gage, and W. Greatbatch, "A transistorized, self-contained, implantable pacemaker for the long-term correction of complete heart block," *Surgery* 48 (1960): 643–654.

69. P. D. White, *Heart Disease*, 4th ed. (New York: Macmillan, 1951), quote p. 944.

70. S. M. Spencer, "Making a heartbeat behave," *Saturday Evening Post* (4 March 1961): 13–14, 48, 50.

71. Earl Bakken, interview by W. Bruce Fye, 12 November 1991, Anaheim, Calif. Several pioneers of pacemakers contributed to a 1963 symposium; see W. W. L. Glenn, ed., "Cardiac pacemakers," *Ann. N.Y. Acad. Sci.* 111 (1964): 813–1122. See also V. Parsonnet and M. Manhardt, "Permanent pacing of the heart: 1952 to 1976," *Am. J. Cardiol.* 39 (1977): 250–256.

72. Several brands of early permanent pacemakers are described and pictured in H. Siddons and E. Sowton, *Cardiac Pacemakers* (Springfield, Ill.: Charles C. Thomas, 1967), pp. 269–326.

73. D. E. Harken, "Pacemakers, past-makers, and the paced: An informal history from A to Z (Aldini to Zoll)," *Biomed. Instrum. Technol.* 25 (1991): 299–321.

74. Minutes, ACC BOT, 9 March 1980, ACC Archives. See also V. Parsonnet, "Cardiac pacing as a subspecialty," *Am. J. Cardiol.* 59 (1987): 989–991.

75. Minutes, ACC BOT, 9 March 1980, ACC Archives.

76. S. B. Foote, *Managing the Medical Arms Race: Public Policy and Medical Device Innovation* (Berkeley: Univ. of California Press, 1992), quote p. 109. See also J. D. Bronzino, V. H. Smith, and M. L. Wade, *Medical Technology and Society: An Interdisciplinary Perspective* (Cambridge: The MIT Press, 1990), esp. pp. 170–175.

77. L. B. Russell, *Technology in Hospitals: Medical Advances and Their Diffusion* (Washington, D.C.: Brookings Institution, 1979).

78. J. Turow, *Playing Doctor: Television, Storytelling, and Medical Power* (New York: Oxford Univ. Press, 1989).

79. K. T. Jackson, *Crabgrass Frontier: The Suburbanization of the United States* (New York: Oxford Univ. Press, 1985).

80. A. R. Henderson, R. R. Meijer, H. Black, and G. Oteifa, "Some nontechnical aspects of open-heart surgery in the community hospital," *JAMA* 170 (1959): 28–32,

quote p. 93. A more accurate estimate of the number of infants born with congenital defects of the cardiovascular system is 20,000. See Moriyama et al., *Cardiovascular Diseases in the United States,* p. 257. Cardiac surgery would not be necessary (or possible) in all of these individuals; it would depend on the type and severity of the defect.

81. Crocetti, "Cardiac diagnostic and surgical facilities."

82. K. L. White and M. A. Ibrahim, "The distribution of cardiovascular disease in the community," *Ann. Intern. Med.* 58 (1963): 627–636.

83. Appendix 2 [attached to summary minutes], Inter-Society Commission for Heart Disease Resources, first Advisory Committee meeting, 16 January 1969, Burch Papers. According to a member of the commission, their "guidelines have been widely quoted and used by some groups, [but] they were never implemented to any great degree at the local level, which was the original plan." F. H. Adams to W. B. Fye, 5 June 1992.

84. Foote, *Managing the Medical Arms Race,* table 3, page 90. See Russell, *Technology in Hospitals,* esp. pp. 30–31.

85. D. B. Effler, "Introduction," in *Surgical Treatment of Coronary Arteriosclerosis,* R. G. Favaloro (Baltimore: Williams & Wilkins, 1970), pp. xi–xvi, quote p. xi.

86. The technique of multiple bypass grafts was especially significant because it could be used to treat patients with severe, multivessel coronary disease. W. D. Johnson, R. J. Flemma, D. Lepley Jr., and E. H. Ellison, "Extended treatment of severe coronary disease: A total surgical approach," *Ann. Surg.* 170 (1969): 460–470.

87. I. S. Wright and D. T. Fredrickson, eds., *Cardiovascular Diseases: Guidelines for Prevention and Care. Reports of the Inter-Society Commission for Heart Disease Resources* (Washington, D.C.: GPO, 1973), quote p. 78. The committee members are listed on p. xi.

88. W. W. L. Glenn, "Some reflections on the coronary bypass operation," *Circulation* 45 (1972): 869–877.

89. A. Ribicoff and P. Danaceau, *The American Medical Machine* (New York: Saturday Review Press, 1972), pp. 90–91.

90. Russell, *Technology in Hospitals,* esp. pp. 136–141.

91. Z. Y. Dyckman, *A Study of Physicians' Fees* (Washington, D.C.: GPO, 1979).

92. R. G. Petersdorf, "Internal medicine 1976: Consequences of subspecialization and technology," *Ann. Intern. Med.* 84 (1976): 92–94.

93. J. A. Barondess, "Technology in medicine: Some associated problems," *Forum on Medicine* (April 1978): 26–27, 31–33.

94. T. A. Preston and R. G. Petersdorf, "Are there too many cardiologists and are they doing the wrong thing?" in *Current Controversies in Cardiovascular Disease,* ed. E. Rapaport (Philadelphia: W. B. Saunders, 1980), pp. 3–20, quote p. 15.

95. D. M. Fox, *Health Policies, Health Politics: The British and American Experience, 1911–1965* (Princeton: Princeton Univ. Press, 1986), quote p. 191.

96. Quoted in Ribicoff and Danaceau, *American Medical Machine,* pp. 87–88.

97. Ibid., pp. 12, 71.

98. *Source Book of Health Insurance Data, 1993* (Washington, D.C.: Health Insurance Association of America, 1994), table 4.6, p. 84.

99. For Certificate-of-Need legislation, see S. S. Blume, *Insight and Industry: On the Dynamics of Technological Change in Medicine* (Cambridge: MIT Press, 1992).

100. L. T. Coggeshall, *Planning for Medical Progress through Education* (Washington, D.C.: Association of American Medical Colleges, 1965), esp. pp. 14–31. See also J. D. Howell, "Lowell T. Coggeshall and American medical education: 1901–1987," *Acad. Med.* 67 (1992): 711–718.

101. J. S. Millis, ed., *The Graduate Education of Physicians: The Report of the Citizens Commission on Graduate Medical Education* (Chicago: AMA, 1966), quotes pp. 39, 30.

102. W. G. Rothstein, *American Medical Schools and the Practice of Medicine, a History* (New York: Oxford Univ. Press, 1987), p. 285.

103. Richard S. Ross, interview by W. Bruce Fye, 11 June 1993, Baltimore. See also V. W. Lippard and E. Purcell, *Case Histories of Ten New Medical Schools* (New York: Josiah Macy, Jr. Foundation, 1972).

104. *The President's Commission on Heart Disease, Cancer and Stroke. Report to the President. Volume 2* (Washington, D.C.: GPO, 1965), quote p. 90.

105. Hearings Before a Subcommittee of the [House] Committee on Appropriations. *Departments of Labor and Health, Education, and Welfare Appropriations for 1967, 89th Cong., 2nd sess. Part 4. Department of Health, Education, and Welfare. National Institutes of Health* (Washington, D.C.: GPO, 1966), p. 473. See also Minutes, NAHC, 13–14 March 1969, NHLBI Archives.

106. Senate Committee on Appropriations. *Report to Accompany HR13111. Calendar No. 607. 91st Cong., 1st sess. Report No. 91–610* (Washington, D.C.: GPO, 1969).

107. H. Margulies and L. S. Bloch, *Foreign Medical Graduates in the United States* (Cambridge: Harvard Univ. Press, 1969). See also I. Butter and R. G. Sweet, "Licensure of foreign medical graduates: An historical perspective," *Milbank Q.* 55 (1977): 315–340. For a recent perspective, see M. E. Whitcomb, "Correcting the oversupply of specialists by limiting residencies for graduates of foreign medical schools," *N. Engl. J. Med.* 333 (1995): 454–456.

108. Ribicoff and Danaceau, *American Medical Machine*, quote p. 30.

109. W. G. Menke, "Divided labor: The doctor as specialist," *Ann. Intern. Med.* 72 (1970): 943–950.

110. S. M. Shortell, "Occupational prestige differences within the medical and allied health professions," *Soc. Sci. Med.* 8 (1974): 1–9. Emphasis in original.

111. E. M. Kennedy, *In Critical Condition: The Crisis in America's Health Care* (New York: Simon & Schuster, 1972), quote p. 190.

112. J. K. Iglehart, "Health report: Kennedy effort to revise health manpower carries over to '75," *Natl. Journal Reports* 6 (1974): 1949–1952.

113. R. S. Daniels and R. W. Vilter, "President Nixon's budget proposals and the medical colleges," *Ann. Intern. Med.* 79 (1973): 127–129, quote p. 129.

114. Ross interview.

115. William D. Nelligan, interview by W. Bruce Fye, 28 December 1993, Bethesda, Md.

116. Minutes, ACC BOT, 14 February 1973, ACC Archives.

117. Ross interview.

118. R. H. Ebert, "Biomedical research policy: A re-evaluation," *N. Engl. J. Med.* 289 (1973): 348–351, quote p. 351. See Chapter 7 for Wright's statements regarding physician workforce included in the 1965 report of the President's Commission on Heart Disease, chaired by DeBakey.

119. Ribicoff and Danaceau, *American Medical Machine,* quote p. 166.

120. A. G. Swanson, "Graduate education: Once for the exceptional, now essential for all," *J. Med. Educ.* 48 (1973): 183–185, quote p. 184.

121. F. H. Adams and R. C. Mendenhall, "Profile of the cardiologist: Training and manpower requirements for the specialist in adult cardiovascular disease," *Am. J. Cardiol.* 34 (1974): 389–456.

122. W. H. Pritchard and W. H. Abelmann, "Future manpower needs in cardiology," *Am. J. Cardiol.* 34 (1974): 444–448.

123. A. Relman, "The responsible role of a chairman of the department of medicine in postgraduate training," *Am. J. Cardiol.* 36 (1975): 563–564.

124. H. D. McIntosh to W. D. Nelligan, 13 November 1974, in general correspondence 1974 file, ACC Archives.

125. R. D. Cotton, "Pending federal legislation and postgraduate training," *Am. J. Cardiol.* 36 (1975): 558–559.

126. "Washington news," *Cardiology* 3, no. 3 (1974): 4.

127. *Health Professions Educational Assistance Act of 1976. PL 94–484* (Washington, D.C.: GPO, 1976).

128. J. C. Burnham, "American medicine's golden age: What happened to it," *Science* 215 (1982): 1474–1479. See, for example, J. Barzun, "The professions under siege," *Harper's Magazine* (October 1978): 61–68.

129. T. Cooper, "The government's concerns regarding postgraduate training and health care delivery," *Am. J. Cardiol.* 36 (1975): 555–557.

130. E. Ginzberg, "Manpower for cardiology: No easy answers," *Am. J. Cardiol.* 37 (1976): 955–958.

131. F. H. Adams, "Who is a cardiologist?" *Am. J. Cardiol.* 35 (1975): 761–762.

132. J. G. Scannell, G. E. Brown, M. J. Buckley, P. A. Ebert, H. Laufman, C. E. Rackley, et al., "Report of the Inter-Society Commission for Heart Disease Resources: Optimal resources for cardiac surgery guidelines for program planning and evaluation," *Circulation* 52 (1975): A23–A41.

133. E. J. Levit and W. D. Holden, "Special board certification rates: A longitudinal tracking study of U.S. medical school graduates," *JAMA* 239 (1978): 407–412.

134. P. H. Futcher, *Activities of the American Board of Internal Medicine, 1967–1975* (Philadelphia: ABIM, 1988), esp. pp. 37–42.

135. Ibid., p. 41.

136. "Cardiology manpower. Ninth Bethesda conference," *Am. J. Cardiol.* 37 (1976): 941–983, quote p. 977.

137. Ibid., quotes pp. 963, 983.

138. J. F. Burnum, "What one internist does in his practice: Implications for the internist's disputed role and education," *Ann. Intern. Med.* 78 (1973): 437–444.

139. R. C. Mendenhall ed., *Cardiology Practice Study Report* (Hyattsville, Md.: DHEW, Health Resources Administration, 1978), table 3.7.2, pp. 94–95.

140. R. A. Chase, "Proliferation of certification in medical specialties: Productive or counterproductive," *N. Engl. J. Med.* 294 (1976): 497–499.

141. E. Ginzberg, "Manpower for cardiology: No easy answers," *Am. J. Cardiol.* 37 (1976): 955–958.

142. Minutes, ACC BOT, 22 February 1976, ACC Archives.

143. E. C. Rosenow Jr., *History of the American College of Physicians: Executive Perspectives 1959–1977* (Philadelphia: ACP, 1984), quote p. 341.

144. F. J. Ingelfinger, "League for beleagured internists," *N. Engl. J. Med.* 292 (1975): 589–590.

145. Rosenow, *History of the American College of Physicians,* quote p. 350.

146. R. H. Moser, *A Decade of Decision: A Physician Remembers the American College of Physicians, 1977–1986* (Philadelphia: ACP, 1991), quote p. 11.

147. For tensions among ABIM members regarding this tendency toward fragmentation of internal medicine, see Futcher, *Activities of the American Board of Internal Medicine,* pp. 37–42.

148. "Federated Council for Internal Medicine statement on manpower," *Ann. Intern. Med.* 90 (1979): 108–109.

149. B. Surawicz, "Should we reduce graduate cardiovascular training programs?" *Am. J. Cardiol.* 43 (1979): 870–871.

150. *Report of the Graduate Medical Education National Advisory Committee. September 1980. Vol. 1. GMENAC Summary Report. DHHS Pub. No. (HRA) 81–651* (Washington, D.C.: U.S. Dept. of Health and Human Services, 1981). See also D. R. McNutt, "GMENAC: Its manpower forecasting framework," *Am. J. Public Health* 71 (1981): 1116–1124.

151. U. E. Reinhardt, "The GMENAC forecast: An alternative view," *Am. J. Public Health* 71 (1981): 1149–1157, quote p. 1149.

152. M. Menken, "The coming oversupply of neurologists in the 1980s: Implications for neurology training programs," *Neurology* 32 (1982): 510–512.

153. J. E. Hoopes, "Health manpower legislation," *Plast. Reconstr. Surg.* 68 (1981): 253–258, quote p. 258.

154. *GMENAC Summary Report.*

155. "GMENAC projects 18% reduction in cardiologists needed for 1990," *Cardiology* 9, no. 4 (1980): 4.

156. "Trends in adult cardiology fellowships," *Cardiology* 16, no. 8 (1987): 1.

157. R. Fein, "Health manpower: Challenge for the eighties," *Yale J. Biol. Med.* 54 (1981): 209–218, quote p. 216.

CHAPTER 9   *The Price of Success: Tensions in and around Cardiology*

1. E. Ginzberg, *American Medicine: The Power Shift* (Totowa, N.J.: Rowman & Allanheld, 1985), esp. pp. 14–20.

2. J. F. Goodwin, "The clinical approach: Cui bono?" *European Heart J.* 12 (1991): 751–752.

3. The titles of books published during the past two decades reveal some of these tensions: J. H. Knowles, ed., *Doing Better and Feeling Worse: Health in the United States* (New York: W. W. Norton, 1977); M. J. Lepore, *Death of the Clinician: Requiem or Reveille?* (Springfield, Ill.: Charles C. Thomas, 1982); M. Silverman and P. R. Lee, *Pills, Profits, and Politics* (Berkeley: Univ. of California Press, 1974); E. H. Ahrens Jr., *The Crisis in Clinical Research: Overcoming Institutional Obstacles* (New York: Oxford Univ. Press, 1992); I. J. Lewis and C. G. Sheps, *The Sick Citadel: The American Academic Medical Center and the Public Interest* (Cambridge: Oelgeschlager, Gunn & Hain, 1983); J. T. Bennett and T. J. DiLorenzo, *Unhealthy Charities: Hazardous to Your Health and Wealth* (New York: Basic Books, 1994); R. Stevens, *In Sickness and in Wealth: American Hospitals in the Twentieth Century* (New York: Basic Books, 1989); M. A. Rodwin, *Medicine, Money, and Morals: Physicians' Conflicts of Interest* (New York: Oxford Univ. Press, 1993); S. B. Foote, *Managing the Medical Arms Race: Public Policy and Medical Device Innovation* (Berkeley: Univ. of California Press, 1992); R. W. Moss, *The Cancer Industry: Unraveling the Politics* (New York: Paragon House, 1989); and T. J. Moore, *Heart Failure: A Critical Inquiry into American Medicine and the Revolution in Heart Care* (New York: Random House, 1989).

4. See, for example, O. W. Anderson, *Health Services in the United States: A Growth Enterprise since 1875* (Ann Arbor, Mich.: Health Administration Press, 1985), and E. Ginzberg, *The Medical Triangle: Physicians, Politicians, and the Public* (Cambridge: Harvard Univ. Press, 1990).

5. J. R. E[lkinton], "The image of the American physician," *Ann. Intern. Med.* 55 (1961): 527–528. See also J. C. Burnham, "American medicine's golden age: What happened to it?" *Science* 215 (1982): 1474–1479.

6. E. Hill, "The American doctor: End of a legend," *Saturday Evening Post* (15 June 1963): 30–37.

7. G. Rosen, "Whither specialization," in *Medicine and Society: Contemporary Medical Problems in Historical Perspective* (Bryn Mawr, Pa.: Bryn Mawr College, 1971), pp. 196–219.

8. Discussing the health care needs of the elderly in cities, Kennedy wrote, "Their problem is that they need a family physician to make house calls." E. M. Kennedy, *In Critical Condition: The Crisis in America's Health Care* (New York: Simon & Schuster, 1972), quote p. 110. See pp. 234–252 for his prescription for reforming American health care.

9. R. C. Fox, "A sociological perspective on organ transplantation and hemodialysis," *Ann. N.Y. Acad. Sci.* 169 (1970): 406–428, quote p. 422.

10. F. W. Hastings and L. T. Harmison, *Artificial Heart Program Conference Proceedings, Washington, DC, 9–13 June 1969* (Washington, D.C.: GPO, 1969). See also D. P. Lubeck and J. P. Bunker, "Considering an artificial heart program," in *The Machine at the Bedside*, ed. S. J. Reiser and M. Anbar (Cambridge: Cambridge Univ. Press, 1984), pp. 247–251, and J. R. Hogness and M. VanAntwerp, eds., *The Artificial Heart: Prototypes, Policies, and Patients* (Washington, D.C.: National Academy Press, 1991).

11. Approximately one million cardiac catheterizations were performed in the United States in 1992, but there were only 557 heart transplants. See *Cardiovascular Specialists and the Economics of Medicine* (Bethesda, Md.: ACC, 1994), figure 8.1, p. 43, and *Source Book of Health Insurance Data, 1993* (Washington, D.C.: Health Insurance Association of America, 1994), figure 5.2, p. 100.

12. For estimates on the prevalence of various forms of cardiovascular disease in the United States at this time, see *Heart Disease in Adults, United States, 1960–1962,* National Center for Health Statistics, series 11, no. 6 (Washington, D.C.: GPO, 1964).

13. See H. H. Fudenberg and V. L. Melnick, eds., *Biomedical Scientists and Public Policy* (New York: Plenum Press, 1978).

14. *Research in the Service of Man. Hearings before the Subcommittee on Government Research of the Committee on Government Operations United States Senate. 90th Cong., 1st sess.* (Washington, D.C.: GPO, 1967), quote p. 46.

15. J. E. Bishop, 26 August 1970, quoted in Moss, *Cancer Industry,* p. [4].

16. J. A. Shannon, "Federal support of biomedical sciences: Development and academic impact," *J. Med. Educ.* 51 (suppl. to July 1976), quote p. 14. See also D. M. Fox, *Power and Illness: The Failure and Future of American Health Policy* (Berkeley: Univ. of California Press, 1993).

17. *Public Law 92–423, 92nd Cong., 2d sess. (19 September 1972) National Heart, Blood Vessel, Lung and Blood Act of 1972* (Washington, D.C.: GPO, 1972), quote pp. 784–785. The government had passed a series of laws (most notably in 1906 and 1938) to regulate the pharmaceutical industry. See J. H. Young, *The Medical Messiahs: A Social History of Health Quackery in Twentieth-Century America* (Princeton: Princeton Univ. Press, 1967), and C. O. Jackson, *Food and Drug Legislation in the New Deal* (Princeton: Princeton Univ. Press, 1970).

18. Foote, *Managing the Medical Arms Race,* quote p. 116. See also Foote, "Assessing medical technology assessment: Past, present, and future," *Milbank Q.* 65 (1987): 59–80, and S. H. Altman and R. Blendon, eds., *Medical Technology: The Culprit Behind Health Care Costs?* (Washington, D.C.: DHEW, 1979).

19. Minutes, ACC BOT, 2 October 1977, ACC Archives.

20. S. Perry and J. T. Kalberer Jr., "The NIH consensus-development program and the assessment of health-care technologies: The first two years," *N. Engl. J. Med.* 303 (1980): 169–172.

21. Minutes, ACC BOT, 8 October 1978, ACC Archives.

22. P. Starr, *The Social Transformation of American Medicine* (New York: Basic Books, 1982), quote p. 405.

23. J. B. Kirsner, *The Development of American Gastroenterology* (New York: Raven Press, 1990), see esp. p. 275.

24. M. A. Strosberg, "Technological innovation, specialization, and specialty societies: The case of endoscopy," *Bull. N.Y. Acad. Med.* 55 (1979): 498–509, quote p. 506. See also H. Dirks, "The role of a national specialty society in the 1980s: Orientation to the Washington scene," *Am. J. Gastroenterol.* 77 (1982): 181–183.

25. L. S. Dreifus, "Membership services," *Am. J. Cardiol.* 42 (1978): 336–338. See also "1978–1979 committee appointments," *Am. J. Cardiol.* 41 (1978): 1319–1322.

26. L. S. Dreifus, "Implementation of American College of Cardiology goals," *Am. J. Cardiol.* 42 (1978): 1063–1064.

27. W. R. Harlan, P. E. Parsons, and J. W. Thomas, *Health Care Utilization and Costs of Adult Cardiovascular Conditions, United States, 1980. National Medical Care Utilization and Expenditure Survey* (Washington, D.C.: GPO, 1989).

28. R. D. Cotton, "Washington report on legislation and regulation," *Cardiology* 10, no. 2 (1981): 1.

29. S. Knoebel, "A message from the president," *Cardiology* 11, no. 3 (1982): 5.

30. W. Winters to trustees, Minutes, ACC BOT, 10 October 1982, ACC Archives.

31. C. R. Conti, "Concerns about fragmentation of adult cardiology," *J. Am. Coll. Cardiol.* 14 (1989): 532–533.

32. A. Grüntzig, "Transluminal dilatation of coronary artery stenosis," *Lancet* 1 (1978): 263. PTCA evolved from a balloon catheter technique reported in 1964 by vascular radiologists Charles Dotter and Melvin Judkins for dilating obstructed peripheral arteries. See C. T. Dotter, "Transluminal angioplasty: A long view," *Radiology* 135 (1980): 561–564, and J. W. Hurst, "History of cardiac catheterization," in *Coronary Arteriography and Angioplasty,* ed. S. B. King III and J. S. Douglas Jr. (New York: McGraw-Hill, 1985), pp. 1–9. Pediatric cardiologists had already used special catheters to treat some congenital heart defects. See W. J. Rashkind and W. W. Miller, "Creation of an atrial septal defect without thoracotomy," *JAMA* 196 (1966): 991–992.

33. A. R. Grüntzig, Å. Senning, and W. E. Siegenthaler, "Nonoperative dilatation of coronary-artery stenosis: Percutaneous transluminal coronary angioplasty," *N. Engl. J. Med.* 301 (1979): 61–68.

34. R. K. Myler and S. H. Stertzer, "Coronary and peripheral angioplasty: Historical perspective," in *Textbook of Interventional Cardiology,* ed. E. J. Topol (Philadelphia: W.B. Saunders, 1990), pp. 187–198.

35. "Blowup in the arteries," *Time* (3 July 1978): 85.

36. T. R. Engel and S. G. Meister, "Coronary percutaneous transluminal angioplasty," *Ann. Intern. Med.* 90 (1979): 268–269.

37. See N. O. Borhani, "Magnitude of the problem of cardiovascular-renal diseases," in *Chronic Diseases and Public Health,* eds. A. M. Lilienfeld and A. J. Gifford (Baltimore: Johns Hopkins Univ. Press, 1966), pp. 492–526, figure 9, p. 501; R. H. Kennedy, M. A. Kennedy, R. L. Frye, E. R. Giuliani, D. C. McGoon, J. R. Pluth, et al., "Cardiac-catheterization and cardiac-surgical facilities: Use, trends, and future requirements," *N. Engl. J. Med.* 307 (1982): 986–993, table 5, p. 989; and T. Killip, "Changing medical and surgical therapy in coronary artery disease: Need for prospective studies," in *Coronary Heart Surgery,* eds. H. Roskamm and M. Schmuziger (New York: Springer-Verlag, 1979), pp. 2–9.

38. Harlan et al., *Health Care Utilization and Costs,* table W, p. 23.

39. Grüntzig et al., "Nonoperative dilatation of coronary-artery stenosis," quote p. 65. See also J. P. Vandenbroucke, "A short note on the history of the randomized controlled trial," *J. Chron. Dis.* 40 (1987): 985–987.

40. Minutes, National Heart, Lung, and Blood Advisory Council, 13–14 September 1979, NHLBI Archives. See also S. M. Mullin, E. R. Passamani, and M. B. Mock, "Historical background of the National Heart, Lung, and Blood Institute registry for percutaneous transluminal coronary angioplasty," *Am. J. Cardiol.* 53 (1984): 3C–6C.

41. See Myler and Stertzer, "Coronary and peripheral angioplasty," figure 9-8, p. 192, which depicts approximately 200 people at Grüntzig's last PTCA demonstra-

tion course in Zurich. By 1982 PTCA courses were also being offered by some Americans.

42. D. O. Williams, A. Grüntzig, K. M. Kent, R. K. Myler, S. H. Stertzer, L. Bentivoglio, et al., "Guidelines for the performance of percutaneous transluminal coronary angioplasty," *Circulation* 66 (1982): 693–694. The guidelines have become more stringent in recent years. See J. S. Douglas Jr., C. J. Pepine, P. C. Block, J. A. Brinker, W. L. Johnson Jr., W. P. Klinke, et al., "Recommendations for development and maintenance of competence in coronary interventional procedures," *J. Am. Coll. Cardiol.* 22 (1993): 629–631.

43. The Cardiology Working Group, "Cardiology and the quality of medical practice," *JAMA* 265 (1991): 482–485. See also G. O. Hartzler, "PTCA or aortocoronary bypass surgery: Perspectives," *Z. Kardiol.* 74, suppl. 6 (1985): 111–115.

44. E. J. Topol, ed., *Textbook of Interventional Cardiology* (Philadelphia: W. B. Saunders, 1990).

45. See B. Lüderwitz, *History of the Disorders of Cardiac Rhythm* (Armonk, N.Y.: Futura, 1995); W. B. Fye, "The history of cardiac arrhythmias," in *Textbook of Cardiac Arrhythmias,* ed. J. A. Kastor (Philadelphia: W. B. Saunders, 1993), pp. 1–24; and L. J. Acierno, *The History of Cardiology* (Pearl River, N.Y.: Parthenon Publishing Group, 1994), esp. pp. 335–398.

46. Leonard S. Dreifus, interview by W. Bruce Fye, 16 November 1992, New Orleans. See also P. Denes and M. D. Ezri, "Clinical electrophysiology—A decade of progress," *J. Am. Coll. Cardiol.* 1 (1983): 292–305.

47. J. A. Kastor, "Michel Mirowski and the automatic implantable defibrillator," *Am. J. Cardiol.* 63 (1989): 977–982, 1121–1126.

48. E. P. Steinberg and R. S. Lawrence, "Where have all the doctors gone?" *Ann. Intern. Med.* 93 (1980): 619–623.

49. T. A. Preston and R. G. Petersdorf, "Are there too many cardiologists and are they doing the wrong thing?" In *Current Controversies in Cardiovascular Disease,* ed. E. Rapaport (Philadelphia: W. B. Saunders, 1980), pp. 3–20, quote p. 14.

50. M. K. Schleiter and A. R. Tarlov, "National study of internal medicine manpower: IX. Internal medicine residency and fellowship training: 1984 update," *Ann. Intern. Med.* 102 (1985): 681–685, esp. tables 4 and 5, p. 684.

51. R. G. Petersdorf, "Academic medicine: No longer threadbare or genteel," *N. Engl. J. Med.* 304 (1981): 841–843. See also W. B. Fye, "The origin of the full-time faculty system: Implications for clinical research," *JAMA* 265 (1991): 1555–1562; L. Resnekov, "Issues and challenges for academic cardiology," *Chest* 81 (1982): 137–138; and L. E. Cluff, "Economic incentives of faculty practice: Are they distorting the medical school's mission?" *JAMA* 250 (1983): 2931–2934.

52. D. E. Rogers and R. J. Blendon, "The academic medical center today," *Ann. Intern. Med.* 100 (1984): 751–754.

53. J. B. Wyngaarden, "The clinical investigator as an endangered species," *Bull. N.Y. Acad. Med.* 57 (1981): 415–426.

54. Rogers and Blendon, "Academic medical center," p. 751.

55. R. G. Petersdorf, "How to cope with the doctor glut in the United States," *Am. J. Roentgenol.* 145 (1985): 1128–1130.

56. R. W. Campbell, "The objective of a current cardiology training program: Community-based," *Am. J. Cardiol.* 36 (1975): 569–570.

57. Statistics provided by the Indiana State Department of Health to the ACC, 3 August 1994. Based on 1990 data that reflect only inpatient procedures. Although it is possible some outpatient catheterizations were included, the data are complete for PTCA and CABG.

58. Richard S. Ross, interview by W. Bruce Fye, 11 June 1993, Baltimore.

59. Kennedy, et al., "Cardiac-catheterization and cardiac-surgical facilities."

60. For medical schools and training programs, see Tables A8 and A9. For procedures, see *Cardiovascular Specialists and the Economics of Medicine,* figure 5.4, p. 31. There were 5,384 community hospitals in 1990. *Source Book of Health Insurance Data, 1993,* table 5.2, p. 104.

61. G. Bjork, "Cardiovascular diseases as a problem of medical organization," *World Medical Association Bulletin* 4 (1952): 9–13.

62. J. V. Warren, "The future of internal medicine," *Clin. Res.* 9 (1961): 111–113.

63. Ross interview. See also A. M. Harvey, V. A. McKusick, and J. D. Stobo, *Osler's Legacy: The Department of Medicine at Johns Hopkins, 1889–1989* (Baltimore: Johns Hopkins Univ. Press, 1990), esp. pp. 122–123, 149.

64. W. W. Engstrom, "Residency training in internal medicine, for what; Subspecialty boards, what for?" *Ann. Intern. Med.* 70 (1969): 621–633.

65. W. G. Menke, "Divided labor: The doctor as specialist," *Ann. Intern. Med.* 72 (1970): 943–950, quote p. 943. Two clinician historians recently warned that the "durability of general medicine as a field of professional practice is [threatened by] the rise of hyperspecialism." See R. C. Maulitz and P. B. Beeson, "The inner history of internal medicine," in *Grand Rounds: One Hundred Years of Internal Medicine,* ed. R. C. Maulitz and D. E. Long (Philadelphia: Univ. of Pennsylvania Press, 1988), pp. 15–54, quote p. 46.

66. E. Braunwald, "Future shock in academic medicine," *N. Engl. J. Med.* 286 (1972): 1031–1035. See also R. M. Magraw, *Ferment in Medicine: A Study of the Essence of Medical Practice and of Its New Dilemmas* (Philadelphia: W. B. Saunders, 1966), and J. R. Krevans and P. G. Condliffe, eds., *Reform of Medical Education: The Effect of Student Unrest* (Washington, D.C.: National Academy of Sciences, 1970).

67. John C. Beck, interview by John A. Benson Jr., 27 February 1984, Los Angeles. In *Oral Histories,* ed. J. A. Benson, Jr. (Philadelphia: ACP, 1994), pp. 65–87, quote p. 73. For a recent recapitulation of these themes, see R. M. Glickman, J. C. Bennett, J. P. Nolan, J. D. Stobo, A. H. Rubenstein, and M. A. Mufson, "United we stand," *Ann. Intern. Med.* 118 (1993): 903–904.

68. Beck interview by Benson, quotes pp. 73–74. See also P. H. Futcher, *Activities of the American Board of Internal Medicine, 1967–1975* (Philadelphia: ABIM, 1988), esp. pp. 37–42.

69. E. D. Pellegrino, "The identity crisis of an ideal," in *Controversy in Internal Medicine II,* ed. F. J. Ingelfinger, R. V. Ebert, M. Finland, and A. S. Relman (Philadelphia: W. B. Saunders, 1974), pp. 41–50, quotes p. 43.

70. D. T. Mason, "The department of cardiology: A functional concept that has come of age," *Am. J. Cardiol.* 40 (1977): 1013–1014.

71. Ibid. See also I. J. Lewis and C. G. Sheps, *The Sick Citadel: The American Academic Medical Center and the Public Interest* (Cambridge: Oelgeschlager, Gunn & Hain, 1983). The NHI budget figures are from *National Heart, Lung, and Blood Institute Fact Book. Fiscal Year 1993* (Bethesda, Md.: NHLBI, 1994), p. 63.

72. Mason, "Department of cardiology." See also W. C. Hilles and S. K. Fagan, *Medical Practice Plans at U.S. Medical Schools: A Review of Current Characteristics and Trends* (Washington, D.C.: AAMC, 1977).

73. Mason, "Department of cardiology." A few multispecialty group practices allowed cardiologists to form departments in this era. The Marshfield Clinic (Wisconsin) did so reluctantly in 1979; the cardiologists used Mason's article to help to justify their request.

74. E. Braunwald, "The present state and future of academic cardiology," *Circulation* 66 (1982): 487–490, quotes p. 488.

75. Ibid., p. 487.

76. S. A. Halpern, *American Pediatrics: The Social Dynamics of Professionalism, 1880–1980* (Berkeley: Univ. of California Press, 1988), quote p. 7. See also K. Davis, "Implications of an expanding supply of physicians: Evidence from a cross-sectional analysis," *Johns Hopkins Med. J.* 150 (1982): 55–64.

77. Braunwald, "The present state," quote p. 489.

78. Stephen Reeders in Minutes, NHLBI Advisory Council, 2–3 September 1993, NHLBI Archives.

79. See, for example, R. Roberts, V. J. Dzau, and J. L. Swain, *Molecular Cardiology: Unlocking the Secrets of the Heart* [videotape] (Bethesda, Md.: ACC, 1993).

80. In 1989 Leonard Geddes, Robert O'Rourke, Arnold Katz, Barry Zaret, Burton Sobel, and William Parmley served on a committee that organized the new society, which was formally established the next year during the annual ACC meeting. See "Report. Interim organizational meeting: Association of Cardiology Professors," 1 November 1989, copy kindly supplied by R. O'Rourke. Additional insights into APC came from Barry L. Zaret, interview by W. Bruce Fye, 11 November 1993, Atlanta.

81. B. L. Zaret, W. B. Hood, and R. A. O'Rourke, "Cardiovascular medicine: Subspecialty or specialty," *Am. J. Cardiol.* 72 (1993): 968–970. See also R. A. O'Rourke, "Current trends in clinical cardiology: A march of folly?" *Circulation* 75 (1987): 1097–1101, and "Structure and function of academic divisions of cardiology: Task force reports from the Association of Professors of Cardiology," *Arch. Intern. Med.* 153 (1993): 2305–2316.

82. E. Braunwald, "Cardiology: Division or department?" *N. Engl. J. Med.* 329 (1993): 1887–1890. See also Braunwald, "Future shock in academic medicine," and Braunwald, "The present state and future of academic cardiology."

83. A. Coats, "The structure of departments of medicine," *N. Engl. J. Med.* 33 (1994): 946. See also Maulitz and Beeson, "The inner history of internal medicine."

84. For a discussion of some of these factors, see J. O. Goodman and V. Siragusa, eds., *Cardiology in Transition* (Torrance, Calif.: John Goodman, 1989). See also M. C. Thornhill, "Physician income: Historic and recent changes in payment sources, income levels, and professional autonomy," in *The Business of Medicine*, ed. G. Gitnick, F. Rothenburg, and J. L. Weiner (New York: Elsevier, 1991), pp. 7–17.

For a historical perspective on the advantages and disadvantages of group practice, see R. Fein, *The Doctor Shortage: An Economic Diagnosis* (Washington, D.C.: Brookings Institution, 1967), esp. pp. 94–111.

85. C. M. Matenaer to J. Folz, 26 September 1990, copy in author's possession.

86. It is acknowledged that medical graduates choose specialties partly on the basis of economic considerations. See M. H. Ebell, "Choice of specialty: It's money that matters in the USA," *JAMA* 262 (1989): 1630; Funkenstein, *Medical Students;* and E. C. Shapiro and L. M. Lowenstein, eds., *Becoming a Physician: Development of Values and Attitudes in Medicine* (Cambridge: Ballinger Publishing Company, 1979).

87. M. Kirchner, "Non-surgical practice: What's the key to higher earnings?" *Med. Econ.* 58 (1981): 182–193.

88. G. C. Pope and J. E. Schneider, "Trends in physician income," *Health Aff.* (Spring 1992): 181–193.

89. "Update on physician compensation in different practice settings," *[ACC] Affiliates in Training* 11, no. 3 (April-May 1994): 1–2.

90. E. Braunwald, "Tensions between academic cardiology and internal medicine," *Int. J. Cardiol.* 5 (1984): 223–228, quote p. 225.

91. See "What's new in physician compensation," *Group Practice Journal* 41 (1992): 18–25, table 1, p. 20, and W. C. Smith Jr., *Report on Medical School Faculty Salaries, 1992–1993* (Washington, D.C.: AAMC, 1993).

92. W. W. Parmley, "Emergence of the cardiologist-entrepreneur," *J. Am. Coll. Cardiol.* 21 (1993): 840–841.

93. See W. F. Vogt, "Physician clinical productivity: A comparison of university-based and private multispecialty medical groups," *College Review* 4 (1987): 63–83.

94. L. G. Horan and N. C. Flowers, "Does role dictate response of chiefs and chairmen?" *Int. J. Cardiol.* 6 (1984): 639–644.

95. Kennedy, *In Critical Condition,* quote p. 190.

96. F. Mullan, M. L. Rivo, and R. M. Politzer, "Doctors, dollars, and determination: Making physician work-force policy," *Health Aff.,* suppl. 12 (1993): 138–151. See also J. Hurley, "Simulated effects of incomes-based policies on the distribution of physicians," *Med. Care* 28 (1990): 221–238. For a Marxist interpretation of specialization in American medicine, see V. Navarro, *Medicine under Capitalism* (New York: Prodist, 1976), esp. pp. 140–145.

97. D. J. McCarty, "Why are today's medical students choosing high-technology specialties over internal medicine?" *N. Engl. J. Med.* 317 (1987): 567–569, quote p. 568.

98. "Minutes, ACP Board of Regents, 14 April 1953," *Ann. Intern. Med.* 39 (1953): 404–423, quote p. 415.

99. J. F. Williams Jr., "The involvement of the College in health care policy," *J. Am. Coll. Cardiol.* 4 (1984): 848–849. For the ACP's growing involvement in socioeconomic issues, see R. H. Moser, *A Decade of Decision: A Physician Remembers the American College of Physicians, 1977–1986* (Philadelphia: ACP, 1991).

100. "ACC establishes key contact system," *Cardiology* 15, no. 9 (1986): 8.

101. "ACC leaders attend health policy retreat in Washington, D.C.," *Cardiology* 18, no. 7 (1989): 1. See also J. A. Morone and G. S. Belkin, *The Politics of Health Care Reform: Lessons from the Past, Prospects for the Future* (Durham, N.C.: Duke Univ. Press, 1994).

102. Marie E. Michnich, interview by W. Bruce Fye, 16 March 1994, Atlanta.

103. See R. Stevens, *In Sickness and in Wealth*, esp. pp. 322–327.

104. P. R. Lee, ed., *Medicare Physician Payment: An Agenda for Reform* (Washington, D.C.: Physician Payment Review Commission, 1987). See also W. C. Hsiao, P. Braun, D. L. Dunn, E. R. Becker, D. Yntema, D. K. Verrilli, E. Stamenovic, and S.-P. Chen, "An overview of the development and refinement of the Resource-Based Relative Value Scale," *Med. Care* 30, no. 11, suppl. (1992): NS1–NS12; "Resource-Based Relative Value Scale" [Several articles reprinted from *JAMA*, 28 October 1988] (Chicago: AMA, 1988); and S. A. Lightfoot, "A history of physician payment policies under Medicare," *Bull. Am. Coll. Surg.* 78 (1993): 32–35.

105. C. R. Conti to W. B. Fye, 3 June 1992.

106. "CV specialists get 10% of the 1987 Medicare pie," *Cardiology* 18, no. 10 (1989): 7.

107. W. C. Hsiao, D. L. Dunn, and D. K. Verrilli, "Assessing the implementation of physician-payment reform," *N. Engl. J. Med.* 328 (1993): 928–933, quote p. 928. See also W. C. Hsiao, P. Braun, E. R. Becker, D. L. Dunn, N. Kelly, N. Causino, et al., "Results and impacts of the resource-based relative value scale," *Med. Care* 30 suppl. (November 1992): NS61–NS79, table 4, p. NS68. See also P. Braun, "The resource-based relative value scale: Its further development and reform of physician payment," *Med. Care* 30 suppl. (November 1992): NS1–NS94.

108. "Board of governors address RBRVS," *Cardiology* 21, no. 1 (1992): 1. See also J. M. Levy, M. Borowitz, S. McNeill, W. J. London, and G. Savord, "Understanding the Medicare fee schedule and its impact on physicians under the final rule," *Med. Care* 30 suppl. (November 1992): NS80–NS93, table 1, p. NS87.

109. L. Luciano, "A cure your M.D. won't like," *Money* (Money Extra 1990): 54–59, quotes pp. 56, 59. A recent comparison of the incomes of physicians with those of other professional groups revealed that the "hours-adjusted internal rate of return on the educational investment over a working lifetime" was more favorable for people in business and law than for specialists or primary care physicians. See W. B. Weeks, A. E. Wallace, M. M. Wallace, and H. G. Welch, "A comparison of the educational costs and incomes of physicians and other professionals," *N. Engl. J. Med.* 330 (1994): 1280–1286, figure 3, p. 1285. See also M. J. Prashker and R. F. Meenan, "Subspecialty training: Is it financially worthwhile?" *Ann. Intern. Med.* 115 (1991): 715–719.

110. L. D. Young, "My back hurts, too," *Medical Tribune for the Internist and Cardiologist* 35, no. 12 (1994): 20.

111. M. LaCombe, "What is internal medicine?" *Ann. Intern. Med.* 118 (1993): 384–387.

112. "Congress cuts EKG interpretation payment in 1992." *Cardiology* 19, no. 12 (1990): 1.

113. This letter to Congress was "signed" by more than twenty professional societies and health care organizations, see "ECG legislative update; new legal opinion issued," *ACC Washington Update on Legislation and Regulation* (1992): 3–5. See

also "ECG legislation forwarded to president; veto likely," *Cardiology* 21, no. 11 (1992): 1, and A. M. Hutter Jr. to Dear Colleague, *ACC Washington Update* (May 1992): 1. For a chronology of the ACC's efforts to restore payments for electrocardiogram interpretation, see "ECG non-payment repealed," *ACC Washington Update on Legislation and Regulation* (August 1993): 1–2.

114. R. L. Frye to G. R. Wilensky, 5 August 1991, copy in author's possession.

115. R. L. Frye, "A visit to the physician payment review commission," *J. Am. Coll. Cardiol.* 19 (1992): 114–115.

116. Minutes, ACC BOT, 14 October 1984, ACC Archives.

117. ACC president Henry McIntosh had proposed developing state chapters in 1974, in part, because he was impressed that the AMA and ACP had "strong state organizational structure[s]." His successor and other college leaders did not share his enthusiasm for the concept and the idea lapsed for a decade. H. D. McIntosh to B. S. Maniscalco, 9 March 1994, in *Newsletter, Florida Chapter of the ACC,* 8, no. 1 (May 1994): 9–10. The ACC once had almost two dozen state chapters; they were abolished in 1954. See A. Graybiel, "Report from the president," *Am. Coll. Cardiol. Bull.* (November–December 1954): 1–2, and S. Dack, form letter, 21 November 1956, in Reichert general correspondence 1955–59 file, Reichert Papers, ACC Archives.

118. William D. Nelligan, interviews by W. Bruce Fye, 16–17 March 1993, Anaheim, Calif., and 28 December 1993, Bethesda, Md.

119. Ibid.

120. Minutes, ACC BOG, 9 March 1986, ACC Archives. See also C. R. Conti, "The American College of Cardiology and the development of chapters," *J. Am. Coll. Cardiol.* 14 (1989): 1393–1394.

121. M. Angell, "The doctor as double agent," *Kennedy Institute of Ethics Journal* 3 (1993): 279–286, quotes pp. 279, 282.

122. J. P. Kassirer, "Access to specialty care," *N. Engl. J. Med.* 331 (1994): 1151–1153. See also Kassirer, "Managed care and the morality of the marketplace," *N. Engl. J. Med.* 333 (1995): 50–52.

123. For concerns about the impact of health care reform and managed care on academic medical centers, see J. P. Kassirer, "Academic medical centers under siege," *N. Engl. J. Med.* 331 (1994): 1370–1371, and A. M. Katz, "Health care reform: A threat to research and education in the academic health center," *Circulation* 90 (1994): 1572–1573.

124. A. N. DeMaria, "News from the private sector," *Cardiology* 21, no. 1 (1992): 2.

125. See A. M. Hutter Jr., "Access to cardiovascular care," *Am. Coll. Cardiol.* 21 (1993): 276–278, and D. J. Ullyot, "President's page: The campaign theme—choice," *J. Am. Coll. Cardiol.* 24, no. 3 (1994): 841–842. See also B. C. Fuchs and M. Merlis, "Health care reform: President Clinton's Health Security Act," *CRS Report for Congress* (Washington, D.C.: Library of Congress, 1993); J. K. Iglehart, "Republicans and the new politics of health care," *N. Engl. J. Med.* 332 (1995): 972–975; T. R. Marmor, *Understanding Health Care Reform* (New Haven: Yale Univ. Press, 1994); and P. Starr, "Look who's talking health care reform now," *New York Times Magazine* (3 September 1995): 42–43.

126. C. Kilgore and S. Brown, "'Cream of Crop' C-V doctors form huge national network," *Int. Med. News & Cardiology News* 26 (1993): 1, 16, 38. See also A. N. DeMaria, M. A. Engle, D. C. Harrison, R. D. Judge, N. T. Kouchoukos, T. H. Lee, et al., "Managed care involvement by cardiovascular specialists: Prevalence, attitudes and influence on practice," *J. Am. Coll. Cardiol.* 23 (1994): 1245–1253, and American College of Cardiology, *The Cardiovascular Specialist's Guide to Managed Care,* 5 vols. (Bethesda, Md.: ACC, 1993).

127. D. Morgan, "HMO trend squeezes big-fee medical specialists," *Washington Post* (18 July 1994).

128. J. P. Weiner, "Forecasting the effects of health reform on U.S. physician workforce requirement: Evidence from HMO staffing patterns," *JAMA* 272 (1994): 222–230, table 2, p. 224.

129. Minutes, ACC BOT, 3 March 1986 ACC Archives. See also ACC Member and Non-member Surveys: 1986 (Bethesda, Md.: ACC, 1986).

130. Nelligan interview. See also E. P. Schloss, "Beyond GMENAC: Another physician shortage from 2010 to 2030?" *N. Engl. J. Med.* 318 (1988): 920–922.

131. R. C. Schlant, W. H. Abelmann, R. A. O'Rourke, S. H. Rahimtoola, J. A. Ronan Jr., F. I. Moore, et al., "Task force VII: Summary: A look at the future," *J. Am. Coll. Cardiol.* 12 (1988): 862–868. The conference participants (and their professional affiliations) are listed in R. C. Schlant, W. H. Abelmann, R. A. O'Rourke, and S. H. Rahimtoola, "Trends in the practice of adult cardiology: Implications for manpower," *J. Am. Coll. Cardiol.* 12 (1988): 822–826. See also W. H. Abelmann, "Report of the 1985 American College of Cardiology Survey of Cardiovascular Medicine Manpower," *J. Am. Coll. Cardiol.* 10 (1987): 1361–1364, and W. B. Schwartz, F. A. Sloan, and D. N. Mendelson, "Why there will be little or no physician surplus between now and the year 2000," *N. Engl. J. Med.* 318 (1988): 892–897.

132. J. L. Ritchie, M. D. Cheitlin, M. A. Hlatky, T. J. Ryan, and R. G. Williams, "Task force 5: Profile of the cardiovascular specialist: Trends in needs and supply and implications for the future," *J. Am. Coll. Cardiol.* 24 (1994): 275–328, quotes pp. 320, 321.

133. L. O. Langdon and M. D. Cheitlin, "Downsizing cardiology: Getting the process started," *Circulation* 90 (1994): 1101–1102. See also F. Unger, "European survey on open heart surgery PTCA heart catheterization 1992," *Academia Scientiarum et Artium Europaea* 6 (1993): 1–120; R. J. Carroll, S. D. Horn, B. Soderfeldt, B. C. James, and L. Malmberg, "International comparison of waiting times for selected procedures," *J. Am. Coll. Cardiol.* 25 (1995): 557–563; and R. H. Brook, R. E. Park, C. M. Winslow, J. B. Kosecoff, M. R. Chassin, and J. R. Hampton, "Diagnosis and treatment of coronary disease: Comparison of doctors' attitudes in the USA and the UK," *Lancet* 1 (1988): 750–753. For a discussion that focuses on intensive care, see D. Terres and J. Rapoport, eds., "Cost Containment—A Multicultural Approach," *New Horizons* 2, no. 3 (1994): 273–412.

134. S. A. Schroeder, "Cost containment," in *Annual Report for 1994 of the Robert Wood Johnson Foundation: Cost Containment.* (Princeton: Robert Wood Johnson Foundation, 1995), pp. 6–21, quotes pp. 8, 13. See also L. K. Gunzburger, "Foundations that support medical education and health care: Their missions, accomplishments, and unique role," *Acad. Med.* 69 (1994): 8–17.

135. W. W. Parmley, "Back to the future: Primary care," *J. Am. Coll. Cardiol.* 23 (1994): 822–823. Members of what may be termed the "generalist lobby" have

seized the opportunity to reinforce points they have made for two decades. See S. A. Schroeder, "The latest forecast: Managed care collides with physician supply," *JAMA* 272 (1994): 239–240. See also S. A. Schroeder and L. G. Sandy, "Specialty distribution of U.S. physicians: The invisible driver of health care costs," *N. Engl. J. Med.* 328 (1993): 961–963; J. A. Barondess, "The future of generalism," *Ann. Intern. Med.* 119 (1993): 153–160; "Generating more generalists: An agenda of renewal for internal medicine," *Ann. Intern. Med.* 119 (1993): 1125–1129; and R. G. Petersdorf and L. Goitein, "The future of internal medicine," *Ann. Intern. Med.* 119 (1993): 1130–1137.

136. "Managed care reducing opportunities for CV specialists in some markets," *ACC Affiliates in Training* 12 (January 1995): 1–4, 6. See also S. Goldstein and J. S. Alpert, "The cardiovascular work force: Too large for the future?" *Am. J. Cardiol.* 74 (1994): 394–395.

137. The number of cardiology job offers dropped from 83 to 41; see *N. Engl. J. Med.* 329 (1993): lxii–lxvi, and *N. Engl. J. Med.* 331 (1994): li–lii.

138. ACC executive committee. "Physician workforce statement," 5 December 1994 (Bethesda, Md.: ACC, 1994).

139. A summary of the potential legal implications of any coordinated effort to downsize cardiology training programs is F. M. Northam to K. J. Collishaw, 12 November 1992. ACC, Bethesda, Md.

140. A. S. Relman, "The changing demography of the medical profession," *N. Engl. J. Med.* 321 (1989): 1540–1542.

141. P. J. Carr, J. Noble, R. H. Friedman, B. Starfield, and C. Black, "Choices of training programs and career paths by women in internal medicine," *Acad. Med.* 68 (1993): 219–223.

142. "Status of women in cardiology and in the American College of Cardiology," 21 May 1992, in "Scientific Advisory Meeting II Testimony" (Washington, D.C.: Society for the Advancement of Women's Health Research, 1992). Marian Limacher kindly provided this typescript. Twenty-two other professional societies and organizations participated in this conference. See also *Women's Health Research. Scientific Advisory Meeting II Testimony, 21 May 1992* (Washington, D.C.: Society for the Advancement of Women's Health Research, 1992), and D. I. Allen, "Women in medical specialty societies," *JAMA* 262 (1989): 3439–3443. The author thanks Rita Redberg for providing references and valuable perspective on women in cardiology.

143. "The future of adult cardiology," *JAMA* 262 (1989): 2874–2878. For concerns about the impact of managed care and health care reform on specialists, see D. P. Moynihan, "We shouldn't phase out medical specialists," *New York Times* (28 August 1994): E14, and L. Rawls and R. F. Perry, "Health care reform and graduate medical education," *N. Engl. J. Med.* 331 (1994): 879. A perceptive essay on the changing role of the hospital in American health care is J. D. Stoeckle, "The citadel cannot hold: Technologies go outside the hospital, patients and doctors too." *Milbank Q.* 73 (1995): 3–17.

144. Cardiologists hailed a recent study which indicated that "internists and family practitioners are less aware of or less certain about key advances in the treatment of myocardial infarction than are cardiologists." See J. Z. Ayanian, P. J. Hauptman, E. Guadagnoli, E. M. Antman, C. L. Pashos, and B. J. McNeil, "Knowledge and practices of generalist and specialist physicians regarding drug therapy for acute myocardial infarction," *N. Engl. J. Med.* 331 (1994): 1136–1142. See also T. L. Schreiber, A. Elkhatib, C. L. Grimes, and W. W. O'Neill, "Cardiologist versus internist

management of patients with unstable angina: Treatment patterns and outcomes," *J. Am. Coll. Cardiol.* 26 (1995): 577–582. For a critical perspective on cardiologists' failure to focus on prevention, see J. C. Stevenson, I. F. Godsland, and V. Wynn, "Cardiologists rebuked," *Lancet* 344 (1994): 1557. See also H. Blackburn, "Medical economics, professional attitudes and chronic disease prevention," *Minnesota Med.* 60 (1977): 821–823.

145. American Heart Association, "Invest in biomedical research," (Dallas: AHA, 1994). See also T. J. Thom and F. H. Epstein, "Heart disease, cancer, and stroke mortality trends and their interrelations: An international perspective," *Circulation* 90 (1994): 574–582. See also D. L. Lee, G. E. Dinse, and D. G. Hoel, "Decreasing cardiovascular disease and increasing cancer among whites in the United States from 1973 through 1987," *JAMA* 271 (1994): 431–437.

146. *Continuing Medical Education Resource Catalog 1994* (Bethesda, Md.: ACC, 1994). Statistics from ACC archives. The college launched its own journal, the *Journal of the American College of Cardiology,* in 1983. See "College to publish new official journal," *Cardiology* 11 (July 1982): 1–5.

147. A. M. Hutter Jr., "ACC committees: Structure and appointments," *J. Am. Coll. Cardiol.* 20 (1992): 509–511.

148. J. S. Alpert, "Guidelines for training in adult cardiovascular medicine: Core cardiology training symposium," *J. Am. Coll. Cardiol.* 25 (1995): 1–34. See also W. W. Parmley, "Changing requirements for training in cardiovascular disease," *J. Am. Coll. Cardiol.* 22 (1993): 1548.

149. J. C. Burnham, "The past of the future of medicine," *Bull. Hist. Med.* 67 (1993): 1–27.

150. W. Osler, "Medicine," in *The Progress of the Century* (New York: Harper & Bros: 1901), pp. 173–214, quote p. 178.

Bibliography

Manuscript Collections

ACC Archives. American College of Cardiology Headquarters, Bethesda, Md.

AHA Archives. American Heart Association National Center, Dallas, Tex.

Baruch Papers. Simon Baruch Papers, Seeley G. Mudd Manuscript Library, Princeton University Archives, Princeton, N.J.

Bishop Papers. Louis F. Bishop Papers, Special Collections and Archives, Rutgers University Libraries, New Brunswick, N.J.

Blalock Papers. Alfred E. Blalock Papers, Alan Mason Chesney Medical Archives, Johns Hopkins Medical Institutions, Baltimore, Md.

Burch Papers. George E. Burch Papers, National Library of Medicine, History of Medicine Division, Bethesda, Md.

Cohn Papers. Alfred E. Cohn Papers, Rockefeller Archive Center, Pocantico Hills, North Tarrytown, N.Y.

Hewlett Papers. Albion Walter Hewlett Papers, Lane Medical Library, Stanford University Medical School, Palo Alto, Calif.

Lewis Papers. Sir Thomas Lewis Papers, Contemporary Medical Archives Centre, Wellcome Institute for the History of Medicine, London, England.

NHLBI Archives. Office of the Director, National Heart, Lung, and Blood Institute, Bethesda, Md.

Reichert Papers [Bethesda]. Philip Reichert Papers, American College of Cardiology Headquarters, Bethesda, Md..

Reichert Papers [NYH]. Philip Reichert Papers, Medical Archives, New York Hospital–Cornell Medical Center, New York, N.Y.

Roosevelt Papers. Franklin D. Roosevelt Papers, Franklin D. Roosevelt Library Research Department, Hyde Park, N.Y.

Rutstein Papers. David D. Rutstein Papers, Rare Books and Manuscript Division, Francis A. Countway Library of Medicine, Boston, Mass.

Sprague Papers. Howard A. Sprague Papers, Rare Books and Manuscript Division, Francis A. Countway Library of Medicine, Boston, Mass.

Virchow Society Archives. Rudolf Virchow Society Archives, Special Collections, The New York Academy of Medicine, New York, N.Y.

White Papers. Paul D. White Papers, Rare Books and Manuscript Division, Francis A. Countway Library of Medicine, Boston, Mass.

Wood Papers. Francis C. Wood Papers, Library of the College of Physicians of Philadelphia, Philadelphia, Pa.

Wright Papers. Irving S. Wright Papers, Medical Archives, New York Hospital–Cornell Medical Center, New York, N.Y.

Oral History Sources

I formally interviewed almost fifty people who provided different perspectives on the emergence of American cardiology and cardiovascular surgery. Several former presidents of the ACC and AHA were interviewed. Some of the interviewees have made important contributions to the science and technology of medicine. Others were chosen because they could provide insight into the organization of the specialty. They included doctors (internists, cardiologists, and cardiovascular surgeons) in private practice and academic medicine as well as administrators. The book is not biographical, so very little of the oral history material was incorporated into it directly. My concepts and conclusions reflect many valuable insights gained from the interviews, however. The following list is an oversimplified summary of the individuals interviewed. Each interview was audio taped, and most lasted thirty to ninety minutes. The location and date of each interview are listed. The tapes are stored at the ACC Archives at the college's headquarters (Heart House) in Bethesda, Md.

SUMMARY OF THE ORAL HISTORY INTERVIEWS

Earl Bakken (b. 1924). Founder of Medtronic, Inc., a pioneering biomedical instrument firm based in Minneapolis that initially focused on pacemakers. Bakken described the emergence of modern cardiovascular medicine and surgery from an industry perspective. *Anaheim, Calif., 12 November 1991.*

Arthur Bernstein (b. 1909). A longtime ACC and AHA member who represents the generation of cardiologists trained in the "EKG era." His practice at Newark (N.J.) Beth Israel Hospital spanned half a century. *Newark, N.J., 19 May 1992.*

Richard J. Bing (b. 1909). Medical scientist who left Nazi Germany in 1933. He worked with physiologist Homer Smith in New York and was invited by Alfred Blalock to organize the world's first diagnostic cardiac catheterization laboratory at Johns Hopkins in 1946. *Pasadena, Calif., 11 February 1992.*

Eugene Braunwald (b. 1929). Prominent academic cardiologist, author, and investigator who trained in New York in the early 1950s. He worked at the NHI during its early "Golden Age" and is currently Hersey Professor of Medicine at Harvard. *Anaheim, Calif., 13 November 1991.*

Howard B. Burchell (b. 1907). A Canadian physiological cardiologist who came to the United States in the 1930s, Burchell was a pioneer of cardiac catheterization. He was at the Mayo Clinic during the introduction of open-heart surgery. A prolific author and investigator, Burchell was an influential AHA leader and served as editor of *Circulation. Minneapolis, Minn., 13 January 1991.*

David B. Carmichael (b. 1923). California cardiologist who trained with Paul White and was involved in the early stages of cardiac catheterization. He represented cardiology (through the ACC) in the AMA's house of delegates for seventeen years. *Bethesda, Md., 18 September 1991.*

C. Richard Conti (b. 1934). Academic cardiologist (University of Florida) and former ACC president (1989–90) who trained at Johns Hopkins. He provided a perspective on the growth of cardiology training programs and the impact of technology on practice. *Atlanta, Ga., 8–9 November 1993.*

Denton A. Cooley (b. 1920). Pioneering Houston cardiovascular surgeon who, as an intern, assisted Alfred Blalock with the first "blue-baby" operation. Cooley provided a surgeon's perspective on the emergence of modern cardiology and cardiovascular surgery. *Houston, Tex., 11 April 1992.*

Eliot Corday (b. 1913). Los Angeles cardiologist trained in New York in the "EKG era." Corday, ACC president in 1965–1966, catalyzed the college's entry into the area of government relations. With Grey Dimond, he organized the ACC's "International Circuit Courses," an overseas educational program. *Anaheim, Calif., 13 November 1991.*

Simon Dack (b. 1908, d. 1994). At the time of the interview, the oldest living "influential" of the ACC. He trained in New York in the "EKG era." He was president of the college in 1956–1957 and edited the college's official journal for more than 35 years. *New York, N.Y., 21 October 1991.*

Michael E. DeBakey (b. 1908). Pioneering Houston cardiovascular surgeon who played an important role in the Surgeon General's Office during World War II. DeBakey was an influential member of the "heart lobby," which urged the government to generously support biomedical research. *Houston, Tex., 10 April 1992.*

Lewis Dexter (b. 1910). A pupil of Paul White, Dexter was affiliated with Harvard throughout his professional career. He organized one of the first cardiac catheterization laboratories in America (at the Peter Bent Brigham Hospital) and emphasized the clinical utility of this technique. *Boston, Mass., 15 November 1992.*

E. Grey Dimond (b. 1918). Academic cardiologist and former ACC president (1961–1962) who recruited leading academic cardiologists to join the college. An innovator in medical education, Dimond conceived some of the ACC's most successful programs. He was responsible for the concept of "Heart House," the ACC's headquarters that also served as a teaching center. *Kansas City, Mo., 28–29 January 1993.*

Leonard S. Dreifus (b. 1924). An academic cardiologist (Hahnemann) and former ACC president (1978–1979) who encouraged the college's entry into the area of government relations in the 1970s. *New Orleans, La., 16 November 1992.*

Harvey Feigenbaum (b. 1933). Academic cardiologist (Indiana University) who pioneered and popularized the noninvasive diagnostic technique of cardiac ultrasound (echocardiography). He founded the American Society of Echocardiography. *Atlanta, Ga., 8 November 1993.*

David Feild (b. 1944). An administrator with a background in advertising, Feild joined the ACC in 1980. He was involved in the development of several practice guidelines the college developed during the 1980s and was appointed executive vice president of the college in 1993. *Crystal City, Va., 27 September 1994.*

Charles Fisch (b. 1924). Academic cardiologist (Indiana University) and two-term ACC president (1975–1977) who, with Leonard Dreifus and Eliot Corday, encouraged the college's entry into the area of government relations. Fisch has held many positions in the college. *New Orleans, La., 16 November 1992.*

Samuel M. Fox (b. 1923). Trained in Philadelphia during the early "catheterization era," Fox was at the NHI for several years. In that capacity, he was influential in encouraging the development of coronary care units throughout the country in the 1960s. He was ACC president in 1972–1973. *Anaheim, Calif., 17 March 1993.*

Peter L. Frommer (b. 1932). On the staff of the NHLBI since 1963, Frommer has been deputy director of the institute since 1978. He has a three-decade perspective on the government's involvement in cardiovascular medicine and surgery. *Atlanta, Ga., 14 April 1994.*

Palmer H. Futcher (b. 1910). Academic internist who served as executive director of the ABIM from 1967 to 1975. This interview focused on the growth and significance of specialty board examinations. *Philadelphia, Pa., 23 October 1991.*

Eli Ginzberg (b. 1911). Academic economist (Columbia) who became interested in health care delivery during World War II. The author of many books on health policy, Ginzberg has a special interest in the socioeconomic aspects of American medicine, the politics of medicine and medical research, and medical workforce issues. *Atlanta, Ga., 14 April 1994.*

Richard Gorlin (b. 1926). Academic cardiologist who was a pioneer in cardiac catheterization techniques. He chaired the Department of Medicine at Mount Sinai Medical Center, New York, from 1974 to 1992. *Atlanta, Ga., 14–15 March 1994.*

Frank J. Gouze (b. 1913). A pupil of pioneering American electrocardiographer George Farr, he joined Marshfield Clinic (Wis.) in 1948. Although he was a trained cardiologist, Gouze's cardiology practice grew slowly until he was elected a fellow in the ACC. *Marshfield, Wis., 27 May 1993.*

Dwight E. Harken (b. 1910, d. 1993). Harvard surgeon who was a major innovator in the field of heart surgery. As ACC president (1964–1965), Harken aggressively recruited leading academic cardiologists to join the college. *Dallas, Tex., 14 April 1992.*

A. McGehee Harvey (b. 1912). Academic internist who chaired the Department of Medicine at Johns Hopkins from 1946 to 1973. He witnessed the emergence of cardiology as a major subspecialty within an academic medical department. He provided a medical perspective on the Blalock-Taussig era at Johns Hopkins. *Baltimore, Md., 10 June 1993.*

Arthur Hollman (b. 1923). British cardiologist who was a student under Thomas Lewis at University College Hospital in 1943. Among the first British cardiologists to perform cardiac catheterization (beginning in 1957 at Hammersmith Hospital, London). *Marshfield, Wis., 2 October 1994.*

J. Willis Hurst (b. 1920). A pupil of Paul White, Hurst is an academic cardiologist (Emory University), prolific author, and former AHA president. He was Lyndon Johnson's cardiologist and provided insight into the history of academic cardiology and the support of cardiovascular research by Congress. *Anaheim, Calif., 11 November 1991.*

Adolph M. Hutter Jr. (b. 1937). Academic cardiologist (Massachusetts General Hospital) and former ACC president (1992–1993) who encouraged the college's increasing involvement in the area of government relations. *Atlanta, Ga., 8–9 November 1993.*

Thomas Killip (b. 1927). Academic cardiologist who was a leader in the coronary care unit movement during the 1960s and 1970s when he was chief of the cardiology division at New York Hospital. *Dallas, Tex., 13 November 1994.*

Charles E. Kossmann (b. 1909). Academic cardiologist (University of Tennessee) who trained in New York during the "EKG era." Kossmann provided valuable insight into the dynamics of cardiology in New York during the 1940s and 1950s. *(Taped responses to questions mailed April 1993.)*

Dennis M. Krikler (b. 1928). British academic cardiologist (Hammersmith Hospital, London) and former editor of the *British Heart Journal* who has been active in the ACC and the AHA. He provided a European perspective on American cardiology. *Atlanta, Ga., 8 November 1993.*

Paul R. Lichtlen (b. 1929). A European cardiologist born in Switzerland, Lichtlen did part of his training at Johns Hopkins in the early 1960s. He developed a coronary care unit in Zurich where he also worked with Andreas Grüntzig during the development of percutaneous transluminal coronary angioplasty (PTCA). *Atlanta, Ga., 10 November 1993.*

Bill L. Martz (b. 1922). Academic cardiologist (Indiana University) and former ACC president (1969–1970) who was largely responsible for the ACC entering the field of audiotape continuing medical education. He also played a major role in the creation of Heart House, the college's administrative and learning center in Bethesda, Md. *(Taped responses to questions mailed March 1993.)*

Ben D. McCallister (b. 1932). McCallister trained in cardiology at the Mayo Clinic where he was codirector of the cardiac catheterization laboratory in the 1960s. In 1969 he moved to Kansas City, Mo., where he and Jim Crockett formed a single-specialty cardiology group practice. This became one of the nation's most successful single-specialty groups and led to the formation of the Mid America Heart Institute. *Atlanta, Ga., 15 March 1994.*

Marie E. Michnich (b. 1947). Associate Executive Vice President for Health Policy at the ACC, Dr. Michnich is a nurse with a doctorate in public health and health services research. She was former legislative assistant to Senator Robert Dole and joined the college in 1987 to direct the health policy program. *Atlanta, Ga., 16 March 1994.*

William D. Nelligan (b. 1926). The college's first professional administrator. His hiring catalyzed the move of the national headquarters from the Empire State Building in New York to Bethesda, Md. During Nelligan's tenure (1965–1992), the ACC matured into a major national organization and cardiology became a technology-oriented, procedural specialty. *Anaheim, Calif., 16–17 March 1993; Bethesda, Md., 28 December 1993.*

Oglesby Paul (b. 1916). Paul White's pupil and biographer, Paul is an academic cardiologist (University of Illinois and Northwestern University) and former AHA president who provided insight into the evolution of academic cardiology and the tensions between the AHA and ACC a quarter of a century ago. *Boston, Mass., 16 June 1992.*

Otakar Pollak (b. 1906). Czechoslovakian scientist who came to America in 1939 and established the American Society for the Study of Arteriosclerosis twelve years later. There are interesting parallels between the formation of that society and of the ACC, organized in 1949. Pollak provided insight into the challenges immigrant physicians confronted in the 1940s. *Wilmington, Del., 21 September 1992.*

Helen F. Reichert (b. 1909). Widow of ACC founder and longtime secretary-treasurer Philip Reichert (he died in 1987). Since none of the college's fourteen founders are alive, Mrs. Reichert, who knew each of them, provided unique insight into the formation and early history of the organization. *New York, N.Y., 13 August 1991.*

Richard S. Ross (b. 1924). Academic cardiologist, dean, and former AHA president whose career at Johns Hopkins coincided with the explosive growth of cardiology. He provided a perspective on the emergence of academic cardiology. *Baltimore, Md., 11 June 1993.*

Donald H. Singer (b. 1929). Academic cardiologist who was a pupil of Louis Katz in Chicago. Katz was an AHA loyalist, and Singer provided insight into the tensions between the AHA and the ACC a quarter of a century ago. *Marshfield, Wis., 20 August 1992.*

H. Jeremy C. Swan (b. 1922). Academic cardiologist (UCLA and Cedars-Sinai Medical Center) who held many positions in the ACC, including president (1973–1974). A pioneer in the field of cardiac catheterization. *(Taped responses to questions mailed September 1993.)*

Warren J. Taylor (b. 1921). Boston cardiothoracic surgeon and pupil of Dwight Harken resigned as president-elect of the ACC when the *Boston Globe* published an article claiming that his open-heart surgery program at Malden Hospital had a high mortality rate. An interesting perspective on the impact of the media on the public's perception of medicine. *Boston, Mass., 15 June 1992.*

Daniel J. Ullyot (b. 1936). A cardiac surgeon who attended the University of Minnesota Medical School when C. Walton Lillehei was at his peak as an innovative cardiac surgeon. Ullyot entered the field of cardiac surgery just as saphenous vein coronary bypass graft surgery was being introduced. He was ACC president 1994–1995. *Bethesda, Md., 28 April 1994.*

Sylvan L. Weinberg (b. 1923). A practicing cardiologist from Dayton, Ohio, who was a pupil of researcher Louis Katz. Weinberg has been a member of the ACC for almost 40 years and played an important role in encouraging the organization to become more active in the area of government relations. He was ACC President during 1993–1994. *Anaheim, Calif., 12 November 1991.*

Lewis Weisblatt (b. 1921). A staff member of the NYHA from 1948 to 1983. He provided insight into the relationship between the NYHA and the AHA as well as the dynamics of medicine in New York City during the 1950s and 1960s. *New York, N.Y., 12 April 1993.*

Richard Allen Williams (b. 1936). Academic cardiologist (UCLA) who trained at Harvard. Williams has a long-standing interest in the health problems of African Americans and founded the Association of Black Cardiologists in 1974. *Atlanta, Ga., 15 March 1994.*

Irving S. Wright (b. 1902). Academic internist (Cornell–New York Hospital) who helped establish vascular medicine as a specialty in the 1930s. Served as AHA president around the time the ACC was founded. With Michael DeBakey and Mary Lasker, an influential member of the "heart lobby." *New York, N.Y., 14 August 1991.*

Barry L. Zaret (b. 1940). Academic cardiologist (Yale) and pioneer in the field of nuclear cardiology. He was a founder of the American Society of Nuclear Cardiology and served as president of the Association of Professors of Cardiology. *Atlanta, Ga., 11 November 1993.*

Secondary Sources

Abbott, A. *The System of Professions: An Essay on the Division of Expert Labor.* Chicago: Univ. of Chicago Press, 1988.

Acierno, L. J. *The History of Cardiology.* Pearl River, N.Y.: Parthenon Publishing Group, 1994.

Ahrens, E. H., Jr. *The Crisis in Clinical Research.* New York: Oxford Univ. Press, 1992.

American Medical Directory. [Various editions]. Chicago: AMA [1906–1994].

Bachman, G. W. *Health Resources in the United States: Personnel, Facilities, and Services.* Washington, D.C.: Brookings Institution, 1952.

Bates, B. *Bargaining for Life: A Social History of Tuberculosis, 1876–1938.* Philadelphia: Univ. of Pennsylvania Press, 1992.

Beeson, P. B. "Changes in medical therapy during the past half century." *Medicine* 59 (1980): 79–99.

Belth, N. C. *A Promise to Keep: A Narrative of the American Encounter with Anti-Semitism.* New York: Schocken Books, 1981.

Ben-David, J. *Scientific Growth: Essays on the Social Organization and Ethos of Science,* ed. G. Freudenthal. Berkeley: Univ. of California Press, 1991.

Benedek, T. G. "A century of American rheumatology." In *Grand Rounds: One Hundred Years of Internal Medicine,* ed. R. C. Maulitz and D. E. Long. Philadelphia: Univ. of Pennsylvania Press, 1988, 159–209.

Bennett, J. T. and T. J. DiLorenzo. *Unhealthy Charities: Hazardous to Your Health and Wealth.* New York: Basic Books, 1994.

Bennett, R. V. *Hope in Heart Disease: The Story of Louis Faugères Bishop.* Philadelphia: Dorrance & Co., 1948.

Benson, J. A., Jr. *Oral Histories: American Board of Internal Medicine Chairmen, 1947–1985.* Philadelphia: ABIM, 1994.

Bigelow, W. G. *Cold Hearts: The Story of Hypothermia and the Pacemaker in Heart Surgery.* Toronto: McClelland and Stewart, 1984.

Bing, R. J. *Cardiology: The Evolution of the Science and the Art.* Chur, Switzerland: Harwood Academic Publishers, 1992.

Bishop, L. F. "History of cardiology." *N.Y. State J. Med.* 28 (1928): 140–141.

Bishop, L. F., Jr. *The Birth of a Specialty: The Diary of an American Cardiologist, 1926–1972.* New York: Vantage Press, 1977.

Bishop, L. F., Jr. "Cardiology as a specialty." *N.Y. State J. Med.* 76 (1976): 1170–1174.

Blank, H. L. "The Responses of Physicians to Medical Reform: Health Care and the Medical Profession in New York City, 1890–1940." Ph.D. diss., State University of New York at Stony Brook, 1983.

Bloomfield, A. L. *A Bibliography of Internal Medicine: Communicable Diseases.* Chicago: Univ. of Chicago Press, 1958.

Blümchen, G. *Beiträge zur Geschichte der Kardiologie.* Leichlingen, Germany: Roder-birken Klinik, 1978.

Boerigter, R. J. "A History of the American College of Sports Medicine." Ph.D. diss., University of Utah, 1978.

Bonner, T. N. *American Doctors and German Universities: A Chapter in International Intellectual Relations, 1870–1914.* Lincoln: Univ. of Nebraska Press, 1963.

Booth, C. C. "Clinical research." In *Companion Encyclopedia of the History of Medicine,* ed. W. F. Bynum and R. Porter. New York: Routledge, 1993, 1: 205–229.

Bowers, J. Z. and E. E. King, eds. *Academic Medicine: Present and Future.* New York: Rockefeller Archive Center, 1983.

Bowers, J. Z. and E. F. Purcell, eds. *The University and Medicine: The Past, the Present, and Tomorrow.* New York: Josiah Macy, Jr. Foundation, 1977.

Braunwald, E. "Thirty-five years of progress in cardiovascular research." *Circulation* 70 (1984): III 8–25.

Braunwald, E. "On future directions for cardiology." *Circulation* 77 (1988): 13–32.

Braunwald, E. "The golden age of cardiology." In *An Era in Cardiovascular Medicine,* ed. S. B. Knoebel and S. Dack. New York: Elsevier Science Publishing, 1991, 1–4.

Brecher, R. and E. Brecher. *The Rays: A History of Radiology in the United States and Canada.* Baltimore: Williams & Wilkins, 1959.

Bronzino, J. D., V. H. Smith, and M. L. Wade. *Medical Technology and Society: An Interdisciplinary Perspective.* Cambridge: MIT Press, 1990.

Brye, D. L., ed. *European Immigration and Ethnicity in the United States and Canada: A Historical Bibliography.* Santa Barbara, Calif.: ABC-Clio Information Services, 1983.

Burch, G. E. "Changing concepts in cardiovascular therapy: A quarter century perspective." *Am. Heart J.* 93 (1977): 413–418.

Burch, G. E. and N. P. DePasquale. *A History of Electrocardiography with a new Introduction by J. D. Howell.* 2d ed. San Francisco: Jeremy Norman, 1990.

Burchell, H. B. "A cardiologist's view of modern cardiovascular surgery." *Dis. Chest* 55 (1969): 323–328.

Burchell, H. B. "Important events in cardiology, 1940–1982." *JAMA* 249 (1983): 1197–1200.

Burnett, J. "The origins of the electrocardiograph as a clinical instrument." *Med. Hist.* suppl. 5 (1985): 53–76.

Bush, V. *Science: The Endless Frontier.* Washington, D.C.: GPO, 1945.

Bynum, W. F. *Science and the Practice of Medicine in the Nineteenth Century.* New York: Cambridge Univ. Press, 1994.

Cabot, R. C. "The historical development and relative value of laboratory and clinical methods of diagnosis," *Boston Med. Surg. J.* 157 (1907): 150–153.

Callahan, J. A. and T. E. Keys, eds. *Classics of Cardiology: A Collection of Classic Works on the Heart and Circulation with Comprehensive Biographic Accounts of the Authors. Volume 3.* Malabar, Fla.: Robert E. Krieger, 1983.

Campbell, M. "The British Cardiac Society and the Cardiac Club: 1922–1961." *Br. Heart J.* 24 (1962): 673–695.

Campion, F. D. *The AMA and U.S. Health Policy Since 1940.* Chicago: Chicago Review Press, 1984.

Carter, R. *The Gentle Legions: A Probing Study of the National Voluntary Health Organizations.* Garden City, N.Y.: Doubleday, 1961.

Chapman, C. B. and J. M. Talmadge. "The evolution of the right to health concepts in the United States." *Pharos* 34 (1971): 30–51.

Chávez, I. "Thirty years' progress in cardiological diagnosis." *Am. J. Cardiol.* 1 (1958): 3–18.

Clark, B. R., ed. *The Academic Profession: National, Disciplinary, and Institutional Settings.* Berkeley: Univ. of California Press, 1987.

Coggeshall, L. T. *Planning for Medical Progress through Education.* Washington, D.C.: Association of American Medical Colleges, 1965.

Cohn, A. E. "The first cardiac clinic." *JAMA* 121 (1943): 70.

Coll, B. D. *Perspectives in Public Welfare: A History.* Washington, D.C.: DHEW, 1969.

Comroe, J. H., Jr. *Exploring the Heart: Discoveries in Heart Disease and High Blood Pressure.* New York: W. W. Norton, 1983.

Comroe, J. H., Jr., and R. D. Dripps. *The Top Ten Clinical Advances in Cardiovascular-Pulmonary Medicine and Surgery 1945–1975.* Washington, D.C.: GPO, 1978.

Cooley, D. A. "Perspectives in cardiac surgery with personal reflections." *Surg. Clin. North Am.* 5 (1978): 895–906.

Cooter, R. *Surgery and Society in Peace and War: Orthopaedics and the Organization of Modern Medicine, 1880–1948.* London: Macmillan Press, 1993.

Cordasco, F. *Medical Education in the United States: A Guide to Information Sources.* Detroit: Gale Research Company, 1980.

Corwin, E. H. L. *The American Hospital.* New York: Commonwealth Fund, 1946.

Coser, L. A. *Refugee Scholars in America: Their Impact and Their Experiences.* New Haven: Yale Univ. Press, 1984.

Cournand, A. F. "Cardiac catheterization: Development of the technique, its contributions to experimental medicine, and its initial applications in man." *Acta Med. Scand.* suppl. 579 (1975): 3–32.

Cournand, A. F. *From Roots to Late Budding: The Intellectual Adventures of a Medical Scientist.* New York: Gardner Press, 1986.

Crane, D. *Invisible Colleges: Diffusion of Knowledge in Scientific Communities.* Chicago: Univ. of Chicago Press, 1972.

Dack, S. "An editor's account of the history of the college." *Am. J. Cardiol.* 13 (1989): 5–11.

Davis, A. B. *Medicine and Its Technology: An Introduction to the History of Medical Instrumentation.* Westport, Conn.: Greenwood Press, 1981.

Day, H. W. "History of coronary care units." *Am. J. Cardiol.* 30 (1972): 405–407.

DeBakey, M. E. "The development of vascular surgery." *Am. J. Surg.* 137 (1979): 697–738.

Deitrick, J. E. and R. C. Berson. *Medical Schools in the United States at Mid-Century.* New York: McGraw-Hill, 1953.

de la Chapelle, C. E., ed. *The New York Heart Association: Origins and Development, 1915–1965.* New York: NYHA, 1966.

Denes, P. and M. D. Ezri. "Clinical electrophysiology—A decade of progress." *J. Am. Coll. Cardiol.* 1 (1983): 292–305.

Dexter, L. "Early days of cardiac catheterization." *J. Applied Cardiol.* 4 (1989): 343–344.

Dimond, E. G. *Take Wing! Interesting Things That Happened on My Way to School.* Kansas City, Mo.: Lowell Press, 1991.

Dinnerstein, L. *Anti-Semitism in America.* New York: Oxford Univ. Press, 1994.

Directory of Medical Specialists Certified by American Boards. [Various Publishers. Various Editions].

Divine, R. A. *American Immigration Policy, 1924–1952.* New Haven: Yale Univ. Press, 1957.

Doby, T. *Development of Angiography and Cardiovascular Catheterization.* Littleton, Mass.: Publishing Sciences Group, 1976.

Dreiling, D. A. "The first fifty years: A history of the evolution of the American College of Gastroenterology as a society for clinical gastroenterology." *Am. J. Gastroenterol.* 78 (1983): 138–139.

Drury, A. N. and R. T. Grant. "Thomas Lewis." *Obituary Notices of Fellows of the Royal Society* 14 (1945): 179–202.

Duffy, J. *A History of Public Health in New York City, 1866–1966.* New York: Russell Sage Foundation, 1974.

Duffy, J. *The Sanitarians: A History of American Public Health.* Urbana, Ill.: Univ. of Chicago Press, 1990.

Duke, M. *The Development of Medical Techniques and Treatment: From Leeches to Heart Surgery.* Madison, Conn.: International Universities Press, 1991.

East, T. *The Story of Heart Disease.* London: William Dawson and Sons, 1957.

Elkin, D. C. and M. E. DeBakey, eds. *Vascular Surgery in World War II.* Washington, D.C.: GPO, 1955.

Engle, M. A. "Growth and development of state of the art care for people with congenital heart disease." *J. Am. Coll. Cardiol.* 13 (1989): 1453–1457.

English, P. C. *Shock, Physiological Surgery, and George Washington Crile: Medical Innovation in the Progressive Era.* Westport, Conn.: Greenwood Press, 1980.

Erlen, J. *The History of the Health Care Sciences and Health Care, 1700–1980. A Selective Annotated Bibliography.* New York: Garland, 1984.

The Evan Bedford Library of Cardiology: Catalogue of Books, Pamphlets and Journals. London: Royal College of Physicians, 1977.

Faber, K. *Nosography: The Evolution of Clinical Medicine in Modern Times.* 2d ed. New York: Paul B. Hoeber, 1930.

Favaloro, R. G. *The Challenging Dream of Heart Surgery: From the Pampas to Cleveland.* Boston: Little, Brown, 1994.

Felch, W. C. and C. C. Greene Jr. *Aspiration and Achievement: The Story of the American Society of Internal Medicine, 1956–1981.* Washington, D.C.: ASIM, 1981.

Fermi, L. *Illustrious Immigrants: The Intellectual Migration from Europe, 1930–41.* 2d ed. Chicago: Univ. of Chicago Press, 1971.

Fifield, J. C., ed. *American Physicians and Surgeons: A Biographical Directory of Practicing Members of the Medical Profession in the United States and Canada.* Minneapolis: Midwest, 1931.

Fishman, A. P. and D. W. Richards, eds. *Circulation of the Blood: Men and Ideas.* New York: Oxford Univ. Press, 1964.

Fitz, R. "The rise of the practice of internal medicine as a specialty." *N. Engl. J. Med.* 242 (1950): 569–574.

Flint, H. L. *The Heart: Old and New Views.* New York: Paul B. Hoeber, 1921.

Foote, S. B. *Managing the Medical Arms Race: Public Policy and Medical Device Innovation.* Berkeley: Univ. of California Press, 1992.

Forssmann, W. *Experiments on Myself: Memoirs of a Surgeon in Germany.* New York: St. Martin's Press, 1974.

Fox, D. M. *Health Policies, Health Politics: The British and American Experience, 1911–1965.* Princeton: Princeton Univ. Press, 1986.

Fox, D. M. *Power and Illness: The Failure and Future of American Health Policy.* Berkeley: Univ. of California Press, 1993.

Fox, R. C. and J. P. Swazey. *Spare Parts: Organ Replacement in American Society.* New York: Oxford Univ. Press, 1992.

Frank, R. G., Jr. "American physiologists in German laboratories, 1865–1914." In *Physiology in the American context, 1850–1940,* ed. G. L. Geison. Bethesda, Md.: American Physiological Society, 1987, 11–46.

Freidson, E. *Profession of Medicine: A Study of the Sociology of Applied Knowledge.* New York: Dodd, Mead, 1974.

Freidson, E. "Foreword." In *The Making of Rehabilitation: A Political Economy of Medical Specialization, 1890–1980.* G. Gritzer and A. Arluke. Berkeley: Univ. of California Press, 1985, xi-xxii.

Freidson, E. *Medical Work in America: Essays on Health Care.* New Haven: Yale Univ. Press, 1989.

Freidson, E. and J. Lorber, eds. *Medical Men and Their Work.* Chicago: Aldine-Atherton, 1972.

Freund, P. A., ed. *Experimentation with Human Subjects.* New York: George Braziller, 1970.

Freymann, J. G. *The American Health Care System: Its Genesis and Trajectory.* Huntington, N.Y.: Krieger, 1977.

Friedman, S. G. *A History of Vascular Surgery.* Mount Kisco, N.Y.: Futura Publishing Company, 1989.

Frohlich, E. D. "Achievements in hypertension: A 25-year overview." *J. Am. Coll. Cardiol.* 1 (1983): 225–239.

Fudenberg, H. H. and V. L. Melnick, eds. *Biomedical Scientists and Public Policy.* New York: Plenum Press, 1978.

Fulton, F. T. *The Story of the Heart Station at the Rhode Island Hospital.* Providence: [Frank T. Fulton], 1955.

Fulton, H. "Sixty years of cardiovascular roentgenology." *Am. J. Roentgenol.* 76 (1956): 657–663.

Fye, W. B. "The historical literature of internal medicine: An annotated bibliography." *Ann. Intern. Med.* 87 (1977): 123–128.

Fye, W. B. "Coronary arteriography: It took a long time." *Circulation* 70 (1984): 781–787.

Fye, W. B. *Bibliography of the History of Cardiovascular Medicine and Surgery.* Bethesda, Md.: National Library of Medicine, 1986.

Fye, W. B. *American Contributions to Cardiovascular Medicine and Surgery.* Bethesda, Md.: NIH, 1986.

Fye, W. B. *The Development of American Physiology: Scientific Medicine in the Nineteenth Century.* Baltimore: Johns Hopkins Univ. Press, 1987.

Fye, W. B. "The origin of the full-time faculty system: Implications for clinical research." *JAMA* 265 (1991): 1555–1562.

Fye, W. B. "Albion Walter Hewlett: Teacher, clinician, scientist, and missionary for 'pathologic physiology'." In *Medical Lives and Scientific Medicine at Michigan, 1891–1969,* ed. J. D. Howell. Ann Arbor: Univ. of Michigan Press, 1993, 45–72.

Fye, W. B. "Disorders of the heartbeat: A historical overview from antiquity to the mid-20th century." *Am. J. Cardiol.* 72 (1993): 1055–1070.

Fye, W. B. "A history of the American Heart Association's Council on Clinical Cardiology." *Circulation* 87 (1993): 1057–1063.

Fye, W. B. "A history of the origin, evolution, and impact of electrocardiography." *Am. J. Cardiol.* 73 (1994): 937–949.

Galdston, I., ed. *The Impact of the Antibiotics on Medicine and Society.* New York: International Universities Press, 1958.

Garcia-Palmieri, M. R. *The International Society and Federation of Cardiology and Its Components: Historical Data, 1950–1990.* San Juan, P.R.: Mario R. Garcia-Palmieri, 1990.

Geiger, R. L. *To Advance Knowledge: The Growth of American Research Universities, 1900–1940.* New York: Oxford Univ. Press, 1986.

Geiger, R. L. *Research and Relevant Knowledge: American Research Universities since World War II.* New York: Oxford Univ. Press, 1993.

Ginzberg, E. *The Medical Triangle: Physicians, Politicians, and the Public.* Cambridge: Harvard Univ. Press, 1990.

Ginzberg, E. "The impact of World War II on U.S. medicine." *Am. J. Med. Sci.* 304 (1992): 268–271.

Ginzberg, E. and A. B. Dutka. *The Financing of Biomedical Research.* Baltimore: Johns Hopkins Univ. Press, 1989.

Ginzberg, E. and A. M. Yohalem, eds. *The University Medical Center and the Metropolis.* New York: Josiah Macy, Jr. Foundation, 1974.

Glaser, W. A. *Paying the Doctor: Systems of Remuneration and Their Effects.* Baltimore: Johns Hopkins Univ. Press, 1970.

Glenn, W. W. L. "Some account of the early years of cardiac surgery." *Conn. Med.* 44 (1980): 338–344.

Gorny, P. *Histoire Illustrée de la Cardiologie.* Paris: Les Éditions Roger Dacosta, 1985.

Goulden, J. C. *The Best Years, 1945–1950.* New York: Atheneum, 1976.

Gritzer, G. and A. Arluke. *The Making of Rehabilitation: A Political Economy of Medical Specialization, 1890–1980.* Berkeley: Univ. of California Press, 1985.

Gunn, S. M. and P. S. Platt. *Voluntary Health Agencies: An Interpretive Study.* New York: Ronald Press Company, 1945.

Hafner, A. W., ed. *Directory of Deceased American Physicians, 1804–1929.* Chicago: AMA, 1994.

Hall, P. D. *Inventing the Non-Profit Sector and Other Essays on Philanthropy, Voluntarism, and Non-Profit Organizations.* Baltimore: Johns Hopkins Univ. Press, 1992.

Halpern, S. A. *American Pediatrics: The Social Dynamics of Professionalism, 1880–1980.* Berkeley: Univ. of California Press, 1988.

Harden, V. A. *Inventing the NIH: Federal Biomedical Research Policy, 1887–1937.* Baltimore: Johns Hopkins Univ. Press, 1986.

Hardy, J. D. *The World of Surgery, 1945–1985: Memoirs of One Participant.* Philadelphia: Univ. of Pennsylvania Press, 1986.

Harris, S. E. *The Economics of American Medicine.* New York: Macmillan, 1964.

Harvey, A. M. *Science at the Bedside: Clinical Research in American Medicine, 1905–1945.* Baltimore: Johns Hopkins Univ. Press, 1981.

Harvey, A. M. *The Association of American Physicians, 1886–1986.* Baltimore: Waverly Press, 1986.

Health in America: 1776–1976. Washington, D.C.: Department of Health, Education and Welfare, 1976.

Herrick, J. B. *A Short History of Cardiology.* Springfield, Ill.: Charles C. Thomas, 1942.

Herrick, J. B. *Memories of Eighty Years.* Chicago: Univ. of Chicago Press, 1949.

Hirshfield, D. S. *The Lost Reform: The Campaign for Compulsory Health Insurance in the United States from 1932 to 1943.* Cambridge: Harvard Univ. Press, 1970.

"The History of the Medical Vascular Section of the Mayo Clinic." Typescript c1957. Mayo Medical Archives, Rochester, Minn.

A History of the Scientific Councils of the American Heart Association. New York: AHA, 1967.

Hogness, J. R. and M. VanAntwerp, eds. *The Artificial Heart: Prototypes, Policies, and Patients.* Washington, D.C.: National Academy Press, 1991.

Hospital Council of Greater New York. *Hospital Staff Appointments of Physicians in New York City.* New York: Macmillan, 1951.

Howell, J. D. "The changing face of twentieth-century American cardiology." *Ann. Intern. Med.* 105 (1986): 772–782.

Howell, J. D. "Cardiac physiology and clinical medicine? Two case studies." In *Physiology in the American Context: 1850–1940,* ed. G. L. Geison. Bethesda, Md.: American Physiological Society, 1987, 279–292.

Howell, J. D., ed. *Technology and American Medical Practice 1880–1930: An Anthology of Sources.* New York: Garland, 1988.

Howell, J. D. "Hearts and minds: The invention and transformation of American cardiology." In *Grand Rounds: One Hundred Years of Internal Medicine,* ed. R. C. Maulitz and D. E. Long. Philadelphia: Univ. of Pennsylvania Press, 1988, 243–275.

Howell, J. D. "Diagnostic technologies: X-rays, electrocardiograms, and CAT scans." *S. Calif. Law Rev.* 65 (1991): 529–564.

Howell, J. D., ed. *Medical Lives and Scientific Medicine at Michigan, 1891–1969.* Ann Arbor: Univ. of Michigan Press, 1993.

Howell, J. D. *Technology in the Hospital: Transforming Patient Care in the Early Twentieth Century.* Baltimore: Johns Hopkins Univ. Press, 1995.

Huddle, T. S. "Science, Practice, and the Reform of American Medical Education." Ph.D. diss., University of Illinois at Urbana-Champaign, 1988.

International Who's Who in World Medicine, 1947. New York: American Universities Medical Research Publications, 1947.

Jackman, J. C. and C. M. Borden, eds. *The Muses Flee Hitler: Cultural Transfer and Adaptation, 1930–1945.* Washington, D.C.: Smithsonian Institution Press, 1983.

Jackson, K. T. *Crabgrass Frontier: The Suburbanization of the United States.* New York: Oxford Univ. Press, 1985.

Johnson, J. A. and W. J. Jones. *The American Medical Association and Organized Medicine: A Commentary and Annotated Bibliography.* New York: Garland, 1993.

Johnson, S. L. *The History of Cardiac Surgery.* Baltimore: Johns Hopkins Univ. Press, 1970.

Kagan, S. R. *Jewish Contributions to Medicine in America from Colonial Times to the Present.* 2d ed. Boston: Boston Medical Publishing Co., 1939.

Karpovich, P. V. *Adventures in Artificial Respiration.* New York: Association Press, 1953.

Kass, E. H. "History of the subspecialty of infectious diseases in the United States." In *Grand Rounds: One Hundred Years of Internal Medicine,* ed. R. C. Maulitz and D. E. Long. Philadelphia: Univ. of Pennsylvania Press, 1988, 87–115.

Kaufman, M., S. Galishoff, and T. L. Savitt, eds. *Dictionary of American Medical Biography.* Westport, Conn.: Greenwood Press, 1984.

Kaufman, S. R. *The Healer's Tale: Transforming Medicine and Culture.* Madison: Univ. of Wisconsin Press, 1993.

Kenney, M. *Biotechnology: The University-Industrial Complex.* New Haven: Yale Univ. Press, 1986.

King, L. S. *Transformations in American Medicine: From Benjamin Rush to William Osler.* Baltimore: Johns Hopkins Univ. Press, 1991.

Kirklin, J. W. "Open-heart surgery at the Mayo Clinic: The 25th anniversary." *Mayo Clin. Proc.* 55 (1980): 339–341.

Kirsner, J. B. *The Development of American Gastroenterology.* New York: Raven Press, 1990.

Kisch, B., ed. *Franz M. Groedel Anniversary Volume on the Occasion of His Seventieth Birthday.* New York: Brooklyn Medical Press, 1951.

Kisch, B. *Wanderungen und Wandlungen: Die Geschichte eines Arztes im 20. Jahrhundert.* Cologne: Greven Verlag, 1966.

Knopf, S. A. *A History of the National Tuberculosis Association: The Anti-Tuberculosis Movement in the United States.* New York: National Tuberculosis Association, 1922.

Knowles, J. H., ed. *Doing Better and Feeling Worse: Health in the United States.* New York: W. W. Norton, 1977.

Kohrman, C. H., R. M. Andersen, and M. M. Clements. *Training Physicians: The Case of Internal Medicine.* San Francisco: Jossey-Bass, 1994.

Knowles, J. H., ed. *Hospitals, Doctors, and the Public Interest.* Cambridge: Harvard Univ. Press, 1985.

Koren, N. *Jewish Physicians: A Biographical Index.* Jerusalem: Israel Universities Press, 1973.

Lape, E. E., ed. *Medical Research: A Midcentury Survey.* Boston: Little, Brown, 1955.

Larson, M. S. *The Rise of Professionalism: A Sociological Analysis.* Berkeley: Univ. of California Press, 1977.

Lawrence, C. "Incommunicable knowledge: Science, technology and the clinical art in Britain, 1850–1914." *J. Contemp. Hist.* 20 (1985): 503–520.

Lawrence, C. "Moderns and ancients: The 'new cardiology' in Britain 1880–1930." *Med. Hist.* suppl. 5 (1985): 1–33.

Lawrence, C. "'Definite and material': Coronary thrombosis and cardiologists in the 1920s." In *Framing Disease*, ed. C. E. Rosenberg and J. Golden. New Brunswick, N.J.: Rutgers Univ. Press, 1992, 50–82.

Lederer, S. E. *Subjected to Science: Human Experimentation in America Before the Second World War.* Baltimore: Johns Hopkins Univ. Press, 1995.

Lee, T. H. and L. Goldman. "The coronary care unit turns 25: Historical trends and future directions." *Ann. Intern. Med.* 108 (1988): 887–894.

Leibowitz, J. O. *The History of Coronary Heart Disease.* London: Wellcome Institute of the History of Medicine, 1970.

Lepore, M. J. *Death of the Clinician: Requiem or Reveille?* Springfield, Ill.: Charles C. Thomas, 1982.

Levitan, T. *Islands of Compassion: A History of the Jewish Hospitals of New York.* New York: Twayne Publishers, 1964.

Lightfoot, S. A. "A history of physician payment policies under Medicare." *Bull. Am. Coll. Surg.* 78 (1993): 32–35.

Lippard, V. W. *A Half-Century of American Medical Education: 1920–1970.* New York: Josiah Macy, Jr. Foundation, 1974.

Lock, S. and F. Wells, eds. *Fraud and Misconduct in Medical Research.* London: BMJ Publishing Group, 1993.

Logan, V. W. "The American Board of Internal Medicine, 1936–1966." Philadelphia: ABIM, 1970.

Long, D. and J. Golden, eds. *The American General Hospital: Communities and Social Contexts.* Ithaca, N.Y.: Cornell Univ. Press, 1989.

Longmire, W. P., Jr. *Alfred Blalock: His Life and Times* [Los Angeles]: William P. Longmire Jr., 1991.

Lowe, T. E., H. B. Kay, and H. A. Luke. *The Practical Significance of Modern Cardiological Investigations.* Melbourne: Melbourne Univ. Press, 1951.

Lüderitz, B. *History of the Disorders of Cardiac Rhythm.* Armonk, N.Y.: Futura, 1995.

Ludmerer, K. M. "The rise of the teaching hospital in America." *J. Hist. Med. Allied Sci.* 38 (1983): 389–414.

Ludmerer, K. M. *Learning to Heal: The Development of American Medical Education.* New York: Basic Books, 1985.

Ludmerer, K. M. "The medical schools of New York and the national enterprise of biomedical research, 1850–1987." *Bull. N.Y. Acad. Med.* 64 (1988): 216–236.

Ludmerer, K. M. "The origins of Mount Sinai School of Medicine." *J. Hist. Med. Allied Sci.* 45 (1990): 469–489.

Lyden, F. L., H. J. Geiger, and O. L. Peterson. *The Training of Good Physicians: Critical Factors in Career Choices.* Cambridge: Harvard Univ. Press, 1968.

Mackenzie, J. "The position of medicine at the beginning of the twentieth century illustrated by the state of cardiology," *N.Y. Med. J.* 115 (1922): 61–66.

Magraw, R. M. *Ferment in Medicine: A Study of the Essence of Medical Practice and of Its New Dilemmas.* Philadelphia: W. B. Saunders, 1966.

Mair, A. *Sir James Mackenzie, M.D. 1853–1925, General Practitioner.* Edinburgh: Churchill Livingstone, 1973.

Mannebach, H. *Hundert Jahre Herzgeschichte: Entwicklung der Kardiologie 1887–1987.* Berlin: Springer-Verlag, 1988.

Margulies, H. and L. S. Bloch. *Foreign Medical Graduates in the United States.* Cambridge: Harvard Univ. Press, 1969.

Marion, P. *Afin que Batte le Coeur: L'Epopée de la Chirurgie Cardiaque.* Lyon: Presses Universitaires de Lyon, 1990.

Marks, H. M. "Notes from the underground: The social organization of therapeutic research." In *Grand Rounds: One Hundred Years of Internal Medicine,* ed. R. C. Maulitz and D. E. Long. Philadelphia: Univ. of Pennsylvania Press, 1988, 297–336.

Marks, H. M. "Medical technologies: Social contexts and consequences." In *Companion Encyclopedia of the History of Medicine,* ed. W. F. Bynum and R. Porter. New York: Routledge, 1993, 2: 1592–1618.

Marrus, M. R. *The Unwanted: European Refugees in the Twentieth Century.* New York: Oxford Univ. Press, 1985.

Martin, S. C. and J. D. Howell. "One hundred years of clinical preventive medicine in America." *Prim. Care* 16 (1989): 3–8.

Master, A. M. "Reminiscences of fifty years in cardiology at Mount Sinai with special reference to the two-step test." *Mt. Sinai J. Med.* 39 (1972): 486–505.

Matthews, D. N. *Fighting Heart Disease: The History of the British Heart Foundation, 1961–1988.* Oxford: Blackwell Scientific Publications, 1990.

Maulitz, R. C. "Grand rounds: An introduction to the history of internal medicine." In *Grand Rounds: One Hundred Years of Internal Medicine,* ed. R. C. Maulitz and D. E. Long. Philadelphia: Univ. of Pennsylvania Press, 1988, 3–13.

Maulitz, R. C., ed. *Unnatural Causes: The Three Leading Killer Diseases in America.* New Brunswick, N.J.: Rutgers Univ. Press, 1988.

McIntosh, H. D. and J. A. Garcia. "The first decade of aortocoronary bypass grafting, 1967–1977." *Circulation* 57 (1978): 405–431.

McKelvey, B. *The Urbanization of America, 1860–1915*. New Brunswick, N.J.: Rutgers Univ. Press, 1963.

Means, J. H. *The Association of American Physicians: Its First Seventy-Five Years*. New York: McGraw-Hill, 1961.

Meckel, R. A. *Save the Babies: American Public Health Reform and the Prevention of Infant Mortality, 1850–1929*. Baltimore: Johns Hopkins Univ. Press, 1990.

The Medical Directory of New York, New Jersey and Connecticut. Volume 35. New York: Medical Society of the State of New York, 1933.

Middleton, W. S. "The evolution of modern cardiology, being in some measure the experience of a stethoscope (1908–1968)." In *Values in Modern Medicine*. Madison: Univ. of Wisconsin Press, 1972, 112–123.

Miller, T. G. "The development of specialty medical clinics at the Hospital of the University of Pennsylvania." *Trans. Stud. Coll. Physicians Phila.* 32 (1965): 104–108.

Minetree, H. *Cooley: The Career of a Great Heart Surgeon*. New York: Harper's Magazine Press, 1966.

Monteith, W. B. R., ed. *Bibliography with Synopsis of the Original Papers of the Writings of Sir James Mackenzie*. London: Oxford Univ. Press, 1930.

Moore, T. J. *Heart Failure: A Critical Inquiry into American Medicine and the Revolution in Heart Care*. New York: Random House, 1989.

Moore, W. M. *Fighting for Life: The Story of the American Heart Association 1911–1975*. Dallas: AHA, 1983.

Morgan, W. G. *The American College of Physicians: Its First Quarter Century*. Philadelphia: ACP, 1940.

Moser, R. H. *A Decade of Decision: A Physician Remembers the American College of Physicians, 1977–1986*. Philadelphia: ACP, 1991.

Mueller, R. L. and S. Scheidt. "History of drugs for thrombotic disease: Discovery, development, and directions for the future." *Circulation* 89 (1994): 432–449.

Myers, J. A. *A History of the American College of Chest Physicians, 1935–1959*. [Chicago]: American College of Chest Physicians, 1959.

Myers, R. J. *Medicare*. Bryn Mawr, Pa.: McCahn Foundation, 1970.

Naef, A. P. *The Story of Thoracic Surgery*. Toronto: Hogrefe & Huber, 1990.

Nakamoto, J. and C. Verner. *Continuing Education in the Health Professions: A Review of the Literature, 1960–1970*. Syracuse, N.Y.: ERIC Clearing House on Adult Education, 1973.

National Heart, Lung, and Blood Institute Fact Book. Fiscal Year 1993. Bethesda, Md.: NHLBI, 1994.

Neill, C. A. and E. B. Clark. *The Developing Heart: A 'History' of Pediatric Cardiology*. Boston: Kluwer Academic Publishers, 1995.

Numbers, R. L., ed. *Compulsory Health Insurance: The Continuing American Debate*. Westport, Conn.: Greenwood Press, 1982.

Oleson, A. and J. Voss, eds. *The Organization of Knowledge in Modern America, 1860–1920*. Baltimore: Johns Hopkins Univ. Press, 1979.

Oral History of Twenty-Five Years of American Cardiology. Celebrating the 25th Anniversary of the American College of Cardiology, 1949–1974. Bethesda, Md.: ACC [ACCEL], 1974.

Oren, D. A. *Joining the Club: A History of Jews and Yale*. New Haven: Yale Univ. Press, 1985.

Packard, B. "Changing perspectives: The National Heart, Lung, and Blood Institute programs for research training and career development." *J. Am. Coll. Cardiol.* 12 (1988): 827–828.

Page, I. H. *Hypertension Research: A Memoir, 1920–1960.* New York: Pergamon Press, 1988.

Patterson, J. T. *The Dread Disease: Cancer and Modern American Culture.* Cambridge: Harvard Univ. Press, 1987.

Paul, O. *Take Heart: The Life and Prescription for Living of Dr. Paul Dudley White.* Boston: Francis A. Countway Library of Medicine, 1986.

Pauly, M. V. and W. L. Kissick, eds. *Lessons from the First Twenty Years of Medicare.* Philadelphia: Univ. of Pennsylvania Press, 1988.

Peitzman, S. J. "Nephrology in America from Thomas Addis to the artificial kidney." In *Grand Rounds: One Hundred Years of Internal Medicine,* ed. R. C. Maulitz and D. E. Long. Philadelphia: Univ. of Pennsylvania Press, 1988, 211–241.

Pickstone, J. V., ed. *Medical Innovations in Historical Perspective.* New York: St. Martin's Press, 1992.

Piersol, G. M. *Gateway of Honor: The American College of Physicians 1915–1959.* Philadelphia: ACP, 1962.

Poen, M. M. *Harry S. Truman versus the Medical Lobby: The Genesis of Medicare.* Columbia: Univ. of Missouri Press, 1979.

Porter, R. J. and T. E. Malone, eds. *Biomedical Research: Collaboration and Conflict of Interest.* Baltimore: Johns Hopkins Univ. Press, 1992.

Preston, T. A. "Historical development of operations for coronary artery disease." In *Coronary Artery Surgery: A Critical Review.* New York: Raven Press, 1977, 7–26.

Racker, E. *Science and the Cure of Diseases: Letters to Members of Congress.* Princeton: Princeton Univ. Press, 1979.

Rappleye, W. C., ed. *Graduate Medical Education: Report of the Commission on Graduate Medical Education.* Chicago: Univ. of Chicago Press, 1940.

Rashkind, W. J. "Pediatric cardiology: A brief historical perspective." *Pediat. Cardiol.* 1 (1979): 63–71.

Ravenel, M. P., ed. *A Half Century of Public Health.* New York: American Public Health Association, 1921.

Redman, E. *The Dance of Legislation.* New York: Simon & Schuster, 1973.

Reichert, P. "A history of the development of cardiology as a medical specialty." *Clin. Cardiol.* 1 (1978): 5–15.

Reichert, P. "The American College of Cardiology, Its First Thirty Years." [1980], History file, ACC Archives.

Reichert, P. and L. F. Bishop Jr. "Sir James Mackenzie and his polygraph: The contribution of Louis Faugeres Bishop, Sr." *Am. J. Cardiol.* 24 (1969): 401–403.

Reingold, N. *Science, American Style.* New Brunswick, N.J.: Rutgers Univ. Press, 1991.

Reiser, S. J. *Medicine and the Reign of Technology.* Cambridge: Cambridge Univ. Press, 1978.

Reiser, S. J. "The medical influence of the stethoscope." *Sci. Am.* 240 (1979): 148–156.

Reiser, S. J. and M. Anbar, eds. *The Machine at the Bedside: Strategies for Using Technology in Patient Care.* New York: Cambridge Univ. Press, 1984.

Richards, R. K. *Continuing Medical Education: Perspectives, Problems, Prognosis.* New Haven: Yale Univ. Press, 1978.

Richmond, J. B. *Currents in American Medicine: A Developmental View of Medical Care and Education.* Cambridge: Harvard Univ. Press, 1969.

Rodman, J. S. *History of the American Board of Surgery, 1937–1952.* Philadelphia: J.B. Lippincott, 1956.

Rodwin, M. A. *Medicine, Money, and Morals: Physicians' Conflicts of Interest.* New York: Oxford Univ. Press, 1993.

Romaine-Davis, A. *John Gibbon and His Heart-Lung Machine.* Philadelphia: Univ. of Pennsylvania Press, 1991.

Rosen, G. *The Specialization of Medicine with Particular Reference to Ophthalmology.* New York: Froben Press, 1944.

Rosen, G. "Whither specialization." In *Medicine and Society: Contemporary Medical Problems in Historical Perspective.* Bryn Mawr, Pa.: Bryn Mawr College, 1971, 196–219.

Rosen, G. *Preventive Medicine in the United States, 1900–1975.* New York: Science History Publications, 1975.

Rosen, G. *The Structure of American Medical Practice, 1875–1941.* Philadelphia: Univ. of Pennsylvania Press, 1983.

Rosen, G. *A History of Public Health.* 2d ed. Introduction E. Fee. Biographical essay E. Morman. Baltimore: Johns Hopkins Univ. Press, 1993.

Rosenberg, C., ed. *Medical Care in the United States: The Debate Before 1940.* New York: Garland, 1989.

Rosenberg, C. E. *The Care of Strangers: The Rise of America's Hospital System.* New York: Basic Books, 1987.

Rosenberg, C. F. and J. Golden, eds. *Framing Disease: Studies in Cultural History.* New Brunswick, N.J.: Rutgers Univ. Press, 1992.

Rosenkrantz, B. G. *Public Health and the State: Changing Views in Massachusetts, 1842–1936.* Cambridge: Harvard Univ. Press, 1972.

Rosenow, E. C., Jr. *History of the American College of Physicians: Executive Perspectives 1959–1977.* Philadelphia: ACP, 1984.

Ross, W. S. *Crusade: The Official History of the American Cancer Society.* New York: Arbor House, 1987.

Rothstein, W. G. *American Medical Schools and the Practice of Medicine, a History.* New York: Oxford Univ. Press, 1987.

Rowbottom, M. and C. Susskind. *Electricity and Medicine: History of Their Interaction.* San Francisco: San Francisco Press, 1984.

Russell, L. B. *Technology in Hospitals: Medical Advances and Their Diffusion.* Washington, D.C.: Brookings Institution, 1979.

Safar, P. "History of cardiopulmonary-cerebral resuscitation." In *Cardiopulmonary Resuscitation,* ed. W. Kaye and N. G. Bircher. New York: Churchill Livingstone, 1989, 1–53.

Schechter, D. C. *Exploring the Origins of Electrical Cardiac Stimulation: Selected Works of David Charles Schechter, M.D., F.A.C.S., on the History of Electrotherapy.* Minneapolis: Medtronic, 1983.

Schlepper, M. and S. Dack. "Franz Groedel, Bruno Kisch and the founding of the American College of Cardiology." *Am. J. Cardiol.* 12 (1988): 577–580.

Schneider, D. M. and A. Deutsch. *The History of Public Welfare in New York State, 1867–1940.* Chicago: Univ. of Chicago Press, 1941.

Schwartzman, D. *Innovation in the Pharmaceutical Industry.* Baltimore: Johns Hopkins Univ. Press, 1976.

Schwarz, J. C., ed. *Who's Who Among Physicians and Surgeons. Volume 1.* New York: J. C. Schwarz, 1938.

Segall, H. N. *Pioneers of Cardiology in Canada 1820–1970. The Genesis of Canadian Cardiology.* Willowdale, Ontario: Hounslow Press, 1988.

Selzer, A. "Fifty years of progress in cardiology: A personal perspective." *Circulation* 77 (1988): 955–963.

Sherry, S. "The origin of thrombolytic therapy." *J. Am. Coll. Cardiol.* 14 (1989): 1085–1092.

Sherry, S. *Reflections and Reminiscences of an Academic Physician.* Philadelphia: Lea & Febiger, 1993.

Shonick, W. *Government and Health Services: Government's Role in the Development of U.S. Health Services 1930–1980.* New York: Oxford Univ. Press, 1995.

Shorter, E. *Bedside Manners: The Troubled History of Doctors and Patients.* New York: Simon and Schuster, 1985.

Shryock, R. H. *American Medical Research: Past and Present.* New York: Commonwealth Fund, 1947.

Shryock, R. H. *National Tuberculosis Association, 1904–1954. A Study of the Voluntary Health Movement in the United States.* New York: National Tuberculosis Association, 1957.

Shumacker, H. B., Jr. *The Society for Vascular Surgery. A History: 1945–1983.* Manchester, Mass.: Society for Vascular Surgery, 1984.

Shumacker, H. B., Jr. *The Evolution of Cardiac Surgery.* Bloomington: Indiana Univ. Press, 1992.

Smillie, W. G. *Public Health: Its Promise for the Future.* New York: Macmillan, 1955.

Snellen, H. A. "Birth and growth of the European Society of Cardiology," *Eur. Heart J.* 1 (1980): 5–7.

Snellen, H. A. *Two Pioneers of Electrocardiography: The Correspondence between Einthoven and Lewis from 1908–1926.* Rotterdam: Donker Academic Publications, 1983.

Snellen, H. A. *History of Cardiology.* Rotterdam: Donker Academic Publications, 1984.

Somers, H. M. and A. R. Somers. *Doctors, Patients, and Health Insurance: The Organization and Financing of Medical Care.* Washington, D.C.: Brookings Institution, 1961.

Somers, H. M. and A. R. Somers. *Medicare and the Hospitals: Issues and Prospects.* Washington, D.C.: Brookings Institution, 1967.

Spink, W. W. *Infectious Diseases: Prevention and Treatment in the Nineteenth and Twentieth Centuries.* Minneapolis: Univ. of Minnesota Press, 1978.

Starr, P. *The Social Transformation of American Medicine.* New York: Basic Books, 1982.

Stern, B. J. *Society and Medical Progress.* Princeton: Princeton Univ. Press, 1941.

Stern, B. J. *American Medical Practice in the Perspectives of a Century.* New York: Commonwealth Fund, 1945.

Stern, B. J. *Medical Services by Government: Local, State, and Federal.* New York: Commonwealth Fund, 1946.

Stevens, R. *American Medicine and the Public Interest.* New Haven: Yale Univ. Press, 1971.

Stevens, R. "The curious career of internal medicine: Functional ambivalence, social success." In *Grand Rounds: One Hundred Years of Internal Medicine,* ed. R. C. Maulitz and D. E. Long. Philadelphia: Univ. of Pennsylvania Press, 1988, 339–364.

Stevens, R. *In Sickness and in Wealth: American Hospitals in the Twentieth Century.* New York: Basic Books, 1989.

Stevens, R. and R. A. Stevens. *Welfare Medicine in America: A Case Study of Medicaid.* New York: Free Press, 1974.

Strickland, S. P. *Politics, Science, and Dread Disease: A Short History of United States Medical Research Policy.* Cambridge: Harvard Univ. Press, 1972.

Strickland, S. P. *The Story of the NIH Grants Program.* Lanham, Md.: Univ. Press of America, 1989.

Strosberg, M. A. "Technological innovation, specialization, and specialty societies: The case of endoscopy." *Bull. N.Y. Acad. Med.* 55 (1979): 498–509.

Sturdy, S. "The political economy of scientific medicine: Science, education and the transformation of medical practice in Sheffield, 1890–1922." *Med. Hist.* 36 (1992): 125–159.

Surawicz, B. "Pharmacologic treatment of cardiac arrhythmias: 25 years of progress." *J. Am. Coll. Cardiol.* 1 (1983): 365–381.

Swazey, J. P. and R. C. Fox. "The clinical moratorium: A case study of mitral valve surgery." In *Experimentation with Human Subjects,* ed. P. A. Freund. New York: George Brazillier, 1970, 315–357.

Szekeres, L. and J. G. Papp. "The discovery of antiarrhythmics." In *Discoveries in Pharmacology. Hormones and Inflammation,* ed. M. J. Parnham and J. Bruinvels. New York: Elsevier Science Publishers, 1984, 2: 185–215.

Taylor, L. C., Jr. *The Medical Profession and Social Reform, 1885–1945.* New York: St. Martin's Press, 1974.

Temin, P. *Taking Your Medicine: Drug Regulation in the United States.* Cambridge: Harvard Univ. Press, 1980.

Thom, T. J. and F. H. Epstein. "Heart disease, cancer, and stroke mortality trends and their interrelations: An international perspective." *Circulation* 90 (1994): 574–582.

Thomas, V. T. *Pioneering Research in Surgical Shock and Cardiovascular Surgery: Vivien Thomas and His Work with Alfred Blalock.* Philadelphia: Univ. of Pennsylvania Press, 1985.

Thompson, L. and W. S. Downs, eds. *Who's Who in American Medicine, 1925.* New York: Who's Who Publications, 1925.

Triolo, V. A. and M. B. Shimkin. "The American Cancer Society and cancer research origins and organization: 1913–1943." *Cancer Res.* 29 (1969): 1615–1641.

Tumin, M. M. *An Inventory and Appraisal of Research on American Anti-Semitism.* New York: Freedom Books, 1961.

Turner, T. B. *Heritage of Excellence: The Johns Hopkins Medical Institutions, 1914–1947.* Baltimore: Johns Hopkins Univ. Press, 1974.

Vander Veer, J. B. *Cardiology at the Pennsylvania Hospital (1920–1980).* Philadelphia: Pennsylvania Hospital, 1986.

Veiga-Pires, J. A. and R. G. Grainger, eds. *Pioneers in Angiography: The Portuguese School of Angiography.* Lancaster, U.K.: MTP Press, 1982.

Vevier, C., ed. *Flexner: 75 Years Later. A Current Commentary on Medical Education.* New York: Univ. Press of America, 1987.

Vogel, M. J. *The Invention of the Modern Hospital: Boston 1870–1930.* Chicago: Univ. of Chicago Press, 1980.

Wain, H. *A History of Preventive Medicine.* Springfield, Ill.: Charles C. Thomas, 1970.

Wainwright, M. *Miracle Cure: The Story of Penicillin and the Golden Age of Antibiotics.* Oxford: Basil Blackwell, 1990.

Walsh, J. J. *History of Medicine in New York: Three Centuries of Medical Progress.* New York: National Americana Society, 1919.

Wangensteen, O. H. and S. D. Wangensteen. *The Rise of Surgery from Empiric Craft to Scientific Discipline.* Minneapolis: Univ. of Minnesota Press, 1978.

Warner, J. H. "The fall and rise of professional mystery: Epistemology, authority and the emergence of laboratory medicine in nineteenth-century America." In *The*

Laboratory Revolution in Medicine, ed. A. Cunningham and P. Williams. Cambridge: Cambridge Univ. Press, 1992, 110–141.

Weatherall, M. *In Search of a Cure: A History of Pharmaceutical Discovery.* Oxford: Oxford Univ. Press, 1990.

Weeks, L. E. and H. J. Berman. *Shapers of American Health Care Policy: An Oral History.* Ann Arbor, Mich.: Health Administration Press, 1985.

Weinberg, S. L. "The patient with heart disease and the cardiovascular physician and surgeon: 1958–1983." *Am. J. Cardiol.* 1 (1983): 6–12.

Weisse, A. B. *Conversations in Medicine: The Story of Twentieth-Century American Medicine in the Words of Those Who Created It.* New York: New York Univ. Press, 1984.

Weisz, D. and C. Kruytbosch. *Studies of Scientific Disciplines: An Annotated Bibliography.* Washington, D.C.: National Science Foundation, 1982.

Weisz, G. "The development of medical specialization in 19th-century Paris." In *French Medical Culture in the 19th Century*, ed. A. La Berge and M. Feingold. *Clio Medica.* Atlanta: Editions Rodophi B.V., 1994, 25: 149–188.

Wertenbaker, L. *To Mend the Heart.* New York: Viking Press, 1980.

Wheatley, S.C. *The Politics of Philanthropy: Abraham Flexner and Medical Education.* Madison: Univ. of Wisconsin Press, 1988.

White, P. D. "Heart disease forty years ago and now." *JAMA* 149 (1952): 799–801.

White, P. D. *My Life and Medicine: An Autobiographical Memoir.* Boston: Gambit, 1971.

White, P. D. and H. Donovan. *Hearts: Their Long Follow-Up.* Philadelphia: W. B. Saunders, 1967.

White, P. D., H. B. Sprague, L. N. Katz, and R. W. Wilkins. "A Transcript of the '20th Anniversary Program,' A Special Presentation to the Assembly of the American Heart Association, Nov. 25, 1968." New York: AHA, 1968.

Who's Important in Medicine. New York: Institute for Research in Biography, 1945.

Who's Important in Medicine. 2d ed. Hicksville, N.Y.: Institute for Research in Biography, 1952.

Wiggers, C. J. *Reminiscences and Adventures in Circulation Research.* New York: Grune & Stratton, 1958.

Willius, F. A. and T. J. Dry. *A History of the Heart and Circulation.* Philadelphia: W. B. Saunders, 1948.

Wilson, L. G. *Medical Revolution in Minnesota: A History of the University of Minnesota Medical School.* St. Paul: Midewiwin Press, 1989.

Wilson, R. M. *The Beloved Physician: Sir James Mackenzie.* London: John Murray, 1926.

Wintrobe, M. M. *Blood, Pure and Eloquent: A Story of Discovery, of People, and of Ideas.* New York: McGraw-Hill, 1980.

Wintrobe, M. M. *Hematology, the Blossoming of a Science: A Story of Inspiration and Effort.* Philadelphia: Lea & Febiger, 1985.

Wolstenholme, G. E. W., C. M. O'Connor, and M. O'Connor, eds. *Significant Trends in Medical Research.* Boston: Little, Brown, 1959.

Woodford, F. P., ed. *Medical Research Systems in Europe.* Amsterdam: Elsevier, 1973.

Woodman, W. F., M. C. Shelley, and B. J. Reichel. *Biotechnology and the Research Enterprise: A Guide to the Literature.* Ames: Iowa State Univ. Press, 1989.

Wooley, C. F. *Academic Heritage: The Transmission of Excellence—Cardiology at the Ohio State University.* Mount Kisco, N.Y.: Futura Publishing Company, 1992.

Zollinger, R. M. *Elliott Carr Cutler and the Cloning of Surgeons.* Mount Kisco, N.Y.: Futura Publishing Company, 1988.

Index

AAMC, 86, 87, 278, 325

Abbott, Osler, 204, 205, 206, 207–208

ABIM. *See* American Board of Internal Medicine

ABMS, 91, 92

Academic cardiologists, 13, 50; American College of Cardiology and, 135, 138, 141–143, 148–149, 186, 190–192, 196–197, 200–203, 205, 206–207, 214, 231, 235, 240, 247, 283; American Heart Association and, 34, 51–52, 56, 81, 83, 84, 85, 96, 99, 107, 119–120, 135, 186, 229; Association of American Physicians and, 69–70; certification of, 91; competition and, 307–308, 319; continuing medical education and, 196–197; defined, 14; dependence on professional societies, 327–328; early history of, 33–36; early lack of support for, 77–78; federal funding and, 150–162, 215, 221, 239, 240, 242; federal laws affecting, 243; growth in numbers and prestige, 306; income/reimbursement of, 313–314, 319; influence on development of field, 34; lack of opportunities for, 51; physiological cardiologists differentiated from, 33; practitioner cardiologists differentiated from, 33; practitioner cardiologists versus, 69–70, 117, 119–120; primary interests of, 71; public health cardiologists differentiated from, 35; research and, 105, 150–162; specialist surplus and, 329,

331; taxation of, 316; technologies emphasized by, 301

Academic medical centers, 69–70, 279–280; cardiovascular surgery programs in, 168; competition with private practitioners, 319; federal funding of, 161; internist/cardiologist tensions in, 310; percutaneous transluminal coronary angioplasty in, 304; profitability of training programs in, 306–307; subspecialty faculty defection from, 314

ACC. *See* American College of Cardiology

ACCEL, 214

ACCESS, 213–214

Access to health care, 327–329

Acierno, Louis, 5

ACP. *See* American College of Physicians

Acute myocardial infarction: anticoagulants and, 110; coronary artery bypass graft surgery and, 260; coronary care units and (*see* Coronary care units); current treatment of, 315; early lack of treatment for, 76; Eisenhower's, 188–189, 216; electrocardiography and, 254–255; hospital care of patients with, 255t; identified as distinct syndrome, 65; incidence of, 273; Johnson's, 216, 219; percutaneous transluminal coronary angioplasty and, 303; thrombolytic therapy and, 315

Adams, Forrest, 287–288

Adams, Wright, 211

Fye, Bruce
   American cardiology: the history of a specialty and its college /
W. Bruce Fye.
      p.   cm.
   Includes bibliographical references and index.
   ISBN 0-8018-5292-7 (alk. paper)
   1. Cardiology—United States—History. 2. American College of
Cardiology—History. 3. American College of Cardiology. I. Title.
   [DNLM: 1. Cardiology—history—United States. 2. Societies,
Medical—history—United States. WG 11 AA1 F9a 1996]
RC666.5.F94   1996
616.1'2'00973—dc20
DNLM/DLC
for Library of Congress   95-25523
                                                                                    CIP